Current Treatment Options for Fuchs Endothelial Dystrophy

Claus Cursiefen • Albert S. Jun
Editors

Current Treatment Options for Fuchs Endothelial Dystrophy

Springer

Editors
Claus Cursiefen
Department of Ophthalmology
University of Cologne
Cologne
Germany

Albert S. Jun
Wilmer Eye Institute
Johns Hopkins Medical Institutions
Baltimore
Maryland
USA

ISBN 978-3-319-43019-5 ISBN 978-3-319-43021-8 (eBook)
DOI 10.1007/978-3-319-43021-8

Library of Congress Control Number: 2016956895

Printed on acid-free paper

This Springer imprint is published by Springer Nature
The registered company is Springer International Publishing AG Switzerland
The registered company address is Gewerbestrasse 11, 6330 Cham, Switzerland

Foreword

When Ernst Fuchs described what we now call Fuchs endothelial dystrophy (FED) in 1910, he was so humble to state that the disease origin may in fact later be discovered as not epithelial in nature – as he thought in times without slit-lamp examination.

We nowadays in fact know that FED is primarily an endothelial disease, and we obviously now know much more, as this book tries to define in state-of-the-art fashion. But we certainly should remain as humble as Fuchs in that we still do not understand large aspects of FED pathogenesis and treatment.

Fortunately for our patients, in parallel to the growing knowledge of disease mechanisms of FED, the field of lamellar corneal transplant surgery has undergone a revolution in recent years so that we can offer much better and safer treatment options such as DSAEK and DMEK.

This book aims to provide a thought-provoking overview of all aspects of FED, from pathogenesis to modern surgical and cellular therapy.

We hope that this work even further stimulates progress toward our goals to gain better insights into disease mechanisms and to develop even safer and better treatment options for our patients with corneal endothelial diseases.

Cologne, Germany
Baltimore, MD, USA
October 2016

Claus Cursiefen
Albert S. Jun

Contents

Chapter 1
Epidemiology and Genetic Basis of Fuchs Endothelial Corneal Dystrophy

Guadalupe Villarreal Jr., Laura Kallay, Gustavo Vedana, and Albert S. Jun

1.1 Introduction

Fuchs endothelial corneal dystrophy (FECD) was first described in 1910 by Austrian ophthalmologist Ernst Fuchs. In his report "Dystrophia Epithelialis Corneae," Fuchs described a series of 13 patients that developed progressive central corneal clouding with loss of corneal sensation and formation of epithelial vesicles resulting in eventual vision loss [14]. While he gave the name "Dystrophia epithelialis" based on his hypothesis that the primary site of pathology was at the level of the corneal epithelium, Prof. Fuchs understood that the name could later be "replaced by a better one, when the true nature of the disease [was] discerned" [14, 25]. Since his initial description, significant progress has been made over the past century in our understanding of the epidemiology, genetics, and pathophysiology of this endothelial dystrophy.

G. Villarreal Jr. • L. Kallay • G. Vedana • A.S. Jun, MD, PhD (✉)
Cornea & External Disease Division, Wilmer Eye Institute,
Johns Hopkins Medical Institutions,
600 N. Broadway, Woods 376, Baltimore, MD 21287, USA
e-mail: aljun@jhmi.edu

C. Cursiefen, A.S. Jun (eds.), *Current Treatment Options for Fuchs Endothelial Dystrophy*, DOI 10.1007/978-3-319-43021-8_1

1.2 Epidemiology

FECD is a progressive disease characterized by the loss of endothelial cells, thickening of Descemet membrane, formation of guttae, and development of corneal edema resulting in a significant decrease in visual acuity. In its most severe manifestation, blindness ensues [32]. In a global survey of corneal transplantation and eye banking by Gain et al., FECD was the primary indication for all corneal transplantations performed worldwide, accounting for 39 %, followed by keratoconus (27 %) and infectious keratitis sequelae (20 %) [16]. Data from the Eye Bank Association of America have similarly identified FECD as the most common indication for corneal transplantation, accounting for 22 % of all corneal transplants in the USA [54].

Clinical progression of FECD is typically graded using the Krachmer grading scale, which is divided from Grade 0–5, with Grade 0 indicating 0–12 central guttae; Grade 1, greater than 12 central non-confluent guttae; Grade 2, 1–2 mm of confluent central guttae; Grade 3, 2–5 mm of confluent central guttae; Grade 4, greater than 5 mm of confluent central guttae; and Grade 5, greater than 5 mm of confluent guttae with stromal or epithelial edema [36]. Limitations to the Krachmer grading scale include interobserver variability in grading as well as the development of stromal thickening or edema in stages other than Grade 5 [11].

Another staging system commonly utilized divides FECD into four stages of clinical progression [1]. In Stage 1, the patient is asymptomatic, but slit-lamp biomicroscopy demonstrates the presence of central guttae, variable amount of pigment on the endothelial surface, and a thickening and gray appearance to Descemet membrane. In Stage 2 of the disease, the patient develops a painless decrease in visual acuity and glare, particularly upon awakening, related to the presence of epithelial and stromal edema. In Stage 3, the patient may experience episodes of pain due to the formation and rupture of epithelial and subepithelial bullae. Lastly, in Stage 4, visual acuity is severely compromised and may be reduced to hand motions with the development of avascular subepithelial scarring which limits bullae formation. At this stage, the patient is generally free of painful episodes.

Based on the time of onset of the disease, FECD is divided into two clinical subtypes: an early onset and late-onset forms. The early onset form of FECD is rare and has been associated with autosomal dominant Q455K, Q455V, and L450W mutations in the gene encoding the alpha 2 subunit of collagen 8 (COL8A2) [4, 18, 40, 49]. COL8A2 is an important structural component of Descemet membrane. Patients with early onset FECD can exhibit changes in the first decade of life, with continued progression over the next two to three decades [21]. In contrast to late-onset FECD, in which there is a strong female predominance, men and women are equally affected in the early onset form, a reflection of the autosomal dominant pattern of inheritance.

Late-onset FECD is more common than the early onset form. In a 1967 study of 1,016 people without any known ocular pathology in Jacksonville, Florida, Lorenzetti et al. reported a 3.9 % prevalence of confluent corneal guttae in individuals aged 40 or older [42]. This estimate was based on slit-lamp examination alone. In the Reykjavik Eye Study, the prevalence of any primary central corneal guttae in Icelandic individuals over the age of 55, based on both slit-lamp and specular microscopy, was 11 % for females and 7 % for males [86]. In the Kumejima Study, the prevalence of any central corneal guttae in Japanese residents age 40 years or older, based on specular microscopy alone, was 4.1 % overall [22]. There was a significant difference in the prevalence of central corneal guttae between Japanese men and women, 2.4 % versus 5.8 %, respectively [22]. Interestingly, a retrospective histopathologic study by Santo et al. found that the frequency of FECD in corneal specimens from Japanese patients undergoing keratectomy or keratoplasty over a 34-year period from 1959 through 1992 was only 0.7 % [66]. The low frequency of FECD among Japanese individuals needing corneal transplantation may in part relate to their significantly higher corneal endothelial cell density as compared to an age-matched American population [43].

Unlike early onset FECD, a female predominance of 2.5–3.5:1 has also been reported in late-onset FECD [2, 13, 31, 86]. Patients with late-onset FECD typically manifest changes by the fifth decade of life, with progression over the next two to three decades [21]. Although the median age of onset for the late-onset form of FECD is at least four decades later than that of the early onset form, both display a similar linear rate of disease progression, with advancement in clinical severity grade occurring on average every 5 years [18].

The use of central corneal thickness (CCT) to grade FECD is challenging given the frequent absence of baseline CCT data and variability of CCT in a population. Additionally, the use of ultrasonic pachymetry to measure CCT is limited by the ability to consistently measure corneal thickness at the same location [45]. However, as suggested by data from Kopplin et al., monitoring of CCT changes in patients may be useful in following FECD progression [35]. In contrast to the subjective morphological clinical grading of FECD, for which interobserver agreement is only moderate, work by Repp et al. has suggested that the ratio of the central corneal thickness to the peripheral corneal thickness at 4 mm from the center ($CPTR_4$), which functions as an internal reference, may serve as an objective and repeatable metric to assess the severity of FECD [58]. While the presence of corneal edema has traditionally only been reflected at the end stage of the Krachmer grading scale [36], the presence of corneal edema is not specific to end-stage disease and can be seen in early clinical grades of FECD, underscoring the importance and incorporation of these data into clinical grading schemes [58].

Data from Fujimoto et al. have further suggested that monitoring of guttae in the peripheral zone, 3.7 mm peripheral to the center, was significantly correlated with disease grade in advanced cases of FECD [15]. The degree of guttae in the central and paracentral zones (0.6 mm from center), which are damaged earlier and more severely in FECD, was not found to be useful in distinguishing between advanced cases (grades 3–5), as these areas had nearly complete guttae formation by this stage [15]. Monitoring guttae formation in the periphery may therefore serve an important role for monitoring disease progression in advanced stages of FECD.

Several risk factors in addition to gender have been associated with the development of central guttae and degree of FECD. In the Reykjavik Eye Study, which was a cross-sectional, random, population-based study of individuals 55 years and older, participants with more than a 20 pack/year smoking history had a 2.2-fold increased risk of development of any primary central guttae [86]. Higher weight and body mass index were additionally associated with a 2.5 and 7 % respective decrease in the risk of any central corneal guttae [86]. In the Fuchs Genetics Multi-Center Study, both female sex and smoking were associated with an increased risk, 34 % and 30 %, respectively, of advanced FECD (grades 4–6) [85]. The association of smoking with increased risk of FECD may be explained by increased generation of reactive oxygen species and oxidative damage in the setting of already impaired antioxidant defense [27, 79]. While associations between FECD and age-related macular degeneration [57] as well as cardiovascular disease [53] and angle-closure glaucoma [56] have been reported, subsequent reports have not been able to confirm such associations [5, 86].

1.3 Genetic Basis of FECD

Fuchs corneal endothelial dystrophy (FECD) is a complex and heterogeneous genetic disorder of the corneal endothelium with variable expressivity and incomplete penetrance. Two genetic techniques – linkage analysis and genome-wide association study (GWAS) – have been used to elucidate the genetic basis for FECD. At this time, five causal genes (*TCF4*, *AGBL1*, *LOXHD1*, *SLC4A11*, and *ZEB1*) and four causal loci on chromosomes 5, 9, 13, and 18 have been identified in individuals with late-onset FECD. In addition, mutations in *COL8A2* have been shown to cause early onset FECD.

1.3.1 Causal Mutations

1.3.1.1 *TCF4*

Variations in the transcription factor 4 (*TCF4*) gene are the most significant genetic risk factors associated with FECD. This gene, located on chromosome 18q21.1, is a member of the E-protein family of basic helix-loop-helix (bHLH) transcription factors that function in the regulation of multiple developmental pathways including neurogenesis and lymphocyte development [7, 17, 38, 51]. TCF4 has a complex gene organization with 34 exons that produce tissue-specific isoforms that regulate both positive and negative gene expressions [67]. The full-length 671-amino acid TCF4 isoform has an N-terminal transcriptional activation domain (AD1), followed by a nuclear localization signal (NLS), a second transcriptional activation domain (AD2), and a C-terminal basic helix-loop-helix domain that mediates dimerization and E-box binding. Alternative splicing at the 5-prime end results in TCF4 proteins with 18 different N-termini. All isoforms have AD2 and bHLH domains but may lack the AD1 domain and/or NLS.

In 2012, Wieben et al. demonstrated a strong genetic association between intronic cytosine-thymine-guanine (CTG) trinucleotide repeats (CTG18.1) in the *TCF4* gene of FECD patients [80]. They found that 79 % of FECD patients had greater than 50 repeats in the third intron of the *TCF4* gene compared to just 3 % of unaffected control individuals. This trinucleotide repeat (TNR) expansion was found to be highly predictive of the disorder conferring more than a 30-fold increase in the risk for development of FECD in Caucasians. Cosegregation of the triplet repeat expansion with FECD was found in 15 of 29 Caucasian pedigrees with complete penetrance supporting the triplet repeat expansion as being the likely causal genetic variant [69].

Subsequent genetic studies provide evidence that the *TCF4* CTG18.1 repeat expansion is the major causal variant across ethnic groups. In a Singapore Chinese cohort, expansion at the CTG18.1 locus was the only variant identified within the *TCF4* gene in Fuchs patients suggesting that the expanded CTG18.1 allele was the primary and possibly the sole causal variant at this gene locus in the Chinese population [82]. Genetic analysis of Indian FECD patients also found a highly significant association of CTG18.1 alleles with FECD and a minor association with the single nucleotide polymorphism rs17089887. The study found the disease threshold of 50 trinucleotide repeats present in 34 % of FECD subjects and 5 % of control subjects [52]. Together these studies indicate that expansion of CTG18.1 is likely to be the most significant global cause of FECD. Furthermore, disease severity was found to be greater in FECD cases with the CTG18.1 triplet repeat expansion compared to those without the expansion. The length of CTG triplet repeat also positively correlated with the Krachmer grade of severity. Thus, *TCF4* triplet repeat expansion presence and length has predictive clinical and surgical therapeutic implications [69].

While the expansion of the intronic *TCF4* allele plays a key role in the development of FECD, the molecular mechanism of the disease has not been established fully. Multiple mechanisms have been proposed by which the expansion in the *TCF4* gene may cause susceptibility to FECD. It has been suggested that the expanded allele could interfere with transcription initiation and/or splicing of *TCF4* in corneal endothelial cells altering expression levels of specific TCF4 isoforms. TCF4 also plays a key role in epithelial-to-mesenchymal transition through its regulation of zinc finger E-box binding homeobox 1 (ZEB1) protein also known as transcription factor 8 (TCF8) [65]. ZEB1 has been proposed to regulate expression of extracellular matrix components, such as COL8A2, and to induce epithelial-to-mesenchymal transition (EMT) that drives metastatic cancers. The discovery of repeat-associated non-ATG translation in several microsatellite disorders also raises the possibility that the pathogenesis of FECD may also be due to small peptides generated from the poly(CUG)n RNA [8].

More recent studies point to RNA aggregation and toxicity as the basis for endothelial cell death [10, 50]. Accumulated RNA transcripts with expanded repeats can form stable hairpin structures that bind and sequester RNA interacting proteins [74]. Corneal endothelial cells from FECD patients, like cells from patients with the trinucleotide repeat disorder myotonic dystrophy type 1 (DM1), accumulate poly(CUG) n RNA in foci within the nucleus [10, 50]. Poly(CUG)n RNA foci co-localized with and sequestered the mRNA-splicing factor MBNL1 leading to aberrant processing of essential MBNL1-regulated mRNAs including some mRNAs with roles in EMT. The RNA foci and depletion of RNA-binding proteins trigger aberrant splicing and ultimately stimulate apoptosis. Importantly, RNA nuclear foci were not detected in cells from FECD patients who lack the repeat expansion highlighting the central role that CUG RNA nuclear foci play in the pathogenesis of FECD with the CTG18.1 triplet repeat expansion in *TCF4* [50]. Tissue-specific pathogenesis in FECD patients may be related to the corneal endothelium's exposure to an environment subjected to higher levels of oxidative stress. Oxidative stress, previously implicated in the pathogenesis of FECD [3, 27, 79], may cause somatic instability that further contributes to the expansion of the TNRs [10].

1.3.1.2 *AGBL1*

An additional causal mutation that results in dominant late-onset Fuchs corneal dystrophy was recently identified on the long arm of chromosome 15 at position 25.3, the location of the ATP/GTP-binding protein-like1 (*AGBL1*) gene [61]. Linkage analysis followed by next-generation sequencing uncovered a heterozygous nonsense mutation (R1028X) and a missense mutation (C990S) in the *AGBL1* gene in individuals with FECD. *AGBL1* encodes an isoform of cytosolic carboxypeptidase 4 (CCP4), a metallocarboxypeptidase that mediates deglutamylation of target proteins. CCP enzymes catalyze the deglutamylation of long polyglutamate side chains generated by posttranslational polyglutamylation on proteins such as tubulins and myosin light chain kinase (MYLK) [64]. Studies in Purkinje cells obtained from mice that lack a functional CCP1 isoform display microtubule hyperglutamylation that leads to neurodegeneration [78]. These findings demonstrate that regulation of the length of the polyglutamate side chains on tubulin plays a role in neuronal cell survival. Further study is needed to determine if mutations in *AGBL1* identified in patients with FECD also result in microtubule hyperglutamylation and if *AGBL1* mutations play a role in the survival of corneal endothelial cells. Functional analysis demonstrated that AGBL1 interacts specifically with the FECD-associated protein TCF4 and not TCF8, and that *AGBL1* mutations diminish that interaction [61].

1.3.1.3 *LOXHD1*

The lipoxygenase homology domain-containing 1 (*LOXHD1*) gene encodes a highly conserved protein consisting entirely of polycystin/lipoxygenase/alpha-toxin (PLAT) domains, thought to facilitate protein targeting to the plasma membrane. The cytogenetic location of the *LOXHD1* gene is on chromosome 18q21.1. In 2012,

Riazuddin et al. identified *LOXHD1* as a causal gene within a family whose disease was previously linked to the undefined FCD2 locus [60]. The *LOXHD1* gene is not located in the FCD2 locus region, and expanded linkage analysis and sequencing of a targeted region of chromosome 18 uncovered a missense mutant allele in *LOXHD1* that caused progressive hearing loss as the causal variant leading to Fuchs dystrophy in this pedigree. A screen of a cohort of >200 sporadic FECD-affected individuals identified an additional 15 heterozygous missense mutations not found in over 800 control chromosomes. Mutations were modeled to the surface of the protein and were indicative of impaired protein-protein interactions. Expression of *LOXHD1* mutant alleles in cells produced prominent cytoplasmic aggregates similar to what is seen in the corneal phenotype. Amino acid substitutions found in the protein due to these rare alleles in *LOXHD1* could explain the pathogenesis of FECD and provide an understanding of the mechanism by which mutations in the same locus can produce diverse phenotypes.

1.3.1.4 *SLC4A11*

The *SLC4A11* gene, located on chromosome 20p12, was reported to encode a voltage-regulated, electrogenic sodium-coupled borate cotransporter essential for borate homeostasis, cell growth, and cell proliferation [55]. However, the molecular function of SLC4A11 remains to be clearly elucidated. Recent studies indicate that neither bicarbonate nor borate is a substrate for SLC4A11, but it has been shown to be a NH_3/H^+ cotransporter with unique properties [84]. Mutations in *SLC4A11* have been associated with a number of endothelial corneal dystrophies including recessive congenital hereditary endothelial dystrophy 2 (CHED2), corneal endothelial dystrophy with sensorineural deafness (Harboyan syndrome), and dominant late-onset Fuchs endothelial corneal dystrophy [9, 62, 76, 77].

A series of heterozygous mutations of the *SLC4A11* gene are associated with late-onset FECD [62, 70, 77]. In endothelial cells, the transporter is located in the basolateral membrane and was shown to facilitate transmembrane water movement [75]. FECD causal mutations expressed in cells display defective cell surface localization with correlated endoplasmic reticulum accumulation by biochemical assays and confocal immunolocalization [77]. *SLC4A11* knockout mice did not show any abnormalities in the endothelium and Descemet membrane with the primary phenotypic change observed in the cornea being an increase in the height of basal epithelial cells [41].

1.3.1.5 *ZEB1*

ZEB1 is a zinc finger E-box binding homeobox 1 transcription factor, also known as TCF8, located at chromosome 10p11.22. ZEB1 was first shown to play a role in transcriptional repression of interleukin 2 [71, 81] and later found to be important for the induction of epithelial-mesenchymal transition (EMT) [83]. Pathogenic

ZEB1 mutations were first identified as a cause of posterior polymorphous corneal dystrophy-3 (PPCD3) [37]. Later ZEB1 mutations were found to be associated with FECD when Mehta et al. screened 74 unrelated Chinese individuals with FECD for ZEB1 mutations [46]. A novel variant, p.N696S, was present in only one of the FECD cases and was not present in any of the other FECD cases or in 93 control individuals [46]. A second casual mutation in ZEB1 was uncovered by Riazuddin et al. in a large multigenerational family whose disease also linked to the FCD4 locus [63]. Four additional ZEB1 pathogenic mutations were identified in 384 unrelated FECD-affected individuals by sequence analysis [63]. Comparison of ZEB1 mutations supports a genotype-phenotype correlation where FECD causal mutations are missense mutations in exons of ZEB1 at sites that are moderately to highly evolutionarily conserved in vertebrates, and mutations associated with PPCD3 are more deleterious frameshift, nonsense, or lost-start-codon mutations [39]. In vivo studies in zebra fish embryos showed that two of five FECD causal mutations could partially rescue developmental abnormalities caused by morpholino oligonucleotide knockdown of endogenous ZEB1. The other three variants demonstrated phenotypes identical to morpholino injection alone, while wild-type mRNA completely rescued the phenotype [23]. Expression of ZEB1 nonsense and missense mutations that cause PPCD3 and FECD, respectively, in a corneal endothelial cell line support that haploinsufficiency is a cause of PPCD3. Some of the PPCD3 causative mutations expressed truncated ZEB1 proteins that display decreased protein levels and/or impaired cellular localization. In contrast, FECD-associated ZEB1 missense mutations did not significantly alter protein levels or nuclear localization. The mechanisms by which ZEB1 missense mutations lead to FECD remain to be elucidated [6].

1.3.2 FECD Loci Identified by Genetic Linkage Analysis

An early locus (FCD1) linked to late-onset FECD was localized on chromosome 13 to a 26.4-Mb interval between 13pTel and 13q12.13 in a large four-generation Caucasian pedigree that included 13 affected and three unaffected individuals from three generations [73]. Females were observed with the expected 2:1 sex ratio in affected individuals. Of note, two children in this family whose parents were both affected demonstrated clinical signs of late-onset FECD at a young age. Sundin et al. also identified a second locus, FCD2, at chromosome 18q21.2–18q21.32 using linkage analysis of three large families [72]. However, the disease-linked haplotype was different in each family, suggesting that there may be heterogeneity of this locus. FECD in the families associated with chromosome 18 exhibited an autosomal dominant inheritance biased toward women, with 27 affected women and 19 affected men within the three families. In addition, 10 % of individuals with the disease haplotype were unaffected clinically, suggesting a complex mode of inheritance associated with this locus. A third locus, FCD3, localized to 5q33.1–5q35.2 in a three-generation family [59]. FECD in this family was present in eight females and two males. The FCD4 locus was identified by Riazuddin et al. in the region 9p22.1–9p24.1 [63]. Additional mutations in TCF8 were also discovered in some of these affected family members suggesting interaction between two pathologic alleles in this disease. Additional loci have been identified which may contain alternative rare FECD mutations [12].

FCD1 is linked to the most severe and rapidly progressing form of the disease with individuals experiencing a 24 % annual increase in the number of guttae versus a 5 % annual increase for FCD2. FCD3 causes the mildest form of the disease that progresses more slowly than both FCD1- and FCD2-linked diseases [23]. Cosegregation of the rare, late-onset FCD4 haplotype on chromosome 9p with missense mutations of TCF8 results in severe FECD with poor prognosis [63].

1.3.3 COL8A2 *Early Onset FECD*

In 2001, Biswas et al. studied a multigenerational family with an early onset, autosomal dominant form of FECD and discovered a single nucleotide missense mutation at position 1364 of the coding sequence of the α2 collagen VIII (*COL8A2*) gene [4]. This nucleotide change results in a glutamine to lysine (Q455K) substitution in the triple helical domain of the COL8A2 protein. This mutation was the first characterization of the molecular basis of any corneal endothelial dystrophy and the first pathogenic variant of *COL8A2* in humans [4]. A second autosomal dominant *COL8A2* mutation in families with early onset FECD was uncovered in 2005 [18]. This transversion, also located in the collagen repeat domain of the COL8A2 protein, replaces leucine with tryptophan at residue 450 (L450W). A third heterozygous mutation, resulting in a glutamine to valine substitution at amino acid 455 (Q455V), was found in patients of Korean pedigrees with FECD and not in unaffected individuals. Replacement of a polar glutamine with a nonpolar valine is suggested to disrupt the interaction of COL8A2 and COL8A1 proteins in the hexagonal lattice structure of Descemet membrane (DM) [49]. The female-to-male ratio was found to be 1:1 for *COL8A2* mutations, in contrast to late-onset FECD pedigrees where the disease was more prevalent in females with a female-to-male ratio of 2.5:1 [18].

Type VIII collagen is comprised of α1 and α2 polypeptide chains [20, 24]. Collagen VIII is synthesized, processed, and secreted by corneal endothelial cells and is the major protein of DM [28]. Type VIII collagens contribute to assembly and structural integrity of the hexagonal matrix that serves to support the endothelium. In addition, studies suggest collagen VIII also contributes to cell differentiation and plays a role in determining cell phenotype [68]. In early onset FECD associated with the L450W mutation, an excess of both α1 and α2 collagen VIII proteins are deposited, increasing the thickness of the anterior banded layer of DM more than three times that found in normal DM [19]. The increase in COL8A2 protein is accompanied by increased levels of collagen IV, fibronectin, and laminin that contribute to the increase in membrane thickness [19, 44].

Jun et al. created and analyzed transgenic mice carrying the *Col8a2* Q455K mutation [26]. At 5 and 10 months of age, mutant mice began to display hallmark FECD features seen in human disease, including variations in cell size, deviation from the normal hexagonal shape, cell loss, and the presence of DM guttae. Ultrastructural analysis revealed the presence of extremely dilated endoplasmic reticulum (ER), pointing to the activation of ER stress and unfolded protein response. Further biochemical studies confirmed unfolded protein response (UPR) activation and UPR-associated apoptosis in the mutant corneal endothelium [26]. They concluded that the Q455K mutation in *COL8A2* causes FECD through a mechanism involving the UPR and UPR-associated apoptosis. Features of *Col8a2* L450W transgenic mice have been described [47]. These mice displayed a milder corneal endothelial phenotype than that of homozygous Q455K mice yet still exhibited the hallmarks of FECD. Both mutants displayed dilated rough ER and upregulation of UPR pathway genes and proteins. Reverse transcriptase polymerase chain reaction (RT-PCR) analysis of corneal endothelial cells from L450W and Q455K mutant mice revealed upregulation of DNA damage-regulated autophagy modulator protein 1 (*DRAM1*), a lysosomal membrane autophagy marker. RT-PCR of human FECD endothelium provides evidence for upregulation of *DRAM1* relative to autopsy control corneas. Taken together, these findings suggest that altered autophagy contributes to FECD pathogenesis. While mutations in *COL8A2* are not associated with late-onset FECD, the shared features of the early and late-onset forms of the disease suggest that the study of *COL8A2* mutations may provide insights into pathogenesis and potential therapeutic directions.

1.4 Future Therapies

Since the first description of Fuchs endothelial corneal dystrophy over one century ago, corneal transplantation has remained the only definitive treatment for this disease. To date, medical treatments for FECD have been aimed at reducing corneal edema and associated blurred vision. The use of 5 % sodium chloride eye drops or ointment to draw fluid out of the cornea, as well as directing warm air toward the cornea from a hair dryer at arm's distance to facilitate evaporation of fluid, has assisted with transient symptomatic visual improvement. Over the past few decades, however, significant strides have been made in furthering our understanding of the pathophysiological mechanisms underlying FECD and have highlighted several potentially novel areas of pharmacological treatment.

One avenue of pharmacological treatment has been aimed at inhibition of the Rho/ROCK signaling pathway using the ROCK inhibitor Y-27632. The Rho/ROCK pathway has been shown to play an important role in the regulation of apoptosis, cell proliferation, and cell migration [33]. Both in vitro and in vivo experiments using Y-27632 have suggested that inhibition of the Rho/ROCK signaling pathway can stimulate corneal endothelial cell proliferation and wound healing [33]. Koizumi et al. reported successful treatment of a 52-year-old Japanese man with late-onset FECD who underwent 2 mm transcorneal freezing to remove diseased corneal endothelium in the pre-pupillary region followed by treatment with Y-27632 eye drops six times a day for 1 week [34]. Best-corrected vision improved from 20/63 preoperatively to 20/20 at 2 weeks and 20/16 at 24 months postoperatively. A similar improvement was noted in central corneal thickness from 703 μm preoperatively to 568 μm at 6 months postoperatively. Specular microscopy at 18 months demonstrated smaller cells, present at a high density centrally (1549.3 ± 89.7 cells per mm^2), following the 2 mm endothelial cryoablation. As prior work has suggested that the peripheral corneal endothelium can maintain a high proliferative capacity [48], it remains possible that the observed effect reported by Koizumi et al. could be due to denudation of the diseased corneal endothelium alone [34]. Nonetheless, significant interest remains with the use of ROCK inhibitors for the treatment of FECD, and further investigation is needed.

Lithium is an activator of the canonical Wnt signaling pathway. Work by Kim et al. demonstrated that lithium increases corneal endothelial cell survival and autophagy in a *Col8a2* Q455K mouse model of FECD [29]. Additionally, pretreatment of cultured normal bovine corneal endothelial cells with lithium as compared to control cells was found to significantly increase cell viability following incubation with oxidative stress and ER stress agents, hydrogen peroxide and thapsigargin, respectively [29]. Together, these data provided in vitro and in vivo evidence for the use of lithium as a potential pharmacological treatment for FECD.

Another compound of interest is N-acetylcysteine (NAC), which is a thiol-containing antioxidant. Systemic administration of NAC to a *Col8a2* L450W mouse model of FECD was shown to increase corneal endothelial survival with an associated increase in antioxidant cell markers and decrease in ER stress markers as compared to untreated L450W mice [30]. Pretreatment of bovine corneal endothelial cells with NAC resulted in higher cell viability following incubation with oxidative and ER stress agents as compared to control treated cells [30].

With the identification of CTG trinucleotide repeat expansion (>50 repeats) in the *TCF4* gene in 79 % of FECD patients [80], and subsequent studies associating TNR expansion in FECD with RNA aggregation and cellular toxicity [10, 50], the possibility for gene therapy to correct this mutation in addition to medical therapies to target specific disease mechanisms as they are elucidated may yield future treatments for FECD.

Through continued research into the epidemiology, genetics, and pathophysiology underlying FECD, we have been able to make significant strides over the past century in our understanding of this corneal endothelial dystrophy. These discoveries are paving the way for novel avenues of monitoring disease progression and treatment.

References

1. Adamis AP, Filatov V, Tripathi BJ, et al. Fuchs' endothelial dystrophy of the cornea. Surv Ophthalmol. 1993;38(2):149–68.
2. Afshari NA, Pittard AB, Siddiqui A, et al. Clinical study of Fuchs corneal endothelial dystrophy leading to penetrating keratoplasty: a 30-year experience. Arch Ophthalmol. 2006;124(6):777–80. doi:10.1001/archopht.124.6.777.

3. Azizi B, Ziaei A, Fuchsluger T, et al. p53-regulated increase in oxidative-stress–induced apoptosis in Fuchs endothelial corneal dystrophy: a native tissue model. Invest Ophthalmol Vis Sci. 2011;52(13):9291–7. doi:10.1167/iovs.11-8312.
4. Biswas S, Munier FL, Yardley J, et al. Missense mutations in COL8A2, the gene encoding the alpha2 chain of type VIII collagen, cause two forms of corneal endothelial dystrophy. Hum Mol Genet. 2001;10(21):2415–23.
5. Brooks AM, Grant G, Gillies WE. The significance of anterior chamber depth in Fuchs' corneal dystrophy and cornea guttata. Cornea. 1994;13(2):131–5.
6. Chung DW, Frausto RF, Ann LB, et al. Functional impact of ZEB1 mutations associated with posterior polymorphous and Fuchs' endothelial corneal dystrophies. Invest Ophthalmol Vis Sci. 2014;55(10):6159–66. doi:10.1167/iovs.14-15247.
7. Cisse B, Caton ML, Lehner M, et al. Transcription factor E2-2 is an essential and specific regulator of plasmacytoid dendritic cell development. Cell. 2008;135(1):37–48. doi:10.1016/j.cell.2008.09.016.
8. Cleary JD, Ranum LP. Repeat associated non-ATG (RAN) translation: new starts in microsatellite expansion disorders. Curr Opin Genet Dev. 2014;26:6–15. doi:10.1016/j.gde.2014.03.002.
9. Desir J, Moya G, Reish O, et al. Borate transporter SLC4A11 mutations cause both Harboyan syndrome and non-syndromic corneal endothelial dystrophy. J Med Genet. 2007;44(5):322–6. doi:10.1136/jmg.2006.046904.
10. Du J, Aleff RA, Soragni E, et al. RNA toxicity and missplicing in the common eye disease fuchs endothelial corneal dystrophy. J Biol Chem. 2015;290(10):5979–90. doi:10.1074/jbc.M114.621607.
11. Eghrari AO, Garrett BS, Mumtaz AA, et al. Retroillumination photography analysis enhances clinical definition of severe Fuchs corneal dystrophy. Cornea. 2015;34(12):1623–6. doi:10.1097/ICO.0000000000000656.
12. Eghrari AO, Riazuddin SA, Gottsch JD. Fuchs corneal dystrophy. Prog Mol Biol Transl Sci. 2015;134:79–97. doi:10.1016/bs.pmbts.2015.04.005.
13. Elhalis H, Azizi B, Jurkunas UV. Fuchs endothelial corneal dystrophy. Ocul Surf. 2010;8(4):173–84.
14. Fuchs E. Dystrophia epithelialis corneae. Graefes Arch Clin Exp Ophthalmol. 1910; 76:478–508.
15. Fujimoto H, Maeda N, Soma T, et al. Quantitative regional differences in corneal endothelial abnormalities in the central and peripheral zones in Fuchs' endothelial corneal dystrophy. Invest Ophthalmol Vis Sci. 2014;55(8):5090–8. doi:10.1167/iovs.14-14249.
16. Gain P, Jullienne R, He Z, et al. Global survey of corneal transplantation and Eye banking. JAMA Ophthalmol. 2016;134(2):167–73. doi:10.1001/jamaophthalmol.2015.4776.
17. Ghosh HS, Cisse B, Bunin A, et al. Continuous expression of the transcription factor e2-2 maintains the cell fate of mature plasmacytoid dendritic cells. Immunity. 2010;33(6):905–16. doi:10.1016/j.immuni.2010.11.023.
18. Gottsch JD, Sundin OH, Liu SH, et al. Inheritance of a novel COL8A2 mutation defines a distinct early-onset subtype of fuchs corneal dystrophy. Invest Ophthalmol Vis Sci. 2005;46(6):1934–9. doi:10.1167/iovs.04-0937.
19. Gottsch JD, Zhang C, Sundin OH, et al. Fuchs corneal dystrophy: aberrant collagen distribution in an L450W mutant of the COL8A2 gene. Invest Ophthalmol Vis Sci. 2005;46(12):4504–11. doi:10.1167/iovs.05-0497.
20. Greenhill NS, Ruger BM, Hasan Q, et al. The alpha1(VIII) and alpha2(VIII) collagen chains form two distinct homotrimeric proteins in vivo. Matrix Biol J Int Soc Matrix Biol. 2000;19(1):19–28.
21. Hamill CE, Schmedt T, Jurkunas U. Fuchs endothelial cornea dystrophy: a review of the genetics behind disease development. Semin Ophthalmol. 2013;28(5–6):281–6. doi:10.3109/08820538.2013.825283.
22. Higa A, Sakai H, Sawaguchi S, et al. Prevalence of and risk factors for cornea guttata in a population-based study in a southwestern island of Japan: the Kumejima study. Arch Ophthalmol. 2011;129(3):332–6. doi:10.1001/archophthalmol.2010.372.

23. Iliff BW, Riazuddin SA, Gottsch JD. The genetics of Fuchs' corneal dystrophy. Expert Rev Ophthalmol. 2012;7(4):363–75. doi:10.1586/eop.12.39.
24. Illidge C, Kielty C, Shuttleworth A. Type VIII collagen: heterotrimeric chain association. Int J Biochem Cell Biol. 2001;33(5):521–9.
25. Jun AS. One hundred years of Fuchs' dystrophy. Ophthalmology. 2010;117(5):859–60. doi:10.1016/j.ophtha.2010.03.001. e814.
26. Jun AS, Meng H, Ramanan N, et al. An alpha 2 collagen VIII transgenic knock-in mouse model of Fuchs endothelial corneal dystrophy shows early endothelial cell unfolded protein response and apoptosis. Hum Mol Genet. 2012;21(2):384–93. doi:10.1093/hmg/ddr473.
27. Jurkunas UV, Bitar MS, Funaki T, et al. Evidence of oxidative stress in the pathogenesis of fuchs endothelial corneal dystrophy. Am J Pathol. 2010;177(5):2278–89. doi:10.2353/ajpath.2010.100279.
28. Kapoor R, Sakai LY, Funk S, et al. Type VIII collagen has a restricted distribution in specialized extracellular matrices. J Cell Biol. 1988;107(2):721–30.
29. Kim EC, Meng H, Jun AS. Lithium treatment increases endothelial cell survival and autophagy in a mouse model of Fuchs endothelial corneal dystrophy. Br J Ophthalmol. 2013;97(8):1068–73. doi:10.1136/bjophthalmol-2012-302881.
30. Kim EC, Meng H, Jun AS. N-Acetylcysteine increases corneal endothelial cell survival in a mouse model of Fuchs endothelial corneal dystrophy. Exp Eye Res. 2014;127:20–5. doi:10.1016/j.exer.2014.06.002.
31. Kitagawa K, Kojima M, Sasaki H, et al. Prevalence of primary cornea guttata and morphology of corneal endothelium in aging Japanese and Singaporean subjects. Ophthalmic Res. 2002;34(3):135–8. doi:10.1159/000063656.
32. Klintworth GK. Corneal dystrophies. Orphanet J Rare Dis. 2009;4:7. doi:10.1186/1750-1172-4-7.
33. Koizumi N, Okumura N, Ueno M, et al. New therapeutic modality for corneal endothelial disease using Rho-associated kinase inhibitor eye drops. Cornea. 2014;33 Suppl 11:S25–31. doi:10.1097/ICO.0000000000000240.
34. Koizumi N, Okumura N, Ueno M, et al. Rho-associated kinase inhibitor eye drop treatment as a possible medical treatment for Fuchs corneal dystrophy. Cornea. 2013;32(8):1167–70. doi:10.1097/ICO.0b013e318285475d.
35. Kopplin LJ, Przepyszny K, Schmotzer B, et al. Relationship of Fuchs endothelial corneal dystrophy severity to central corneal thickness. Arch Ophthalmol. 2012;130(4):433–9. doi:10.1001/archopthalmol.2011.1626.
36. Krachmer JH, Purcell Jr JJ, Young CW, et al. Corneal endothelial dystrophy. A study of 64 families. Arch Ophthalmol. 1978;96(11):2036–9.
37. Krafchak CM, Pawar H, Moroi SE, et al. Mutations in TCF8 cause posterior polymorphous corneal dystrophy and ectopic expression of COL4A3 by corneal endothelial cells. Am J Hum Genet. 2005;77(5):694–708. doi:10.1086/497348.
38. Lazorchak AS, Wojciechowski J, Dai M, et al. E2A promotes the survival of precursor and mature B lymphocytes. J Immunol. 2006;177(4):2495–504.
39. Lechner J, Dash DP, Muszynska D, et al. Mutational spectrum of the ZEB1 gene in corneal dystrophies supports a genotype-phenotype correlation. Invest Ophthalmol Vis Sci. 2013;54(5):3215–23. doi:10.1167/iovs.13-11781.
40. Liskova P, Prescott Q, Bhattacharya SS, et al. British family with early-onset Fuchs' endothelial corneal dystrophy associated with p.L450W mutation in the COL8A2 gene. Br J Ophthalmol. 2007;91(12):1717–8. doi:10.1136/bjo.2007.115154.
41. Lopez IA, Rosenblatt MI, Kim C, et al. Slc4a11 gene disruption in mice: cellular targets of sensorineuronal abnormalities. J Biol Chem. 2009;284(39):26882–96. doi:10.1074/jbc.M109.008102.
42. Lorenzetti DW, Uotila MH, Parikh N, et al. Central cornea guttata. Incidence in the general population. Am J Ophthalmol. 1967;64(6):1155–8.
43. Matsuda M, Yee RW, Edelhauser HF. Comparison of the corneal endothelium in an American and a Japanese population. Arch Ophthalmol. 1985;103(1):68–70.

44. Matthaei M, Hu J, Meng H, et al. Endothelial cell whole genome expression analysis in a mouse model of early-onset Fuchs' endothelial corneal dystrophy. Invest Ophthalmol Vis Sci. 2013;54(3):1931–40. doi:10.1167/iovs.12-10898.
45. McLaren JW, Nau CB, Erie JC, et al. Corneal thickness measurement by confocal microscopy, ultrasound, and scanning slit methods. Am J Ophthalmol. 2004;137(6):1011–20. doi:10.1016/j.ajo.2004.01.049.
46. Mehta JS, Vithana EN, Tan DT, et al. Analysis of the posterior polymorphous corneal dystrophy 3 gene, TCF8, in late-onset Fuchs endothelial corneal dystrophy. Invest Ophthalmol Vis Sci. 2008;49(1):184–8. doi:10.1167/iovs.07-0847.
47. Meng H, Matthaei M, Ramanan N, et al. L450W and Q455K Col8a2 knock-in mouse models of Fuchs endothelial corneal dystrophy show distinct phenotypes and evidence for altered autophagy. Invest Ophthalmol Vis Sci. 2013;54(3):1887–97. doi:10.1167/iovs.12-11021.
48. Mimura T, Joyce NC. Replication competence and senescence in central and peripheral human corneal endothelium. Invest Ophthalmol Vis Sci. 2006;47(4):1387–96. doi:10.1167/iovs.05-1199.
49. Mok JW, Kim HS, Joo CK. Q455V mutation in COL8A2 is associated with Fuchs' corneal dystrophy in Korean patients. Eye (Lond). 2009;23(4):895–903. doi:10.1038/eye.2008.116.
50. Mootha VV, Hussain I, Cunnusamy K, et al. TCF4 triplet repeat expansion and nuclear RNA foci in Fuchs' endothelial corneal dystrophy. Invest Ophthalmol Vis Sci. 2015;56(3):2003–11. doi:10.1167/iovs.14-16222.
51. Murre C. Helix-loop-helix proteins and lymphocyte development. Nat Immunol. 2005;6(11):1079–86. doi:10.1038/ni1260.
52. Nanda GG, Padhy B, Samal S, et al. Genetic association of TCF4 intronic polymorphisms, CTG18.1 and rs17089887, with Fuchs' endothelial corneal dystrophy in an Indian population. Invest Ophthalmol Vis Sci. 2014;55(11):7674–80. doi:10.1167/iovs.14-15297.
53. Olsen T. Is there an association between Fuchs' endothelial dystrophy and cardiovascular disease? Graefes Arch Clin Exp Ophthalmol. 1984;221(5):239–40.
54. Park CY, Lee JK, Gore PK, et al. Keratoplasty in the United States: a 10-year review from 2005 through 2014. Ophthalmology. 2015;122(12):2432–42. doi:10.1016/j.ophtha.2015.08.017.
55. Park M, Li Q, Shcheynikov N, et al. NaBC1 is a ubiquitous electrogenic Na+-coupled borate transporter essential for cellular boron homeostasis and cell growth and proliferation. Mol Cell. 2004;16(3):331–41. doi:10.1016/j.molcel.2004.09.030.
56. Pitts JF, Jay JL. The association of Fuchs's corneal endothelial dystrophy with axial hypermetropia, shallow anterior chamber, and angle closure glaucoma. Br J Ophthalmol. 1990;74(10):601–4.
57. Rao GP, Kaye SB, Agius-Fernandez A. Central corneal endothelial guttae and age-related macular degeneration: is there an association? Indian J Ophthalmol. 1998;46(3):145–7.
58. Repp DJ, Hodge DO, Baratz KH, et al. Fuchs' endothelial corneal dystrophy: subjective grading versus objective grading based on the central-to-peripheral thickness ratio. Ophthalmology. 2013;120(4):687–94. doi:10.1016/j.ophtha.2012.09.022.
59. Riazuddin SA, Eghrari AO, Al-Saif A, et al. Linkage of a mild late-onset phenotype of Fuchs corneal dystrophy to a novel locus at 5q33.1-q35.2. Invest Ophthalmol Vis Sci. 2009;50(12):5667–71. doi:10.1167/iovs.09-3764.
60. Riazuddin SA, Parker DS, McGlumphy EJ, et al. Mutations in LOXHD1, a recessive-deafness locus, cause dominant late-onset Fuchs corneal dystrophy. Am J Hum Genet. 2012;90(3):533–9. doi:10.1016/j.ajhg.2012.01.013.
61. Riazuddin SA, Vasanth S, Katsanis N, et al. Mutations in AGBL1 cause dominant late-onset Fuchs corneal dystrophy and alter protein-protein interaction with TCF4. Am J Hum Genet. 2013;93(4):758–64. doi:10.1016/j.ajhg.2013.08.010.
62. Riazuddin SA, Vithana EN, Seet LF, et al. Missense mutations in the sodium borate cotransporter SLC4A11 cause late-onset Fuchs corneal dystrophy. Hum Mutat. 2010;31(11):1261–8. doi:10.1002/humu.21356.

63. Riazuddin SA, Zaghloul NA, Al-Saif A, et al. Missense mutations in TCF8 cause late-onset Fuchs corneal dystrophy and interact with FCD4 on chromosome 9p. Am J Hum Genet. 2010;86(1):45–53. doi:10.1016/j.ajhg.2009.12.001.
64. Rogowski K, van Dijk J, Magiera MM, et al. A family of protein-deglutamylating enzymes associated with neurodegeneration. Cell. 2010;143(4):564–78. doi:10.1016/j.cell.2010.10.014.
65. Sanchez-Tillo E, de Barrios O, Siles L, et al. beta-catenin/TCF4 complex induces the epithelial-to-mesenchymal transition (EMT)-activator ZEB1 to regulate tumor invasiveness. Proc Natl Acad Sci U S A. 2011;108(48):19204–9. doi:10.1073/pnas.1108977108.
66. Santo RM, Yamaguchi T, Kanai A, et al. Clinical and histopathologic features of corneal dystrophies in Japan. Ophthalmology. 1995;102(4):557–67.
67. Sepp M, Kannike K, Eesmaa A, et al. Functional diversity of human basic helix-loop-helix transcription factor TCF4 isoforms generated by alternative 5′ exon usage and splicing. PLoS One. 2011;6(7):e22138. doi:10.1371/journal.pone.0022138.
68. Shuttleworth CA. Type VIII collagen. Int J Biochem Cell Biol. 1997;29(10):1145–8.
69. Soliman AZ, Xing C, Radwan SH, et al. Correlation of severity of Fuchs endothelial corneal dystrophy with triplet repeat expansion in TCF4. JAMA Ophthalmol. 2015;133(12):1386–91. doi:10.1001/jamaophthalmol.2015.3430.
70. Soumittra N, Loganathan SK, Madhavan D, et al. Biosynthetic and functional defects in newly identified SLC4A11 mutants and absence of COL8A2 mutations in Fuchs endothelial corneal dystrophy. J Hum Genet. 2014;59(8):444–53. doi:10.1038/jhg.2014.55.
71. Stridh P, Thessen Hedreul M, Beyeen AD, et al. Fine-mapping resolves Eae23 into two QTLs and implicates ZEB1 as a candidate gene regulating experimental neuroinflammation in rat. PLoS One. 2010;5(9):e12716. doi:10.1371/journal.pone.0012716.
72. Sundin OH, Broman KW, Chang HH, et al. A common locus for late-onset Fuchs corneal dystrophy maps to 18q21.2-q21.32. Invest Ophthalmol Vis Sci. 2006;47(9):3919–26. doi:10.1167/iovs.05-1619.
73. Sundin OH, Jun AS, Broman KW, et al. Linkage of late-onset Fuchs corneal dystrophy to a novel locus at 13pTel-13q12.13. Invest Ophthalmol Vis Sci. 2006;47(1):140–5. doi:10.1167/iovs.05-0578.
74. Tan H, Xu Z, Jin P. Role of noncoding RNAs in trinucleotide repeat neurodegenerative disorders. Exp Neurol. 2012;235(2):469–75. doi:10.1016/j.expneurol.2012.01.019.
75. Vilas GL, Loganathan SK, Liu J, et al. Transmembrane water-flux through SLC4A11: a route defective in genetic corneal diseases. Hum Mol Genet. 2013;22(22):4579–90. doi:10.1093/hmg/ddt307.
76. Vithana EN, Morgan P, Sundaresan P, et al. Mutations in sodium-borate cotransporter SLC4A11 cause recessive congenital hereditary endothelial dystrophy (CHED2). Nat Genet. 2006;38(7):755–7. doi:10.1038/ng1824.
77. Vithana EN, Morgan PE, Ramprasad V, et al. SLC4A11 mutations in Fuchs endothelial corneal dystrophy. Hum Mol Genet. 2008;17(5):656–66. doi:10.1093/hmg/ddm337.
78. Wang T, Parris J, Li L, et al. The carboxypeptidase-like substrate-binding site in Nna1 is essential for the rescue of the Purkinje cell degeneration (pcd) phenotype. Mol Cell Neurosci. 2006;33(2):200–13. doi:10.1016/j.mcn.2006.07.009.
79. Wang Z, Handa JT, Green WR, et al. Advanced glycation end products and receptors in Fuchs' dystrophy corneas undergoing Descemet's stripping with endothelial keratoplasty. Ophthalmology. 2007;114(8):1453–60. doi:10.1016/j.ophtha.2006.10.049.
80. Wieben ED, Aleff RA, Tosakulwong N, et al. A common trinucleotide repeat expansion within the transcription factor 4 (TCF4, E2-2) gene predicts Fuchs corneal dystrophy. PLoS One. 2012;7(11):e49083. doi:10.1371/journal.pone.0049083.
81. Williams TM, Montoya G, Wu Y, et al. The TCF8 gene encoding a zinc finger protein (Nil-2-a) resides on human chromosome 10p11.2. Genomics. 1992;14(1):194–6.

82. Xing C, Gong X, Hussain I, et al. Transethnic replication of association of CTG18.1 repeat expansion of TCF4 gene with Fuchs' corneal dystrophy in Chinese implies common causal variant. Invest Ophthalmol Vis Sci. 2014;55(11):7073–8. doi:10.1167/iovs.14-15390.
83. Zhang P, Sun Y, Ma L. ZEB1: at the crossroads of epithelial-mesenchymal transition, metastasis and therapy resistance. Cell Cycle. 2015;14(4):481–7. doi:10.1080/15384101.2015.1006048.
84. Zhang W, Ogando DG, Bonanno JA, et al. Human SLC4A11 Is a Novel NH3/H+ Co-transporter. J Biol Chem. 2015;290(27):16894–905. doi:10.1074/jbc.M114.627455.
85. Zhang X, Igo Jr RP, Fondran J, et al. Association of smoking and other risk factors with Fuchs' endothelial corneal dystrophy severity and corneal thickness. Invest Ophthalmol Vis Sci. 2013;54(8):5829–35. doi:10.1167/iovs.13-11918.
86. Zoega GM, Fujisawa A, Sasaki H, et al. Prevalence and risk factors for cornea guttata in the Reykjavik Eye Study. Ophthalmology. 2006;113(4):565–9. doi:10.1016/j.ophtha.2005.12.014H.

Chapter 2
MicroRNAs in FECD: A New Therapeutic Option?

Mario Matthaei

2.1 Introduction

Studying the gene lin-4 in the nematode *Caenorhabditis elegans* Lee, Feinbaum, and Ambros demonstrated in the early 1990s that its product, a short noncoding RNA, controlled the timing of the larval development of the roundworm by binding to the lin-14 mRNA [1]. Various similar novel small regulatory RNAs have been identified in the following years, and they were termed as microRNAs (miRNAs) [2, 3]. miRNAs are expressed in all multicellular eukaryotes, they are highly conserved among species, and their aberrant regulation is involved in various physiological and pathological conditions [4]. They are small, noncoding 20–24-nucleotides-long RNAs. Their 5′ seed region (reaching from nucleotide 2 to nucleotide 7) is preferably complementary to the highly conserved sites in 3′ untranslated regions (UTRs) of their target mRNAs [5]. A miRNA-mRNA interaction usually requires base pairing of at least five consecutive nucleotides. mRNAs may exhibit binding sites for different miRNAs and individual miRNAs may have hundreds of different mRNA targets [6]. miRNAs cause mRNA destabilization and cleavage or direct translational repression to regulate eukaryotic translation or levels of target mRNA transcripts [5]. miRNAs may function as tuners or binary on/off switches of gene expression [5]. Reports indicate that miRNAs regulate over 60 % of protein-coding genes [6]. The latest update of the miRNA database miRBase lists almost 2600 mature human miRNAs (http://www.mirbase.org), and the detection rate of novel miRNAs is continuously increasing [7].

M. Matthaei, MD, FEBO
University of Cologne, Cologne, Germany
e-mail: mario.matthaei@uk-koeln.de

C. Cursiefen, A.S. Jun (eds.), *Current Treatment Options for Fuchs Endothelial Dystrophy*, DOI 10.1007/978-3-319-43021-8_2

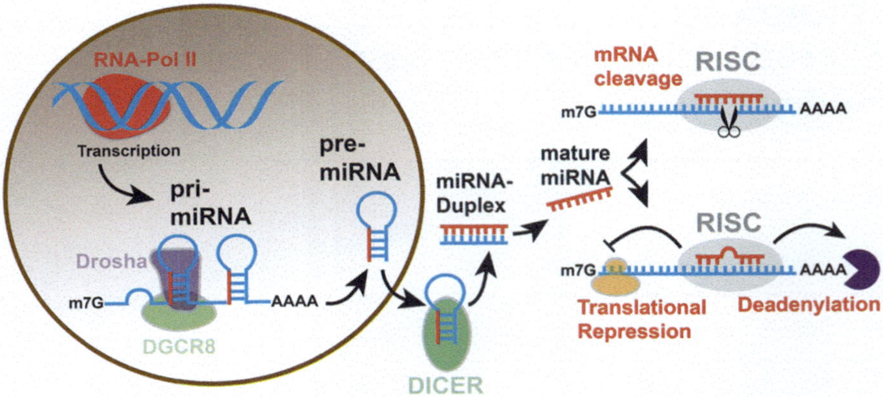

Fig. 2.1 MicroRNA biogenesis and function (figure kindly provided by Professor T. Langmann, University of Cologne)

2.2 MicroRNAs: Biogenesis and Function

Figure 2.1 provides an overview of miRNA biogenesis and function. The miRNA primary transcript (pri-miRNA) is generated by RNA polymerase II [8]. Pri-miRNAs have characteristic local foldback hairpin structures, and their processing starts within the nucleus in a step termed "cropping" [9]. The microprocessor complex consisting of the enzyme Drosha (RNase III) and a cofactor, the DiGeorge syndrome critical region –8 (DGCR8), generates stem-loop structures from the hairpins referred to as precursor miRNAs (pre-miRNAs) [10, 11]. After trafficking to the cytoplasm, the RNase enzyme Dicer (RNase III) cleaves a miRNA duplex from the pre-miRNA consisting of a paired mature miRNA including a guide strand and a passenger strand [12]. The guide strand is loaded into the RNA-induced silencing complex (RISC) [13]. RISC consists of single-stranded miRNA and Argonaute (Ago) proteins. The mature miRNA allows recognition of target mRNAs by partial sequence complementarity. Ago proteins serve as effectors by recruiting factors causing translational repression, mRNA deadenylation (removal of the polyA end), and mRNA decay [9].

2.3 MicroRNAs in Corneal Endothelial Disease

The consistently growing interest in miRNA research has lead to the initiation of the first studies aiming to unravel the involvement of miRNAs in corneal endothelial disorders. Despite the importance of miRNAs in gene regulation under physiological and pathological conditions, the knowledge of miRNAs in the pathogenesis of diseases of the anterior segment of the eye and especially in corneal endothelial disorders is presently extremely limited. Up to date, miR-184 and miR-29 have been identified to be affected in corneal endothelial disorders and were subjected to more detailed analysis [14, 15].

2.3.1 *miR-184*

miR-184 is highly expressed in the central corneal epithelial basal and suprabasal cells as well as in the lens epithelium; its expression was also detected in the corneal endothelium as documented by primary miRNA expression studies in the adult mouse eye [16, 17]. Previous studies found that miR-184 is part of a group of miRNAs that are downregulated in the ischemic retina and that had the potential to reduce retinal neovascularization after intraocular injection [18]. A mutation altering the seed region of miR-184 is responsible for severe familial keratoconus combined with early-onset anterior polar cataract [19]. The same single-base substitution miR-184(+57C>T) is also described in a syndrome characterized by endothelial dystrophy, iris hypoplasia, congenital cataract, and stromal thinning (EDICT syndrome) [14]. Slit-lamp examination of individuals with EDICT syndrome shows corneal haze and a FECD-like beaten-metal appearance of the endothelium [20, 21]. Corneal topography demonstrates nonectatic thinning and uniform steepening of the cornea [20, 21]. Histopathologically, corneas exhibit prominent posterior nodules and attenuated endothelium characteristic of FECD [20, 21]. Pathogenic mechanisms involved in EDICT syndrome may include the miR-184(+57C>T) variant leading to alterations in DICER-binding or RISC assembly reducing expression or activity of mature miR-184 or even resulting in a completely different mature miRNA [14]. The failure of the defective miR-184(+57C>T) variant to sufficiently compete with another miRNA, miR-205, and avoid miR-205 related knockdown of the gene INPPL1 may lead to dysregulation of the Akt signaling pathway and defects in epithelial-mesenchymal transition (EMT) [14, 19, 22]. EMT describes the transition of cells with a polarized character to a migratory phenotype. It is suggested that defective EMT may represent a unifying pathway for corneal endothelial disorders like FECD and EDICT syndrome by irregular migration and replacement of cells particularly from the corneal endothelial periphery to the corneal endothelial center [22].

2.3.2 *miR-29*

A comparative analysis of miRNA expression in corneal endothelial cells from FECD and normal individuals demonstrated downregulation of miRNA levels in FECD endothelium: 87 miRNAs exhibit significantly decreased expression levels in FECD corneal endothelial cells [15]. Such unidirectional alterations in miRNA expression have previously been found in other pathologies including cancer tissue, human and rat cigarette smoke-exposed lung tissue, and cortical tissue affected by neuropsychiatric disorders [15, 23–28], and they may be explained by changes in transcription or epigenetic regulation of primary miRNA transcripts, changes in miRNA biogenesis, alterations in Ago protein expression, or changes in miRNA turnover [15, 23]. miR-29a is among the three most downregulated miRNAs in FECD endothelium, and the spectrum of downregulated mature miRNA transcripts encompasses a total of three members of the miR-29 family [15]. More detailed analyses of putative miR-29 target genes on transcriptional and translational level confirmed increased expression of collagen I, collagen IV, and laminin in FECD endothelial samples [15], suggesting impact of altered miR-29 regulation on subendothelial accumulation of these and other extracellular matrix-associated components in FECD [15]. MiR-29 family members are key modulators of ECM homeostasis and inhibit a variety of ECM-related transcripts and proteins. All miR-29 family members cover a similar spectrum of target genes due to similarities in their sequences and due to their identical seed sequences [29]. Aberrant miR-29 expression is described in hepatic, renal, cardiac, and pulmonary fibrosis [29–34]. These studies in non-ocular tissues are supplemented by an increasing number of reports in ocular tissues like Tenon's capsule or the trabecular meshwork emphasizing the role of miR-29 in ECM modulation [35–37]. Corneal endothelial cells derived from FECD patients exhibit overexpression of EMT-inducing genes ZEB1 and SNAIL1, and it was proposed that ZEB1 and SNAIL1 overexpression may be responsible for increased responsiveness of corneal endothelial cells in FECD to TGF-beta [38]. Activation of TGF-beta pathways causes suppressed miR-29 expression in numerous other ocular and non-ocular tissues [35, 37]. However, the effect of TGF-beta on the expression levels of miR-29 in corneal endothelial cells has so far not been investigated.

2.4 Clinical Potential of miRNAs in Corneal Endothelial Disease

2.4.1 Biomarkers

The expression of miRNAs is altered in human tissues and body fluids under various pathological conditions, and miRNAs represent promising diagnostic and prognostic biomarkers in a multitude of non-ocular diseases including inflammatory diseases, cardiovascular diseases, neurodegenerative diseases, and cancer [39–43]. Future studies need to clarify if these results from studies in non-ocular diseases are transferable also to ocular disorders and confirm practicability of the approach. miRNA expression is not limited to the ocular tissue itself but tear fluid and aqueous and vitreous humor [39, 44–46] also exhibiting miRNA expression represent additional potential sources for diagnostic and prognostic miRNA analysis.

2.4.2 *Therapeutic Potential*

The avascular clear cornea offers the features of an easily accessible tissue which can be clinically examined without difficulties. This allows for the topical application of drugs and a generally uncomplicated clinical evaluation of their therapeutic effects. Alternative modes to topical external application of miRNA modulators by eye drops include subconjunctival, intracameral, or intravitreal injection or even systemic administration. Changes in endothelial miRNA expression or function suggest that miRNAs could be valuable future therapeutic targets in corneal endothelial diseases. Sequence complementarity of miRNAs and their mRNA targets provides the potential to specifically modulate individual miRNAs and genes. However, it must be considered that individual miRNAs have a multitude of target genes, and thus, modulation of a single miRNA may affect numerous cellular processes and pathways. This either beneficial or disadvantageous effect may be even further augmented by individual therapeutics targeting more than one miRNA. miRNA replenishment can be achieved by gene transfer inducing miRNA expression or by administration of miRNA mimics. miRNA mimics feature a guide strand identical to the miRNA of interest and a passenger strand which may be subject to further molecular modifications for optimized functionality [47]. The spectrum of inhibitory miRNA modulators includes antisense oligonucleotides (single-stranded RNAs complementary to target miRNAs), small-molecule inhibitors (small-molecule chemical compounds interfering with miRNA maturation or biogenesis), and miRNA sponges (overexpression of mRNAs with multiple artificial binding sites to a miRNA of interest). Despite the apparently great potential of miRNA therapy for corneal endothelial disorders, future studies will need to refine and increase the spectrum of target miRNAs and of their target genes. Developing therapeutic approaches will bring about challenges including optimizing tropism of therapeutics for corneal endothelial cells, delivery of sufficient therapeutic levels into the corneal endothelial cytosol, and avoidance of off-target effects and unwanted local unphysiological miRNA levels.

2.5 Concluding Remarks

miRNAs are small noncoding RNAs inhibiting gene expression at the posttranscriptional level. They are expressed in all multicellular eukaryotes and highly conserved among species. Studies in ocular and non-ocular tissues and pathologies describe the great potential of this class of endogenous RNAs to serve as biomarkers or treatment targets. Initial studies examining the role of microRNAs in corneal endothelial disorders describe changes in miRNA expression in FECD and EDICT syndromes [14, 15]. Reduced corneal endothelial expression of miR-29 in FECD may be involved in excessive subendothelial ECM deposition [15]. A single-base substitution miR-184(+57C>T) was found in EDICT syndrome and may cause defective EMT [14].

However, the discovery of changes in these two miRNAs/miRNA families represents only a first step toward a new and exciting research field, and improved understanding of the role of miRNAs in physiological and pathological conditions of the corneal endothelium may provide us with a new approach to treat FECD.

References

1. Lee RC, Feinbaum RL, Ambros V. The C. elegans heterochronic gene lin-4 encodes small RNAs with antisense complementarity to lin-14. Cell. 1993;75(5):843–54.
2. Lagos-Quintana M, Rauhut R, Lendeckel W, Tuschl T. Identification of novel genes coding for small expressed RNAs. Science. 2001;294(5543):853–8.
3. Lee RC, Ambros V. An extensive class of small RNAs in Caenorhabditis elegans. Science. 2001;294(5543):862–4.
4. Raghunath A, Perumal E. Micro-RNAs and their roles in Eye disorders. Ophthalmic Res. 2015;53(4):169–86. doi:10.1159/000371853.
5. Bartel DP. MicroRNAs: target recognition and regulatory functions. Cell. 2009;136(2):215–33. doi:10.1016/j.cell.2009.01.002. S0092-8674(09)00008-7 [pii].
6. Friedman RC, Farh KK, Burge CB, Bartel DP. Most mammalian mRNAs are conserved targets of microRNAs. Genome Res. 2009;19(1):92–105. doi:10.1101/Gr.082701.108.
7. Kozomara A, Griffiths-Jones S. miRBase: annotating high confidence microRNAs using deep sequencing data. Nucleic Acids Res. 2014;42(Database issue):D68–73. doi:10.1093/nar/gkt1181.
8. Lee Y, Kim M, Han JJ, Yeom KH, Lee S, Baek SH, Kim VN. MicroRNA genes are transcribed by RNA polymerase II. Embo J. 2004;23(20):4051–60. doi:10.1038/sj.emboj.7600385.
9. Ha M, Kim VN. Regulation of microRNA biogenesis. Nat Rev Mol Cell Bio. 2014;15(8):509–24. doi:10.1038/nrm3838.
10. Lee Y, Ahn C, Han JJ, Choi H, Kim J, Yim J, Lee J, Provost P, Radmark O, Kim S, Kim VN. The nuclear RNase III Drosha initiates microRNA processing. Nature. 2003;425(6956):415–9. doi:10.1038/nature01957.
11. Denli AM, Tops BB, Plasterk RH, Ketting RF, Hannon GJ. Processing of primary microRNAs by the microprocessor complex. Nature. 2004;432(7014):231–5. doi:10.1038/nature03049.
12. Hutvagner G, McLachlan J, Pasquinelli AE, Balint E, Tuschl T, Zamore PD. A cellular function for the RNA-interference enzyme Dicer in the maturation of the let-7 small temporal RNA. Science. 2001;293(5531):834–8. doi:10.1126/Science.1062961.
13. Liu JD, Carmell MA, Rivas FV, Marsden CG, Thomson JM, Song JJ, Hammond SM, Joshua-Tor L, Hannon GJ. Argonaute2 is the catalytic engine of mammalian RNAi. Science. 2004;305(5689):1437–41. doi:10.1126/science.1102513.
14. Iliff BW, Riazuddin SA, Gottsch JD. A single-base substitution in the seed region of miR-184 causes EDICT syndrome. Invest Ophthalmol Vis Sci. 2012;53(1):348–53. doi:10.1167/iovs.11-8783. iovs.11-8783 [pii].
15. Matthaei M, Hu J, Kallay L, Eberhart CG, Cursiefen C, Qian J, Lackner EM, Jun AS. Endothelial cell MicroRNA expression in human late-onset Fuchs dystrophy. 2013. doi:10.1167/iovs.13-12689. Invest Ophthalmol Vis Sci, iovs.13-12689 [pii].
16. Ryan DG, Oliveira-Fernandes M, Lavker RM. MicroRNAs of the mammalian eye display distinct and overlapping tissue specificity. Mol Vis. 2006;12:1175–84.
17. Karali M, Peluso I, Marigo V, Banfi S. Identification and characterization of microRNAs expressed in the mouse eye. Invest Ophthalmol Vis Sci. 2007;48(2):509–15. doi:10.1167/iovs.06-0866.
18. Shen J, Yang X, Xie B, Chen Y, Swaim M, Hackett SF, Campochiaro PA. MicroRNAs regulate ocular neovascularization. Mole Therapy J Am Soc Gene Therapy. 2008;16(7):1208–16. doi:10.1038/mt.2008.104.

19. Hughes AE, Bradley DT, Campbell M, Lechner J, Dash DP, Simpson DA, Willoughby CE. Mutation altering the miR-184 seed region causes familial keratoconus with cataract. Am J Hum Genet. 2011;89(5):628–33. doi:10.1016/j.ajhg.2011.09.014.
20. Akpek EK, Jun AS, Goodman DF, Green WR, Gottsch JD. Clinical and ultrastructural features of a novel hereditary anterior segment dysgenesis. Ophthalmology. 2002;109(3):513–9.
21. Jun AS, Broman KW, Do DV, Akpek EK, Stark WJ, Gottsch JD. Endothelial dystrophy, iris hypoplasia, congenital cataract, and stromal thinning (EDICT) syndrome maps to chromosome 15q22.1-q25.3. Am J Ophthalmol. 2002:134(2):172–6. Pii S0002-9394(02)01401-0. doi:10.1016/S0002-9394(02)01401-0.
22. Iliff BW, Riazuddin SA, Gottsch JD. The genetics of Fuchs' corneal dystrophy. Expert Rev Ophthalmol. 2012;7(4):363–75. doi:10.1586/eop.12.39.
23. Smalheiser NR, Lugli G, Rizavi HS, Torvik VI, Turecki G, Dwivedi Y. MicroRNA expression is down-regulated and reorganized in prefrontal cortex of depressed suicide subjects. Plos One. 2012;7(3), e33201. doi:10.1371/journal.pone.0033201. PONE-D-11-06021 [pii].
24. Beveridge NJ, Gardiner E, Carroll AP, Tooney PA, Cairns MJ. Schizophrenia is associated with an increase in cortical microRNA biogenesis. Mol Psychiatry. 2010;15(12):1176–89. doi:10.1038/mp.2009.84. mp200984 [pii].
25. Graff JW, Powers LS, Dickson AM, Kim J, Reisetter AC, Hassan IH, Kremens K, Gross TJ, Wilson ME, Monick MM. Cigarette smoking decreases global microRNA expression in human alveolar macrophages. Plos One. 2012;7(8), e44066. doi:10.1371/journal.pone.0044066. PONE-D-12-05332 [pii].
26. Schembri F, Sridhar S, Perdomo C, Gustafson AM, Zhang X, Ergun A, Lu J, Liu G, Bowers J, Vaziri C, Ott K, Sensinger K, Collins JJ, Brody JS, Getts R, Lenburg ME, Spira A. MicroRNAs as modulators of smoking-induced gene expression changes in human airway epithelium. Proc Natl Acad Sci U S A. 2009;106(7):2319–24. doi:10.1073/pnas.0806383106. 0806383106 [pii].
27. Izzotti A, Calin GA, Arrigo P, Steele VE, Croce CM, De Flora S. Downregulation of microRNA expression in the lungs of rats exposed to cigarette smoke. FASEB J. 2009;23(3):806–12. doi:10.1096/fj.08-121384. fj.08-121384 [pii].
28. Lu J, Getz G, Miska EA, Alvarez-Saavedra E, Lamb J, Peck D, Sweet-Cordero A, Ebert BL, Mak RH, Ferrando AA, Downing JR, Jacks T, Horvitz HR, Golub TR. MicroRNA expression profiles classify human cancers. Nature. 2005;435(7043):834–8. doi:10.1038/nature03702. nature03702 [pii].
29. Kriegel AJ, Liu Y, Fang Y, Ding X, Liang M. The miR-29 family: genomics, cell biology, and relevance to renal and cardiovascular injury. Physiol Genomics. 2012;44(4):237–44. doi:10.1152/physiolgenomics.00141.2011. physiolgenomics.00141.2011 [pii].
30. Qin W, Chung AC, Huang XR, Meng XM, Hui DS, Yu CM, Sung JJ, Lan HY. TGF-beta/Smad3 signaling promotes renal fibrosis by inhibiting miR-29. J Am Soc Nephrol. 2011;22(8):1462–74. doi:10.1681/ASN.2010121308. ASN.2010121308 [pii].
31. He Y, Huang C, Lin X, Li J. MicroRNA-29 family, a crucial therapeutic target for fibrosis diseases. Biochimie. 2013. doi:S0300-9084(13)00098-9. [pii] 10.1016/j.biochi.2013.03.010.
32. Roderburg C, Urban GW, Bettermann K, Vucur M, Zimmermann H, Schmidt S, Janssen J, Koppe C, Knolle P, Castoldi M, Tacke F, Trautwein C, Luedde T. Micro-RNA profiling reveals a role for miR-29 in human and murine liver fibrosis. Hepatology. 2011;53(1):209–18. doi:10.1002/hep.23922.
33. Pandit KV, Milosevic J, Kaminski N. MicroRNAs in idiopathic pulmonary fibrosis. Transl Res. 2011;157(4):191–9. doi:10.1016/j.trsl.2011.01.012. S1931-5244(11)00044-2 [pii].
34. van Rooij E, Sutherland LB, Thatcher JE, DiMaio JM, Naseem RH, Marshall WS, Hill JA, Olson EN. Dysregulation of microRNAs after myocardial infarction reveals a role of miR-29 in cardiac fibrosis. Proc Natl Acad Sci U S A. 2008;105(35):13027–32. doi:10.1073/pnas.0805038105. 0805038105 [pii].
35. Li N, Cui J, Duan X, Chen H, Fan F. Suppression of type I collagen expression by miR-29b via PI3K, Akt, and Sp1 pathway in human Tenon's fibroblasts. Invest Ophthalmol Vis Sci. 2012;53(3):1670–8. doi:10.1167/iovs.11-8670. iovs.11-8670 [pii].

36. Luna C, Li GR, Qiu JM, Epstein DL, Gonzalez P. Cross-talk between miR-29 and transforming growth factor-betas in trabecular meshwork cells. Invest Ophth Vis Sci. 2011;52(6):3567–72. doi:10.1167/Iovs.10-6448.
37. Villarreal Jr G, Oh DJ, Kang MH, Rhee DJ. Coordinated regulation of extracellular matrix synthesis by the microRNA-29 family in the trabecular meshwork. Invest Ophthalmol Vis Sci. 2011;52(6):3391–7. doi:10.1167/iovs.10-6165. iovs.10-6165 [pii].
38. Okumura N, Minamiyama R, Ho LT, Kay EP, Kawasaki S, Tourtas T, Schlotzer-Schrehardt U, Kruse FE, Young RD, Quantock AJ, Kinoshita S, Koizumi N. Involvement of ZEB1 and Snail1 in excessive production of extracellular matrix in Fuchs endothelial corneal dystrophy. Lab Invest. 2015. doi:10.1038/labinvest.2015.111.
39. Weber JA, Baxter DH, Zhang SL, Huang DY, Huang KH, Lee MJ, Galas DJ, Wang K. The MicroRNA spectrum in 12 body fluids. Clin Chem. 2010;56(11):1733–41. doi:10.1373/clinchem.2010.147405.
40. Sheinerman KS, Umansky SR. Circulating cell-free microRNA as biomarkers for screening, diagnosis, and monitoring of neurodegenerative diseases and other neurologic pathologies. Front Cell Neurosci. 2013;7:150. doi:10.3389/Fncel.2013.00150.
41. Brase JC, Wuttig D, Kuner R, Sultmann H. Serum microRNAs as non-invasive biomarkers for cancer. Mol Cancer. 2010;9:306. doi:10.1186/1476-4598-9-306.
42. van Rooij E, Olson EN. MicroRNA therapeutics for cardiovascular disease: opportunities and obstacles. Nat Rev Drug Discov. 2012;11(11):860–72. doi:10.1038/nrd3864.
43. O'connell RM, Rao DS, Chaudhuri AA, Baltimore D. Physiological and pathological roles for microRNAs in the immune system. Nat Rev Immunol. 2010;10(2):111–22. doi:10.1038/nri2708.
44. Ragusa M, Caltabiano R, Russo A, Puzzo L, Avitabile T, Longo A, Toro MD, Di Pietro C, Purrello M, Reibaldi M. MicroRNAs in vitreus humor from patients with ocular diseases. Mol Vis. 2013;19:430–40.
45. Dunmire JJ, Lagouros E, Bouhenni RA, Jones M, Edward DP. MicroRNA in aqueous humor from patients with cataract. Exp Eye Res. 2013;108:68–71. doi:10.1016/j.exer.2012.10.016.
46. Karali M, Peluso I, Gennarino VA, Bilio M, Verde R, Lago G, Dolle P, Banfi S. miRNeye: a microRNA expression atlas of the mouse eye. Bmc Genomics. 2010;11:715. doi:10.1186/1471-2164-11-715.
47. van Rooij E, Kauppinen S. Development of microRNA therapeutics is coming of age. Embo Mol Med. 2014;6(7):851–64. doi:10.15252/emmm.201100899.

Chapter 3
Clinical Phenotypes of Fuchs Endothelial Corneal Dystrophy (FECD), Disease Progression, Differential Diagnosis, and Medical Therapy

Berthold Seitz and Tobias Hager

3.1 When to Talk About Fuchs Endothelial Corneal Dystrophy (FECD): A Short Recourse to History

It is important to separate mere clinical findings from real diseases. Doing so, it is necessary to draw a clear distinction between "cornea guttata" and "Fuchs endothelial corneal dystrophy (FECD)." Therefore, a short recourse to the first descriptions of the disease may precede this chapter. For the first description of the eponymous dystrophy, the Austrian ophthalmologist Professor Ernst Fuchs had no slit lamp available. Therefore, it was only possible for him to describe the final stage of the disease with central corneal opacity, decreased visual acuity, and reduced corneal sensitivity (Fig. 3.1). Because of the changes of the ocular surface, he kept it for a dystrophy of the corneal epithelium [1]. It can be assumed that not all of the first 13 patients described by Fuchs suffered from a pure FECD according to our present understanding. The term "cornea guttata" (guttata is Latin for "drop-like") for the changes of the endothelial basement membrane in FECD was introduced in 1921 by the Swiss ophthalmologist Alfred Vogt, the decreased corneal sensitivity was abandoned as a diagnostic criterion, and for the first time the slit-lamp image was designated as "hammered bronze" [2]. Based on a series of patients, the American citizens Harry and Jonas Friedenwald in 1925 concluded that changes in the corneal endothelial layer precede changes in the corneal epithelium and thus must be considered in the etiological context [3]. Later it was shown that a thickening of Descemet's membrane and a dilution of the endothelial cell layer in the area of the excrescences that we call guttae accompany these changes [4], so that the excrescences seemed to

B. Seitz, ML, FEBO (✉) • T. Hager
Department of Ophthalmology, Saarland University Medical Center UKS, Kirrbergerstraße 100, D-66424 Homburg/Saar, Germany
e-mail: berthold.seitz@uks.eu

C. Cursiefen, A.S. Jun (eds.), *Current Treatment Options for Fuchs Endothelial Dystrophy*, DOI 10.1007/978-3-319-43021-8_3

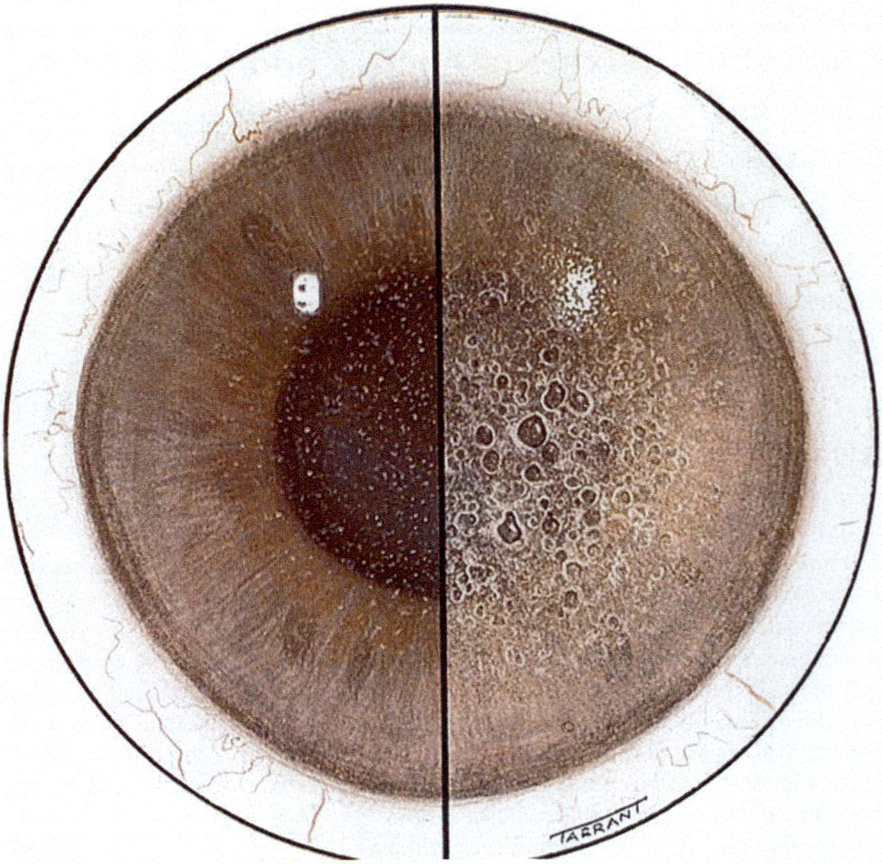

Fig. 3.1 Hand-drawn picture in Prof. Ernst Fuchs' original paper showing epithelial bullae on the right side (Fuchs [1])

be no longer covered by the endothelium [5]. The number of endothelial cells remaining in the cornea is, therefore, inversely proportional to the number of guttae excrescences. However, thickening of the endothelial basement membrane and a loss of corneal endothelial cells also occur in the context of the normal aging processes [6, 7].

Cornea guttata (Fig. 3.2) is thus a typical finding in FECD [8], but not each cornea guttata will progress to FECD [9]. In its strict sense, cornea guttata represents an isolated clinical sign of the endothelial basement membrane (also called Descemet's membrane) without affecting the microscopic tangible architecture of corneal endothelium and corneal stroma [10]. FECD in contrast is a bilateral, often asymmetric dystrophy of the corneal endothelium characterized by morphological changes in corneal endothelial mosaic leading to corneal edema and secondary stromal and epithelial changes [11].

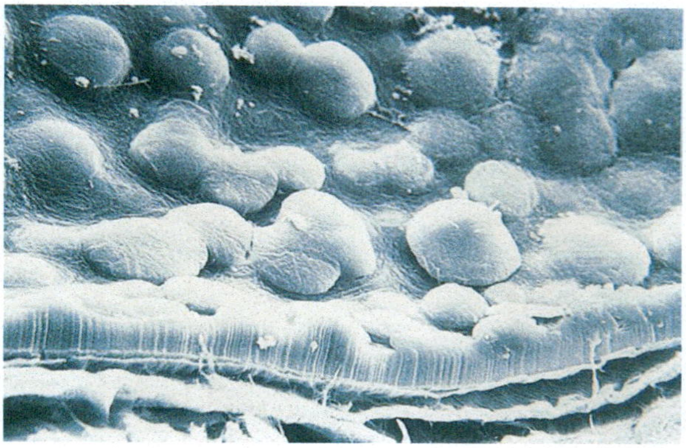

Fig. 3.2 Cornea guttata: excrescences of Descemet's membrane as seen in scanning electron microscopy

3.2 Clinical Phenotypes of FECD

There are two variants of FECD, early-onset FECD and late-onset FECD [9]. Most cases begin in the fourth decade of life or later, but the early variant that counts for 1 % of all FECD patients may start in the first decade [6]. The early form can be attributed to a specific genetic defect, i.e., alpha 2 collagen VIII (*COL8A2*) on the 1p34.3-p32 gene locus [12]. The guttae may develop already in the first decade of life. They are typically small and monomorphic and tend to spread almost from limbus to limbus. This indicates a several-fold more rapid deposition of DM extracellular matrix, supported by the fact that Descemet's membrane in these patients is thicker (up to 38 μm) compared to normal controls where secretion of extracellular matrix by corneal endothelial cells extends tonu lo lypsis throughout the whole life [7]. The inheritance of early-onset FECD is autosomal dominant [9, 13].

The more typical late-onset form of FECD progresses through four clinically defined stages [14]. Here, larger and different-sized guttae start to develop in the central area of the cornea. Late-onset FECD has female predominance and the disease can need decades to develop [15]. Patients complain about intermittent reduced vision from epithelial/stromal edema. Typically, visual acuity is worse in the morning due to increased stromal/epithelial edema after an overnight period of eye closure [9]. However, best-corrected visual acuity typically increases during the day during the first years and even decades after the onset of the disease.

Guttae are best diagnosed at the slit lamp after dilation of the pupil in retroillumination of focusing on Descemet's level (Fig. 3.3) and/or using a broad slit and directing the investigator's gaze next to the slit (Fig. 3.4).

Guttae alone may not cause corneal edema and mild corneal edema may not result in decreased vision [16]. On the other side, corneal guttae without edema may cause the quality of vision to deteriorate. Intraocular forward light scatter caused by corneal guttae alone may result in visual disturbances [17]. In a study to differentiate cornea guttata and FECD, Jackson et al. discovered pigment deposits on the posterior endothelial surface in all but one examined eye [18].

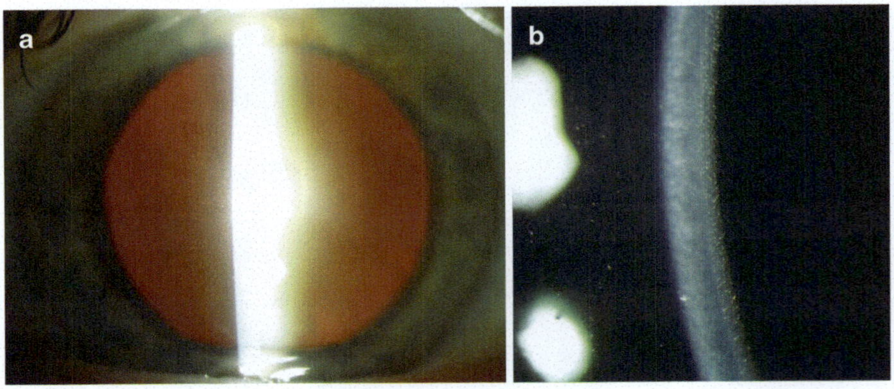

Fig. 3.3 Right eye of a 67-year-old male with late-onset cornea guttata +++. Guttae are best diagnosed at the slit lamp after dilation of the pupil in retroillumination (**a**) of focusing directly on Descemet's membrane (**b**)

Fig. 3.4 In advanced stages, guttae may also be well visualized using a broad slit beam and directing the investigator's gaze next to the slit (*arrows*). Please note typical melanin deposits in the endothelial layer, in the area of the broad beam

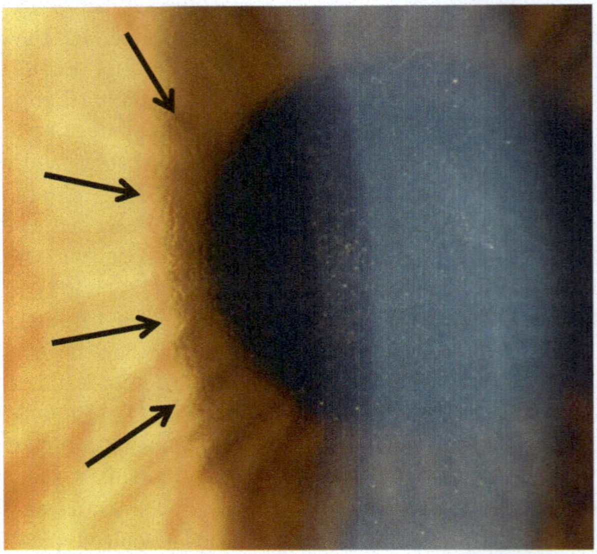

Recently, Amin SR et al. stressed that anterior corneal cellular and structural abnormalities begin early in the course of FECD, before the onset of clinically evident edema. The chronicity of these changes can explain their incomplete resolution after endothelial keratoplasty [19].

Increasing epithelial and stromal edema in more severe stages of the disease is associated with decreased vision (Fig. 3.5). Pain, photophobia, and epiphora are common in advanced stages due to epithelial erosions resulting from burst epithelial bullae occurrence [9]. In addition to pain, these patients are at risk of infectious keratitis having lost their protecting epithelial barrier.

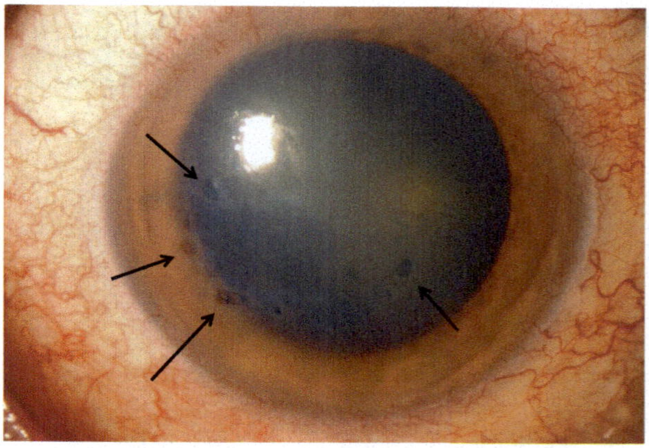

Fig. 3.5 Severe epithelial and stromal edema in FECD associated with decreased vision and multiple epithelial bullae (*arrows*) ("bullous keratopathy")

Typically FECD does not recur on the graft after lamellar or penetrating keratoplasty. Thus, guttae on the graft are typically transplanted, because they were not detected in the eye bank during processing of the donor tissue [9].

3.3 Interpretation of Morphological Examinations

Because FECD is a clinical entity for more than 100 years, several technical devices have been established to aid the slit-lamp-based diagnosis. These may be helpful in determining the clinical stage and, therefore, determining the appropriate time for surgery. Whether a cornea guttata with a best-corrected visual acuity of 20/25 without any endothelial decompensation should be treated surgically with Descemet's membrane endothelial keratoplasty (DMEK) remains at least questionable! Due to their noninvasive nature, all examinations may be performed at all stages of the disease. These include:

1. Noncontact specular microscopy
2. Pachymetry
3. Anterior segment OCT
4. In vivo confocal microscopy

3.3.1 Noncontact Specular Microscopy

Corneal endothelium is – in combination with the excrescences from Descemet's membrane – the key histological layer for diagnosis of FECD. In the morphological picture, two main entities may be estimated:

1. Pattern of corneal guttae
2. Morphology of endothelial cell mosaic

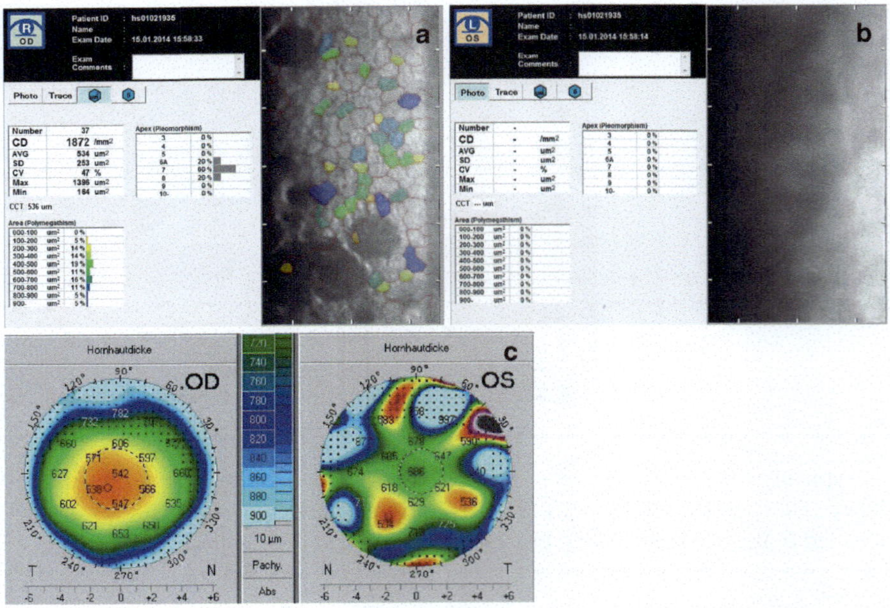

Fig. 3.6 An 80-year-old male with asymmetrical expression of FECD. (**a**) OD: specular microscopic image of the endothelium with few guttae of different sizes, normal tomographic central thickness of 542 μm (Pentacam, **c**), and VA of 20/20. (**b**) OS: no specular microscopic image possibly due to major edema, increased tomographic central thickness of 686 μm (Pentacam, **c**), and VA of 20/100

Typically modern (semi)automated specular microscopes display (1) number of analyzed cells; (2) density of cells per 1 mm^2; (3) average size of analyzed cells; (4) standard deviation of analyzed cell size; (5) coefficient of variance of the analyzed cells, depending on the relation of the mean cell size and the standard deviation; (6) size of the largest analyzed cell; and (7) size of the smallest analyzed cell (Fig. 3.6).

Interestingly, cornea guttata can be seen on the slit lamp before it can be demonstrated in the specular microscopy [20]. The extent of cornea guttata seems to follow a clinically identifiable pattern course. The endothelial mosaic has firstly a strawberry pattern [21] which is the first sign for cornea guttata. This strawberry pattern can present small hyperreflective dots suggestive of protrusions of Descemet's membrane in the center of hyporeflective areas [22]. As cornea guttata progresses, these hyporeflective areas get larger resulting in a craterlike appearance [23]. According to Zoega, the specular image can be divided in five grades. In the fifth grade, guttae occupy more than 50 % of the image [20].

Healthy corneal endothelial cells appear as a regular array of mainly hexagonal cells which exhibit bright cell bodies and dark cell borders [24]. The appearance of guttae in specular microscopy and confocal microscopy is similar [22]. Endothelial cell morphology is one key for the diagnosis of FECD: the main changes include polymegalism (variation in cell size) and pleomorphism (variation in cell shape) [25].

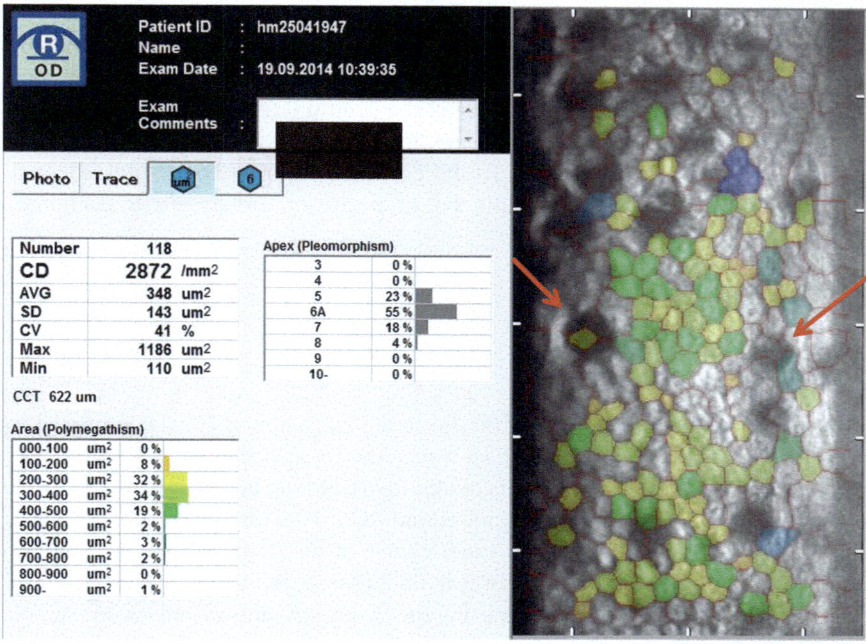

Fig. 3.7 Automated endothelial cell in specular microscopy count will not give valid results in case of unevenly distributed guttae. Especially in large guttae and large endothelial cells, the automatic algorithms result in a too high number of endothelial cells, because too many cell borders are typically falsely introduced, even within the area of a large gutta (*arrows*)

Patients with cornea guttata have reduced proportion of hexagonal cells, but increased proportion of tetragonal, pentagonal, heptagonal, and octagonal cells [23]. This is contradicted by Zoega et al. who did not detect a difference in hexagonality between corneas with and without guttae during a 7-year follow-up [20]. This is in accordance with a study by Kitagawa et al. who also did not detect changes in hexagonality, pachymetry, or visual function in a group of Japanese patients with primary cornea guttata [10]. Therefore, it is insecure whether polymegalism and pleomorphism of the endothelium in the presence of cornea guttata are already diagnostically decisive in order to talk about FECD. Nevertheless, it is a common sense today that in FECD, polymegalism and pleomorphism do increase [26]. The authors attribute this to oxidative stress in general or from hypoxia.

Several attempts have been made to standardize specular microscopy. They focus on the fact that endothelial cell density per square millimeter is notoriously overestimated being very much depending on the individual investigator. It is difficult to find the same area once measured again for a sequential measurement, leading to a considerable variation of images taken from the center of the cornea with guttae [23]. Neither manual nor automated endothelial cell count will give valid results in case of unevenly distributed guttae (Fig. 3.7). There is a possibility to create an effective cell density, correlating the fraction of clear endothelium and the fraction of the image area free of guttae. But this method is based on several assumptions. One assumption is that the scanned area is representative of viable cell density [27]. This depends on the severity of FECD. It could be demonstrated that most of the changes in FECD occur in the central 0.6 mm of the cornea [28]. Corneal edema can lead to light scattering, thus reducing image quality and making central analysis more difficult. In the corneal periphery at 3.7 mm, there is more damage to cells inferotemporally, but no positive correlation with pachymetry could be established so far [28].

3.3.2 Pachymetry

The pachymetry may range up to 1100 μm in the late stage of FECD compared to normal thickness of 530 μm [21, 29]. However, the *change* of central corneal thickness during clinical follow-up visits is more important than the overall value [30]. It is of importance that the thickness measured also depends on the system used. Given the difficulty in defining the exact center of the cornea, separate readings should be obtained if the central corneal thickness is manually measured using ultrasound. Today, tomography (e.g., using the Pentacam) allows better comparison of central corneal thickness values during individual follow-up. A central corneal thickness greater than 640 μm usually indicates corneal edema [31] (Fig. 3.6). Patients with central corneal pachymetry higher than 650 μm have greater than 85 % probability of epithelial edema occurrence [32]. Four millimeters from the center, the cornea is still statistically thicker than normal, but this seems to be clinically much less important. It has been suggested to use a central-to-peripheral thickness ratio (CPTR), i.e., measuring the center of the cornea and at 4 mm to detect individual progression of the disease [31].

3.3.3 Anterior Segment OCT

A theoretical advantage of anterior segment OCT is the possibility to measure corneal thickness layer by layer and not as overall thickness, therefore being able to better differentiate between stromal and epithelial edema. This method holds a second advantage in FECD patients: Descemet's membrane is visualized as a thickened band of two opaque lines. The anterior line is smooth and represents the stromal face of Descemet's membrane, while the posterior line is irregular and wavy with local thickenings strongly corresponding to the histological image [33]. This might allow to determine the progression of the disease. Unfortunately, this clear separation is restricted to ultrahigh-resolution anterior segment OCTs. In contrast, commercially available anterior segment OCTs have limited ability even to depict Descemet's membrane at all.

3.3.4 In Vivo Confocal Microscopy (IVCM)

IVCM is able to demonstrate microstructural changes that correlate well with histological studies. IVCM showed marked diminishment of total nerve number and number of nerve branches in the subbasal corneal nerve plexus with increasing stages of FECD compared to a control group [11]. Corneal sensation is mildly reduced in FECD patients at stage IV when tested with a Cochet-Bonnet esthesiometer [11]. It has to be kept in mind, however, that there is also a decrease of nerve density in the subbasal plexus with age [6]. But nerve alterations in the subbasal plexus can already be demonstrated in early stages of FECD [34]. They seem at first not to have an impact on corneal sensitivity. But in a study on 42 eyes after Descemet's stripping endothelial keratoplasty, corneal sensitivity remained lower than in controls for 36 months after surgery [35]. Pleomorphism and polymegalism can be demonstrated in IVCM and noncontact specular microscopy [36–38]. Guttae can be demonstrated in IVCM as hyporeflective round structures with ill-defined borders. Sometimes, there is a sharp hyperreflective spot in the center of a gutta [36, 37]. In addition, IVCM can help to assess endothelial cell count and morphology in analogy to specular microscopy

3.4 Clinical Stages and Disease Progression

Four clinical stages have been described by Adamis et al. [14]. Cornea guttata starts centrally and spreads peripherally, but the vision is not affected (stage I). Some patients demonstrate cornea guttata but never progress to later stages, and others develop stromal edema due to endothelial decompensation with concomitant mild loss of vision (stage II). Corneal endothelium has a beaten metallike appearance with or without pigment dusting. Corneal guttae in adult-onset FECD are larger than those seen in early-onset FECD. Descemet's membrane is thickened. Stromal edema may progress further toward the epithelium causing intra- and interepithelial edema (epithelial bullae) (so-called bullous keratopathy...) with loss of vision (stage III). Patients with central corneal pachymetry higher than 650 μm have a greater than 85 % probability of epithelial edema occurrence [32]. Subepithelial fibrous tissue ("pannus"), stromal scarring, and peripheral superficial vascularization may occur in long-standing cases from chronic edema, and the pain subsides (stage IV) (Fig. 3.8) [14].

This grading system still strongly relies on subjective parameters which are exclusively taken from the slit lamp. Stages I and II can be difficult to differentiate. Therefore, it is no surprise that in a large study with 100 FECD patients, only moderate agreement between two corneal specialists for this clinical grading was found [31].

The two main functions of the endothelium, barrier and water pump, follow different courses of decline. The barrier function depends on the ability of endothelial cells to fully cover the stromal surface and to maintain cell-to-cell tight junctions.

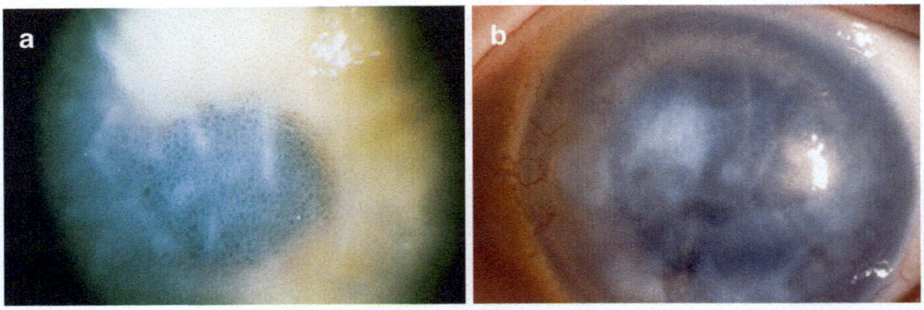

Fig. 3.8 (**a**, **b**) Severe bullous keratopathy with subepithelial fibrosis ("pannus") and peripheral superficial vascularization (**b**) in long-standing FECD (stage IV)

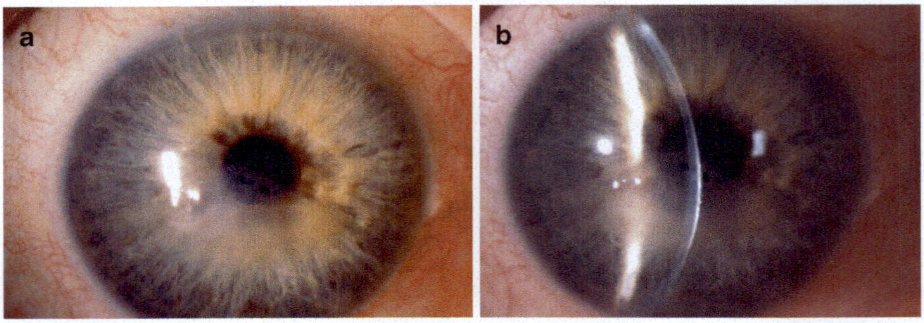

Fig. 3.9 A 73-year-old male with good BCVA of 20/30 (!) despite (para)centrally localized focal bullous keratopathy in FECD. (**a**) Overview and (**b**) slit beam evaluation

Both appear to be intact until end-stage disease. However, the pump function is gradually compromised, as evidenced by reductions in Na+/K+ATPase expression with subsequent stromal edema [30, 39]. The stromal changes are likely to occur secondary to corneal edema rather than due to FECD per se.

Another possibility of staging was presented by Krachmer et al. who focused on the number and confluence of corneal guttae and developed a grading scale from 1 to 6 [40] currently used by the Fuchs endothelial dystrophy genetics multicenter study group [30]. It has been reported that guttae are larger in the center of the cornea compared to paracentral areas [23].

Significant differences in central corneal thickness are also detectable at early grades of FECD; especially 1–2 mm of confluent guttae may begin to develop central corneal thickening [30] – even resulting in localized (para)central bullous keratopathy (Fig. 3.9). In a large multicenter study, female sex and smoking were associated significantly with higher stages of cornea guttata, but not with increased central corneal thickness [41]. It has been suggested to use central corneal thickness to determine the grade of disease progression, but this alone might not be unequivocal because of well-known interindividual variety of central corneal thickness [31].

Concerning contact lens wearing, it was shown that morphology of the endothelial cells is changing toward increasing proportions of polymegalism and pleomorphism during increasing corneal thickness [42]. This phenomenon points toward the conclusion that a deviation of the endothelial morphology from a homogeneous hexagonal shape goes along with a deterioration of the endothelial pumping function.

From our point of view, *progression* should be defined by looking at the following criteria:

1. Best-corrected visual acuity (BCVA)
2. Difference of BCVA between morning (typically worse due to closed eyelids overnight) and afternoon
3. Subjective glare (0, +, ++, +++) especially at night
4. Corneal thickness profile (tomography, e.g., Pentacam or anterior segment OCT)
5. Endothelial cell morphology (pleomorphism, polymegalism) (specular microscopy or confocal microscopy)
6. BUT NOT "endothelial cell count," because this very much depends on the investigator and is notoriously overestimating the amount of the endothelium, strongly depending on where the "region of interest (ROI)" is placed [25]

These criteria are also important for judging whether cataract surgery is still a reasonable option in FECD. Some authors state that below a corneal thickness of 640 μm, modern phacoemulsification would be feasible [43, 44], although Afshari NA et al. found that pachymetry-determined corneal thickness was a poor predictor of visual acuity until extreme levels of corneal edema were reached. At a corneal thickness of approximately 775 μm and greater, mean BCVA was 20/100, compared with a BCVA of 20/60 below that thickness level [43].

3.5 Differential Diagnosis

Differential diagnosis of endothelial dystrophies is typically an easy task. It includes:

1. Posterior polymorphous corneal dystrophy (PPCD)
2. Congenital hereditary endothelial dystrophy (CHED)
3. X-linked endothelial corneal dystrophy (XECD)

3.5.1 Posterior Polymorphous Corneal Dystrophy (PPCD)

In posterior polymorphous dystrophy, the endothelial cells undergo a transformation to epithelial-like cells [45] (Fig. 3.10a, b). Scattered endothelial vesicles can be shown with retroillumination [46]. Of note is that the vesicles in retroillumination can be visualized in IVCM as large oval structures that contain abnormal endothelial cells [37] which allow a clear distinction from FECD corneas. A railroad-shaped

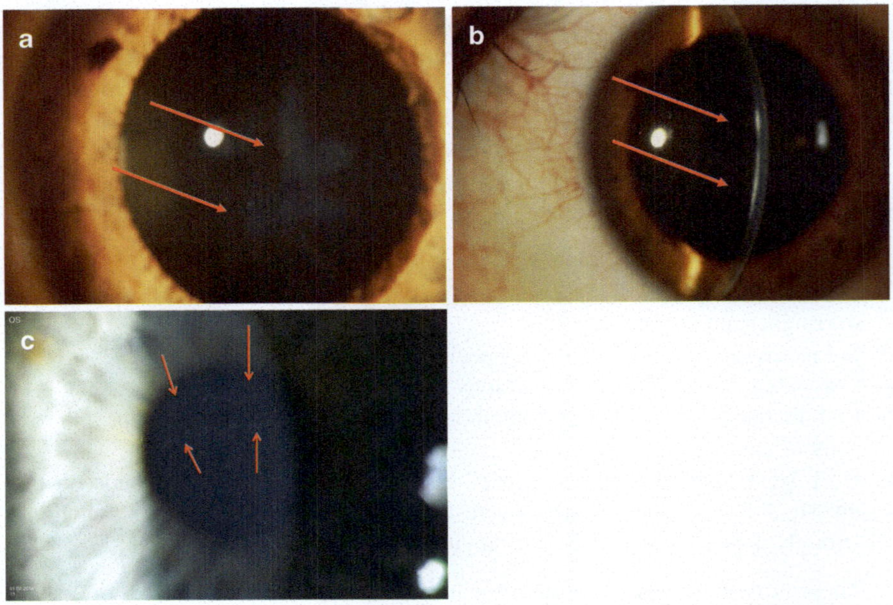

Fig. 3.10 In posterior polymorphous corneal dystrophy (PPCD), the endothelial cells undergo a transformation to epithelial-like cells (**a** overview. **b** slit beam). Often a railroad-shaped pattern (*arrows*) of the corneal endothelium can be seen at the slit lamp which is almost pathognomonic (**c**)

pattern of the corneal endothelium can be seen at the slit lamp and is almost pathognomonic [37] (Fig. 3.10c). Eyes with posterior polymorphous corneal dystrophy (PPCD) often need no therapy for decades. However, the intraocular pressure has to be monitored on a regular basis.

3.5.2 Congenital Hereditary Endothelial Dystrophy (CHED)

Congenital corneal clouding in the form of a milky ground glass appearance is the landmark of CHED, usually already present at birth [47] (Fig. 3.11). Specular microscopy in patients only mildly affected has not yet been published. But specular microscopy in parents of CHED patients may show cornea guttata [47].

3.5.3 X-linked Endothelial Corneal Dystrophy (XECD)

According to the heredity, only males are affected [48]. The so-called endothelial moon craters are the hallmark of this disease (Fig. 3.12a) that can also be demonstrated in female carriers. These alterations compromise the whole corneal

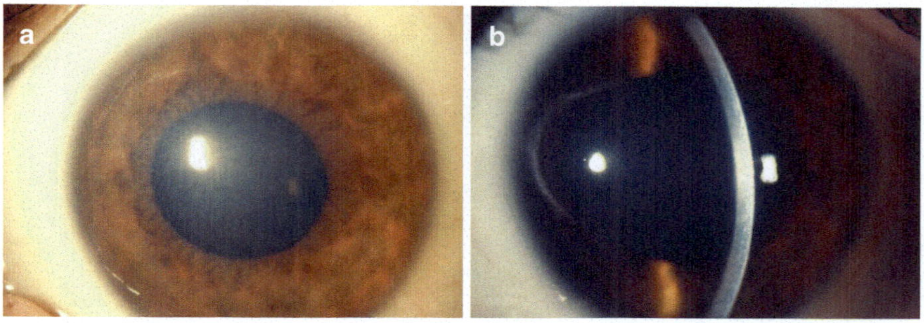

Fig. 3.11 Congenital hereditary endothelial dystrophy (CHED). (**a**) Overview, and (**b**) slit beam

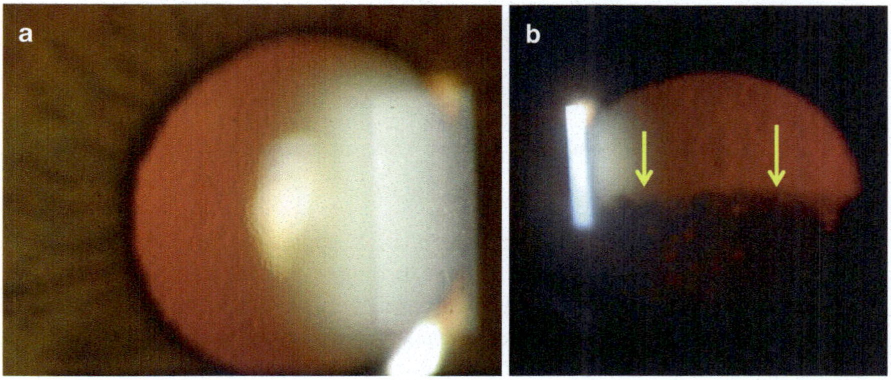

Fig. 3.12 X-linked endothelial corneal dystrophy (XECD). (**a**) "Moon craters." (**b**) Band-shaped keratopathy (*arrows*) in later stages

endothelium. In later life, a band keratopathy (Fig. 3.12b) may develop. Congenital corneal clouding can occur. Until now, no data on noncontact specular microscopy or corneal thickness are available in the literature because of the rarity of this disease.

Differential diagnosis of other alterations of the corneal endothelium include:

1. PEX keratopathy
2. Melanin dispersion syndrome
3. Pseudophakic bullous keratopathy
4. Pseudoguttae

3.5.4 PEX Keratopathy

Whereas fibroblastic metaplasia and the production of abnormal and excess extracellular material by corneal endothelium are believed to be a nonspecific common response to stress, injury, or disease, the production of PEX fibers is a

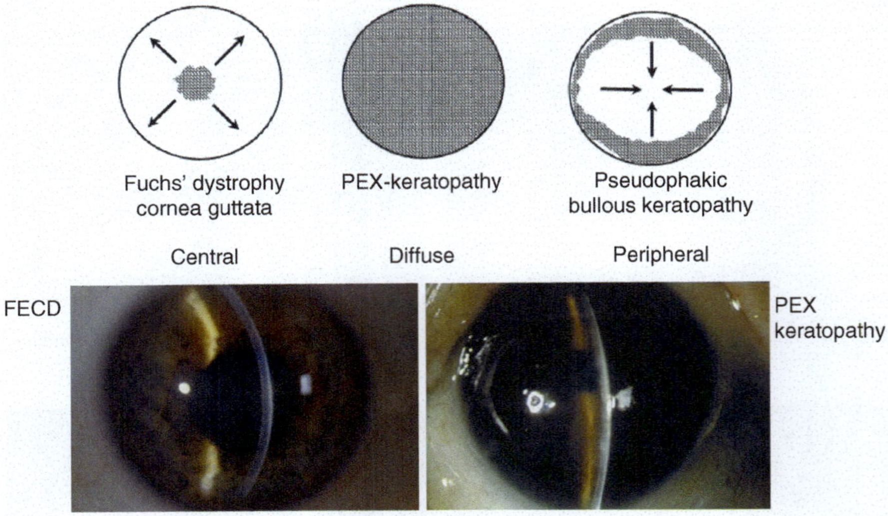

Fig. 3.13 Differential diagnosis of FCED vs. PEX keratopathy (schematic and clinical) [49, 50]

specific and pathognomonic feature of the PEX syndrome. Because, however, this pathognomonic feature is not evident throughout all five stages [49] of the disease, the diagnosis of PEX keratopathy may rely on other clinical and histopathologic criteria, such as diffuse edema, irregular thickening of Descemet's membrane, and pronounced melanin phagocytosis in the presence of an ocular PEX syndrome [49–52].

Circumscribed excrescences of the posterior Descemet's membrane ("guttae") are the clinical and histopathologic hallmark of FECD. The endothelium is attenuated, but mostly intact and shows moderate fibroblastic transformation and moderate amounts of phagocytosed melanin granules. FECD shows obvious similarities and differences with PEX endotheliopathy: the diffuse decompensation pattern on PEX eyes can be easily clinically distinguished from the corneal edema in classical FECD, which usually starts centrally and spreads peripherally, and also from bullous keratopathy (e.g., after anterior chamber lens implantation), which usually starts in the limbal region and spreads centrally (Fig. 3.13). Further clinical differences between Fuchs and PEX endotheliopathies include the presence of typical guttata in FECD which is usually lacking in PEX eyes (Figs. 3.14 and 3.15) and the extent of endothelial loss, which is often more pronounced in PEX eyes (Table 3.1). Besides more severe polymegalism and pleomorphism, PEX eyes may show hyperreflective retrocorneal whitish deposits at slit-lamp examination (Fig. 3.16).

Apart from the corneal endothelial decompensation, both have nuclear cataract that develops sooner or later. But in classical FECD, the iris stroma is not affected, phacodonesis and pseudouveitis are absent, and the incidence of open-angle glaucoma is not significantly increased [14].

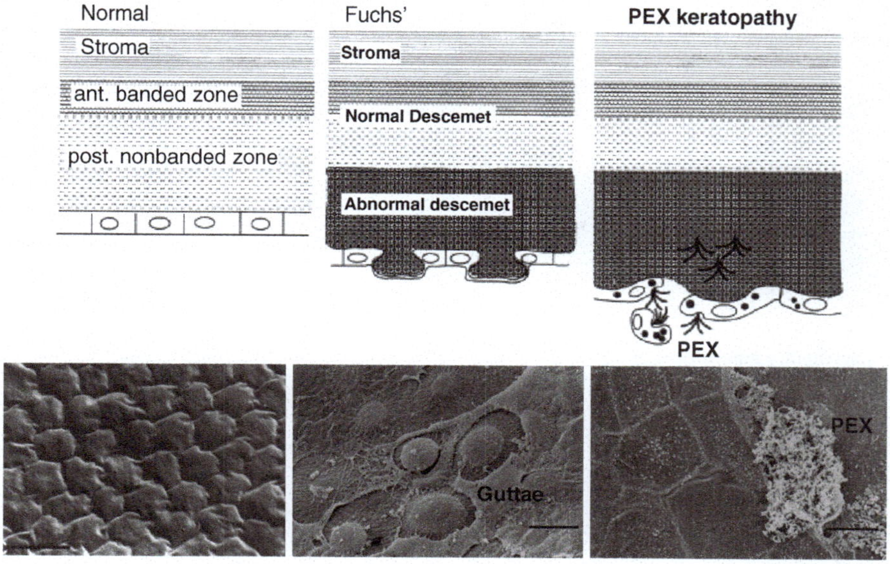

Fig. 3.14 Differential diagnosis of FCED vs. PEX keratopathy (schematic and scanning electron microscopy) [49, 50]

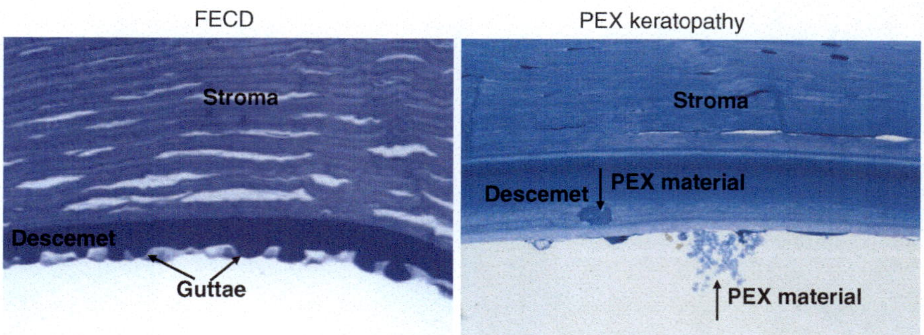

- Cornea guttata (15–30 µm)
- Endothelial cell loss +
- Phagozytosis of Melanin +
- Fibroblastic transformation +

- Diffuse thickening of DM (15–45 µm)
- Endothelial cell loss ++ / +++
- Phagozytosis of Melanin +++
- Fibroblastic transformation +++
- Focal PEX aggregates in and on DM

Fig. 3.15 Differential diagnosis of FCED vs. PEX keratopathy (histopathology) [49, 50]

Differential diagnosis between FECD and PEX keratopathy is not only an academic problem. Concerning microsurgery, FECD is a "friend," while PEX keratopathy is a challenge [52, 53] (Fig. 3.17).

It may be speculated that PEX may be transmitted via a PEX-affected donor to a recipient eye [54, 55].

Table 3.1 Differential diagnosis (DD) of Fuchs endothelial corneal dystrophy and pseudoexfoliation (PEX) keratopathy [49, 50]

	Fuchs dystrophy	PEX keratopathy
I. Clinical DD		
Corneal guttae	+++	(+) Atypical
Endothelial cell loss	+	+>+++
Endothelial decompensation	Central	Diffuse
Nuclear cataract	++	++
Melanin dispersion	+	+++
Iris involvement	–	+>+++
Secondary glaucoma	–	–>+++
II. Histopathologic DD		
Endothelial cell loss	+	+>+++
Fibroblastic transformation	+	+>+++
Melanin phagocytosis	+	+++
Descemet's membrane	Focal guttae formation	Diffuse irregular thickening
Abnormal extracellular matrix	Abnormal posterior banded layer	Abnormal posterior banded layer, PEX material

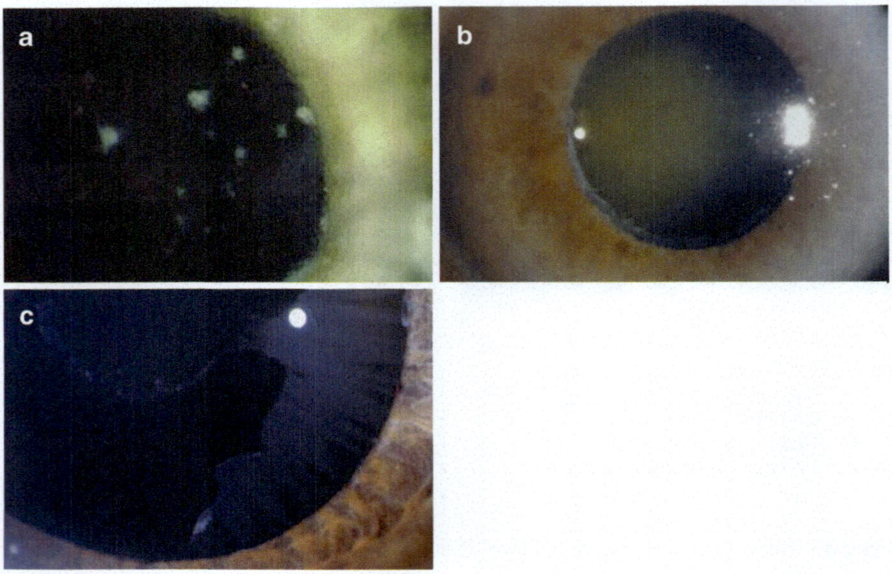

Fig. 3.16 In contrast to FECD, PEX eyes may show hyperreflective whitish deposits (1) retro-corneal (**a**), at the pupillary margin (**b**) and on the anterior lens capsule (**c**) during slit-lamp examination [49, 50]

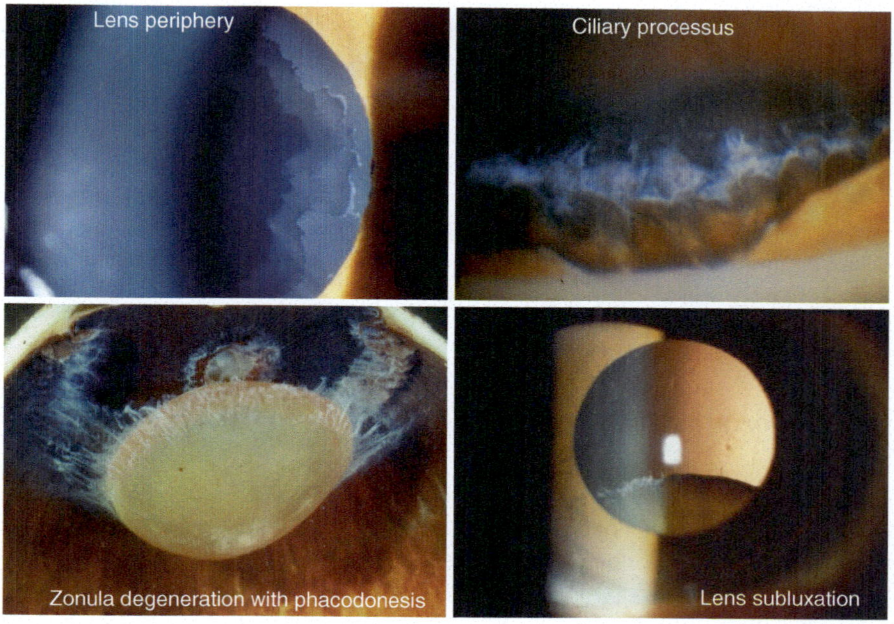

Fig. 3.17 Concerning microsurgery (especially cataract surgery), FECD is a "friend," while PEX keratopathy with associated PEX syndrome is a challenge resulting more often in postoperative elevated pressure, corneal decompensation, zonulolysis with phacodonesis, and eventually lens (sub)luxation [49, 50]

3.5.5 Melanin Dispersion Syndrome

No guttae are present. However, a distinct vertical pattern of pigment can be found on the posterior part of the cornea, forming a Krukenberg spindle. Typically, retroillumination displays radial linear defects of the pigment epithelium of the iris.

3.5.6 Pseudophakic Bullous Keratopathy

Pseudophakic bullous keratopathy is an iatrogenic endothelial damage typically due to suboptimal cataract surgery [56]. It may well appear in eyes with previously normal endothelial cell count and without any guttae. It starts peripherally and goes to the center (FECD starts centrally and goes to the periphery). But in a large study on 137 patients, no differences in the pachymetric profile could be found comparing FECD and pseudophakic bullous keratopathy [29].

3.5.7 *Pseudoguttae*

Pseudoguttae are guttae-like images caused by endothelial edema that may appear in cases of corneal inflammation and disappear upon resolution of the underlying disease [57].

Real guttae are more regular than pseudoguttae, and the endothelial mosaic, if present, is usually relatively normal around the guttae. Although small guttae may occur, if guttae are at all numerous, large ones are also usually present. Inflammatory cells are rarely present in the relief mode with guttae but are always present with blebs associated with uveitis [38].

3.6 Associations with Other Diseases

It remains unclear, whether combinations with various different diseases could be manifestations of a common pathogenetic mechanisms based on a genetic defects or whether these are mere coincidences. A simple coincidence can actually be attributed to single-case descriptions in the literature like coincidence of pre-Descemet's membrane corneal dystrophy and FECD [58]. But it should be kept in mind that combined corneal dystrophies do exist.

There is a known association between increased intraocular pressure and greater central corneal thickness [30]. Several studies have proposed an association between FECD and glaucoma. However, in a large retrospective study with 841 patients, no higher prevalence of glaucoma or ocular hypertension in FECD patients could be demonstrated [59]. In a study with 1610 patients in families with grades IV to VI according to Krachmer [40], a "glaucoma" prevalence of up to 11 % compared to 6 % in a normal population was found [60]. We may suppose that this study included a number of undetected PEX keratopathy eyes in the presumed FECD group [49, 50].

In the Reykjavik Eye Study, an average smoking of one pack/day for 20 years doubled the risk of developing corneal guttae [61].

3.6.1 *Association with Anterior Basement Membrane Dystrophy*

An association of FECD and anterior basement membrane dystrophy has been established in a series of 95 patients with FECD with 25 % having anterior basement membrane dystrophy [62]. However, this might also be a secondary phenomenon.

3.6.2 *Association with Keratoconus*

Although keratoconus and corneal dystrophies are infrequent, there are reported cases of both keratoconus and FECD in the same eye. At first, it seems contradictory with keratoconus being a corneal thinning disease and FECD a corneal thickening disease. Therefore, corneal thinning and concurrent corneal thickening by FECD usually combine in the reported cases to normalize the pachymetry readings to about 557 μm [62]. This double corneal dystrophy seems to be initiated by mutations in the ZEB1 gene [63].

In this context, a triple corneal dystrophy has been described, combining FECD, keratoconus and epithelial basement dystrophy which was negative for ZEB1 [62, 64].

Jurkunas and Azar [65] report on potential complications of ocular surgery with coexistent keratoconus and FECD. Corneal thinning caused by keratoconus and concurrent increase in corneal thickness caused by FECD may combine to "pseudo-normalize" the corneal pachymetry readings. Disease severity of FECD may be underestimated, which may lead to unexpected postoperative visual outcomes. Routine use of preoperative tomography and specular microscopy may help to avert potential surgical complications, especially after cataract surgery [65]. In addition, in progressed combined disease, a penetrating keratoplasty will rather be beneficial to the patient than a posterior lamellar keratoplasty.

3.6.3 Association with Myotonic Dystrophy

Four patients with established diagnosis of myotonic dystrophy and histologically confirmed diagnosis of FECD have been described. Myotonic dystrophy is an autosomal dominant disorder that is the most common inherited muscle disease in adults [66]. It could be demonstrated that some FECD patients have a missense mutation similar to that in myotonic dystrophy [67].

3.7 Medical Therapy

3.7.1 Symptomatic Therapy

The problem in finding an adequate medical therapy is that the pathophysiologic pathway of FECD is only partly understood. We can administer a symptomatic therapy in order to reduce corneal edema. If the tear film is made hypertonic, it will extract water from the cornea according to the phenomenon called osmosis. Clinical experience shows that in particular epithelial edema can be influenced [68]. To decrease the stromal edema, the human cornea would need contact with a fluid of such hypertonicity that treatment would become very painful and damaging [68]. Sodium chloride eye drops penetrate the epithelium poorly and can therefore attract only the water from the epithelial bullae [68]. For more than 40 years, a 5 % sodium chloride solution is in use [69]. The toxic effects of hyperosmolar solutions for the ocular surface are considerably augmented if benzalkonium chloride is used as preservative [70]. Therefore, only hyperosmotic solutions without conservative should be employed. Usually, the recommended drop frequency is four times a day. But this is not the most efficient way in FECD patients. Vision is worst in the morning because there was no evaporation from the tear film overnight due to lid closure. Several applications of these drops during the first waking hours can serve to improve vision. As the day progresses, additional drops may be used as needed [56].

3.7.2 *Causative Therapy*

Causative medical therapeutic approaches are actually at the beginning or still at the clinical horizon. The therapeutic approach depends strongly on the supposed pathophysiological mechanism. Because corneal endothelium does not divide in vivo, loss of endothelial cells seen in FECD is permanent. Given that apoptosis of endothelial cells is the main cause [71, 72], different pathophysiological pathways for a possible medical therapeutic approach have been investigated.

3.7.2.1 Oxidative Stress

H_2O_2 treatments induce a dose-dependent increase in polymegalism and an increase in pleomorphism in corneal endothelial cells of mice [26]. DNA from FECD patients seems to be easier accessible for oxidative stress than that of normal patients. The p53 regulation way which finally leads to apoptosis seems to be involved, too [73]. At the same time, Nrf2 is upregulated. Nrf2 is latent within each cell in the body, unable to move or operate until it is released by an Nrf2 activator. Once released, it migrates into the cell nucleus and binds to the DNA at the location of the antioxidant response element (ARE) which is the master regulator of the total antioxidant system, therefore enhancing the antioxidant system [73]. This contention is partly opposed by Czarny et al., who found evidence that the DNA-repairing system in FECD patients seems to be inhibited [74]. But these results by Czarny et al. were not created in corneal endothelial cells, but in peripheral blood mononuclear cells from FECD patients.

3.7.2.2 Endoplasmic Reticulum (ER) Stress Response

The endoplasmatic reticulum is the main source of intracellular Ca2+ [75] and at the same time the organelle which is responsible for folding of proteins. If there is an excess of proteins to be folded, ER stress is induced. In this case, unfolded protein response is activated which tries to reestablish regular cellular functions by activating different ways [76]:

- Suppression of new protein formation by ribosomes (phospho-eIF2α and CHOP are two proteins participating in this process)
- Intensifying degradation of misfolded proteins
- Creating more chaperones able to correctly fold proteins, for example, GRP78

In a study with ten human FECD corneas, markers for GRP78, phospho-eIF2α, and CHOP compared with non-FECD corneas were increased fourfold [77]. In a murine model used as model for early-onset FECD, ultrastructural analysis showed the predominant defect as dilated endoplasmic reticulum (ER), suggesting ER stress and unfolded protein response (UPR) activation [12].

Both mentioned pathophysiological ways finally lead to apoptosis. Initiation of apoptosis in FECD patients has been proved for caspase-9 [76] and p53 [73].

Kim et al. investigated *lithium* and *N-acetylcysteine* (NAC) in bovine cell culture and a murine model serving as model for early-onset FECD [78]. Experimental approach is causing stress on the endoplasmatic reticulum by application of thapsigargin which leads to a discharge of Ca2+ from the ER and oxidative stress via H_2O_2 [79, 80]. Lithium was tried by Kim et al. because of its capacity to reduce ER stress [79]. The endothelium of lithium-treated mice showed a mild phenotype with few extracellular matrix excrescences compared to untreated mice [79]. N-Acetylcysteine is a thiol-containing antioxidant and radical scavenger. Compared to control mice, NAC-treated mice showed reduced pleomorphism, reduced polymegalism, and preserved hexagonal morphology with fewer extracellular matrix excrescences compared to the untreated group [78].

Ziaei et al. used *sulforaphane*, an Nrf2 agonist, and could demonstrate cytoprotective effects in a cell culture model by decreasing apoptosis and upregulating several ARE elements [81].

3.7.2.3 ROCK Inhibitor

An absolutely different approach has been used by Kinoshita's group in Japan. Rho/Rho kinase (ROCK) promotes actin-myosin-mediated contractile force generation through the phosphorylation of numerous downstream target proteins, thus influencing cell motility [82]. Moreover, during apoptosis, cells undergo significant morphological changes including contraction, dynamic membrane blebbing, and nuclear disintegration, which are driven by ROCK-mediated actin-myosin contractile force [82]. In an animal model, injection of ROCK inhibitor-pretreated cells showed a markedly improved expression of vinculin in contrast to the non-treated cells, suggesting that the inhibitor enhanced the cell adhesion via the induction of focal adhesion complexes and direct injection of pretreated cells in a monkey model found better regenerative capability than with non-pretreated cells [83]. In a case study, Okumura et al. removed the diseased corneal endothelium of a FECD patient in the prepupillary region by transcorneal freezing for 15 s previously used in a rabbit model [84]. Then, they administered ROCK inhibitor eye drops with the specific Rho/Rho kinase (ROCK) inhibitor Y-27632, six times daily for 7 days. After 14 days, a significant reduction of central corneal thickness and improvement of visual acuity could be obtained and could be maintained for at least 2 years [84]. Of note is that the reestablishment of the patient's endothelial function must not be necessarily a direct result of the ROCK inhibitor administration but can at least be helped by the migration of the surrounding sound endothelial cells toward the center. So far, four FECD patients have been treated with this method; of note is that only one had an increase in visual acuity 6 months after treatment compared to pretreatment [85].

3.8 Conclusions

The term FECD should not be used in cornea guttata before endothelial decompensation = "swelling" = "increased central corneal thickness" does occur. Some eyes with cornea guttata will never progress to FECD! FECD must be differentiated from PEX keratopathy with respect to the incidence of secondary glaucoma, therapeutic necessities, and prognosis of corneal transplantation. Concerning microsurgery, FECD is a "friend," while PEX keratopathy is a challenge. Progression of FECD cannot be defined via endothelial cell counts, because numbers are notoriously measured wrong. Progression should be defined via best-corrected visual acuity (worse morning vs afternoon), glare, corneal thickness profile (tomography), and cell morphology. For many decades, symptomatic medical therapy consisted of unpreserved hyperosmolar (5 %) sodium chloride solution. Preclinical causative approaches include lithium, N-acetylcysteine, and the ROCK inhibitor.

References

1. Fuchs E. Dystrophia epithelialis corneae. Graefes Arch Ophthalmol. 1910;76(3):478–508.
2. Vogt A. Weitere Ergebnisse der Spaltlampenmikroskopie des vorderen Bulbusabschnittes. Arch Ophthalmol. 1921;63–113.
3. Friedenwald H, Friedenwald J. Epithelial dystrophy of the cornea. Br J Ophthalmol. 1925;9(1):14–20.
4. Kayes J, Homberg A. The fine structure of the cornea in Fuchs' endothelial dystrophy. IOVS. 1964;3(1):47–67.
5. Bigar F, Schimmelpfennig B, Hürzeler R. Cornea guttata in donor material. Arch Ophthalmol. 1978;96(4):653–5.
6. Gipson IK. Age-related changes and diseases of the ocular surface and cornea. Invest Ophthalmol Vis Sci. 2013;54:ORSF48-53.
7. Zhang C, Bell RW, Sundin OH, De La Cruz Z, Stark WJ, Green WR, Gottsch JD. Immunohistochemistry and electron microscopy of early-onset Fuchs corneal dystrophy in three cases with the same L450W Col8A2 mutation. Trans Am Ophthalmol Soc. 2006;104:85–97.
8. Lisch W, Buob M, Steuhl KP. Cornea guttata und Fuchssche Hornhaut-Endothel-Epithel-Dystrophie. Klin Monatsbl Augenheilkd. 1991;198:83–6.
9. Weiss JS, Moller HU, Aldave AI, Seitz B, Bredrup C, Kivelä T, Munier FL, Rapuano CJ, Nischal KK, Kim EK, Sutphin J, Busin M, Labbé A, Kenyon KR, Kinoshita S, Lisch W. IC3D classification of corneal dystrophies – edition 2. Cornea. 2015;34(2):117–59.
10. Kitagawa K, Fujisaea A, Mizuno T, Sasaki K. Twenty-three cases of primary cornea guttata. Jpn J Ophthalmol. 2000;44(5):572.
11. Bucher F, Adler W, Lehmann HC, Hos D, Steven P, Cursiefen C, Heindl LM. Corneal nerve alterations in different stages of Fuchs' endothelial corneal dystrophy: an in vivo confocal microscopy study. Graefes Arch Clin Exp Ophthalmol. 2014;252:1119–26.

12. Jun AS, Meng H, Ramanan N, Matthaei M, Chakravarti S, Bonshek R, Black GC, Grebe R, Kimos M. An alpha 2 collagen VIII transgenic knock-in mouse model of Fuchs endothelial corneal dystrophy shows early endothelial cell unfolded protein response and apoptosis. Hum Mol Genet. 2012;21(2):384–93.
13. Magovern M, Beauchamp GR, McTigue JW, Fine BS, Baumiller RC. Inheritance of Fuchs' combined dystrophy. Ophthalmology. 1979;86(10):1897–923.
14. Adamis AP, Filatov V, Tripathi RC. Fuchs' endothelial dystrophy of the cornea. Surv Ophthalmol. 1993;38:149–68.
15. Wilson SE, Bourne WM. Fuchs' dystrophy. Cornea. 1988;7(1):2–18.
16. Son H, Villarreal G, Meng H, Eberhart CG, Jun AS. On the origin of "guttae". Br J Ophthalmol. 2014;98(9):1308–10.
17. Watanabe S, Oie Y, Fujimoto H, Soma T, Koh S, Tsujikawa M, Maeda N, Nishida K. Relationship between corneal guttae and quality of vision in patients with mild Fuchs' endothelial corneal dystrophy. Ophthalmology. 2015;122:2103–9.
18. Jackson AJ, Robinson FO, Frazer DG, Archer DB. Corneal guttata: a comparative clinical and specular micrographic study. Eye. 1999;13(6):737–43.
19. Amin SR, Baratz KH, McLaren J, Patel SV. Corneal abnormalities early in the course of Fuchs' endothelial dystrophy. Ophthalmology. 2014;12:2325–33.
20. Zoega GM, Arnarsson A, Sasaki H, Söderberg PG, Jonasson F. The 7-year cumulative incidence of cornea guttata and morphological changes in the corneal endothelium in the Reykjavik Eye Study. Acta Ophthalmol. 2013;91(3):212–8.
21. Alomar TS, Al-Aqaba M, Gray T, Lowe J, Dua HS. Histological and confocal microscopy changes in chronic corneal edema: implications for endothelial transplantation. IOVS. 2011;52:8193–207.
22. Chiou AG, Kaufman SC, Beuerman RW, Ohta T, Soliman H, Kaufman HE. Confocal microscopy in cornea guttata and Fuchs' endothelial dystrophy. Br J Ophthalmol. 1999;83(2):185–9.
23. Giasson CJ, Solomon LD, Polse KA. Morphometry of corneal endothelium in patients with corneal guttata. Ophthalmology. 2007;114:1469–75.
24. Patel DV, McGhee CNJ. Contemporary in vivo confocal microscopy of the living human cornea using white light and laser scanning techniques: a major review. Clin Exp Ophthalmol. 2007;35:71–88.
25. Seitz B, Müller EE, Langenbucher A, Kus MM, Naumann GOH. Reproduzierbarkeit und Validität eines neuen automatisierten Verfahrens der spiegelmikroskopischen Hornhautendothelanalyse. Ophthalmologe. 1997;94:127–35.
26. Jurkunas UV, Bitar MS, Funaki T, Behrooz A. Evidence of oxidative stress in the pathogenesis of Fuchs endothelial corneal dystrophy. Am J Pathol. 2010;177(5):2278–89.
27. McLaren JW, Bachman LA, Kane KM, Patel SV. Objective assessment of the corneal endothelium in Fuchs' Endothelial Dystrophy. IOVS. 2014;55(2):1184–90.
28. Fujimoto H, Maeda N, Soma T, Oie Y, Koh S, Tsujikawa M, Nishida K. Quantitative regional differences in corneal endothelial abnormalities in the central and peripheral zones in Fuchs' Endothelial Corneal Dystrophy. IOVS. 2014;55(8):5090–8.
29. Brunette I, Sherknies D, Terry MA, Chagnon M, Bourges JL, Meunier J. 3-D characterization of the corneal shape in Fuchs dystrophy and pseudophakic keratopathy. IOVS. 2011;52(1):206–14.
30. Kopplin LJ, Przepysnzy K, Schmotzer B, Rudo K, Babineau DC, Patel SV, Verdier DD, Jurkunas U, Iyengar SK, Lass JH. Relationship of Fuchs' Endothelial Corneal Dystrophy severity to central corneal thickness. Arch Ophthalmol. 2012;130(4):1–15.
31. Repp DJ, Hodge DO, Baratz KH, McLaren JW, Patel SV. Fuchs endothelial dystrophy: subjective grading versus objective grading based on the central to peripheral thickness ratio. Ophthalmology. 2013;120(4):687–94.
32. Oh KT, Weil LJ, Oh DM, Mathers WD. Corneal thickness in Fuchs' dystrophy with and without epithelial oedema. Eye. 1998;12:282–4.
33. Shousha MA, Perez VL, Wang J, Ide T, Jiao S, Chen Q, Chang V, Buchser N, Dubovy SR, Feuer W, Yoo SH. Use of ultra-high-resolution optical coherence tomography to detect in vivo characteristics of Descemet's membrane in Fuchs' dystrophy. Ophthalmology. 2010;117(6):1220–7.

34. Schrems-Hoesl LM, Schrems WA, Cruzat A, Shahatit BM, Bayhan HA, Jurkunas UV, Hamrah P. Cellular and subbasal nerve alterations in early stage Fuchs' Endothelial Corneal Dystrophy: an in vivo confocal microscopy study. Eye. 2013;27:42–9.
35. Ahuja YA, Baratz KH, McLAren JW, Bourne WM, Patel SV. Decreased corneal sensitivity and abnormal corneal nerves in Fuchs Endothelial Dystrophy. Cornea. 2012;31(11):1257–63.
36. Cheng LL, Young AL, Wong AK, Law RW, Lam DS. Confocal microscopy of posterior polymorphous endothelial dystrophy. Cornea. 2005;24(5):599–602.
37. Kouassi FX, Touboul D, Schweitzer C, Pinsard L, Garra C, Colin J. In vivo confocal microscopy of posterior polymorphous dystrophy. J Fr Ophtalmol. 2011;34(10):762–4.
38. Brooks AM, Grant GB, Gillies WE. The identification of corneal guttae. Cornea. 1991; 10(3):249–60.
39. Zhang J, Patel DV. The pathophysiology of Fuchs' endothelial dystrophy – a review of molecular and cellular insights. Exp Eye Res. 2015;130:97–105.
40. Krachmer JH, Purcell JJ, Young CW, Bucher KD. Corneal endothelial dystrophy. A study of 64 families. Arch Ophthalmol. 1978;96(11):2036–9.
41. Zhang X, Igo RP, Fondran J, Mootha VV, Oliva M, Hammersmith K, Sugar A, Lass JH, Iyengar SK. Association of smoking and other risk factors with Fuchs' Endothelial Corneal Dystrophy severity and corneal thickness. IOVS. 2013;54(8):5829–35.
42. Nieuwendaal CP, Odenthal MT, Kok JH, Venema HW, Oosting J, Riemslag FC, Kijlstra A. Morphology and function of the corneal endothelium after long-term contact lens wear. IOVS. 1994;35(7):3071–7.
43. Afshari N, Pittard AB, Siddiqui A, Klintworth GK. Clinical study of Fuchs corneal endothelial dystrophy leading to penetrating keratoplasty. Arch Ophthalmol. 2006;124:777–80.
44. Eghrari AO, Daoud Y, Gottsch JD. Cataract surgery in Fuchs corneal dystrophy. Curr Opin Ophthalmol. 2010;21:15–9.
45. Krachmer JH. Posterior polymorphous corneal dystrophy: a disease characterized by epithelial-like endothelial cells which influence management and prognosis. Trans Am Ophthalmol Soc. 1985;83:413–75.
46. Aldave AJ, Ann LB, Frausto RF, Nguyen CK, Yu F, Raber IM. Classification of posterior polymorphous corneal dystrophy as a corneal ectatic disorder following confirmation of associated significant corneal steepening. JAMA Ophthalmol. 2013;131(12):1583–90.
47. Siddiqui S, Zenteno JC, Rice A, Chacon-Camacho O, Naylor SG, Rivera-de la Parra D, Spokes DM, James N, Toomes C, Inglehearn CF, Ali M. Congenital hereditary endothelial dystrophy caused by SLC4A11 mutations progresses to Harboyan syndrome. Cornea. 2014;33(3): 247–51.
48. Schmidt E, Lisch W, Philipp W, Lechner S, Göttinger W, Schlötzer-Schrehardt U, Müller T, Utermann G, Janecke AR. A new X-linked endothelial corneal dystrophy. Am J Ophthalmol. 2006;141(3):478–87.
49. Naumann GOH, Schlötzer-Schrehardt U. Keratopathy in pseudoexfoliation syndrome as a cause of corneal endothelial decompensation: a clinicopathologic study. Ophthalmology. 2000;107(6):1111–24.
50. Schlötzer-Schrehardt UM, Dörfler S, Naumann GOH. Corneal endothelial involvement in pseudoexfoliation syndrome. Arch Ophthalmol. 1993;111:666–74.
51. Seitz B, Müller EE, Langenbucher A, Kus MM, Naumann GOH. Endothelial keratopathy in pseudoexfoliation syndrome: quantitative and qualitative morphometry using automated video image analysis. Klin Monatsbl Augenheilkd. 1995;207:167–75.
52. Conway RM, Schlötzer-Schrehardt U, Küchle M, Naumann GOH. Pseudoexfoliation syndrome: pathological manifestations of relevance to intraocular surgery. Clin Exp Ophthalmol. 2004;32:199–210.
53. Nguyen NX, Lattermann V, Schlötzer-Schrehardt U, Seitz B. Funktionelle Ergebnisse der perforierenden Keratoplastik bei Pseudoexfoliationssyndrom (PEX)-Keratopathie. Klin Monatsbl Augenheilkd. 2004;221:819–24.
54. Küchle M, Naumann GOH. Occurrence of pseudoexfoliation following penetrating keratoplasty for keratoconus. Br J Ophthalmol. 1992;76:98–100.

55. Milioti G, Löw U, Gatzioufas Z, Ninios K, Schirra F, Seitz B. Early manifestation of a pseudoexfoliation syndrome after a corneal transplantation. Klin Monatsbl Augenheilkd. 2011;228:249–51.
56. Levenson JE. Corneal edema: cause and treatment. Surv Ophthalmol. 1975;20(3):190–204.
57. Krachmer JH, Schnitzer JI, Fratkin J. Cornea pseudoguttata: a clinical and histopathologic description of endothelial cell edema. Arch Opthalmol. 1981;99(8):1377–81.
58. Yeh SI, Liu TS, Ho CC, Cheng HC. In vivo confocal microscopy of combined pre-Descemet membrane corneal dystrophy and Fuchs endothelial dystrophy. Cornea. 2011;30(2):222–4.
59. Rice GD, Wright K, Silverstein SM. A retrospective study of the association between Fuchs' endothelial dystrophy and glaucoma. Clin Ophthalmol. 2014;8:2155–9.
60. Nagarsheth M, Singh A, Schmotzer B, Babineau DC, Sugar J, Lee WB, Iyengar SK, Lass JH. The relationship between Fuchs' Endothelial Corneal Dystrophy severity and glaucoma and/or ocular hypertension. Arch Ophthalmol. 2012;130(11):1384–8.
61. Zoega GM, Fujisawa A, Sasaki H, Kubota A, Sasaki K, Kitagawa K, Jonasson F. Prevalence and risk factors for cornea guttata in the Reykjavik Eye Study. Ophthalmology. 2006;113(4):565–9.
62. Cremona FA, Ghosheh FR, Rapuano CJ, Eagle RC, Hammersmith KM, Laibson PR, Ayres BD, Cohen EJ. Keratoconus associated with other corneal dystrophies. Cornea. 2009;28(2):127–35.
63. Lechner J, Dash DP, Muszynska D, Hosseini M, Segev F, Geroge S, Frazer DG, Moore JE, Kaye SB, Young T, Simpson DA, Churchill AJ, Héon E, Willoughby CE. Mutational spectrum of the ZEB1 gene in corneal dystrophies supports a genotype-phenotype correlation. IOVS. 2013;54(5):3215–23.
64. Mazzotta C, Traversi C, Raiskup F, Rizzo CL, Renieri A. First identification of a triple corneal dystrophy association: keratoconus, epithelial basement membrane corneal dystrophy and Fuchs' endothelial corneal dystrophy. Case Rep Ophthalmol. 2014;5(3):281–8.
65. Jurkunas U, Azar DT. Potential complications of ocular surgery in patients with coexistent keratoconus and Fuchs' endothelial dystrophy. Ophthalmology. 2006;113:2187–97.
66. Gattey D, Zhu AY, Stagner A, Terry MA, Jun AS. Fuchs endothelial corneal dystrophy in patients with myotonic dystrophy: a case series. Cornea. 2014;33(1):96–8.
67. Du J, Aleff RA, Soragni E, Kalari K, Nie J, Tang X, Davila J, Kocher JP, Patel SV, Gottesfeld JM, Baratz KH, Wieben ED. RNA toxicity and missplicing in the common eye 5 disease Fuchs Endothelial Corneal Dystrophy. J Biol Chem. 2015;290(10):5979–90.
68. Payrau P, Dohlman CH. Medical treatment of corneal edema. Int Ophthalmol Clin. 1968;8(3):601–10.
69. Green K, Downs S. Reduction of corneal thickness with hypertonic solutions. Am J Ophthalmol. 1973;75:507–10.
70. Clouzeau C, Godefroy D, Riancho L, Rostène W, Baudouin C, Brignole-Baudouin F. Hyperosmolarity potentiates toxic effects of benzalkonium chloride on conjunctival epithelial cells in vitro. Mol Vis. 2012;18:851–63.
71. Broderie VM, Baudrimont M, Vallée A, Ereau TL, Gray F, Laroche L. Corneal endothelial cell apoptosis in patients with Fuchs' dystrophy. IOVS. 2000;41(9):2501–5.
72. Li QJ, Ashraf MF, Shen DF, Green WR, Stark WJ, Chan CC, O'Brien TP. The role of apoptosis in the pathogenesis of Fuchs endothelial dystrophy of the cornea. Arch Ophthalmol. 2001;119(11):1597–604.
73. Azizi B, Ziaei A, Fuchsluger T, Schmedt T, Chen Y, Jurkunas U. p53-regulated increase in oxidative-stress-induced apoptosis in Fuchs endothelial corneal dystrophy: a native tissue model. IOVS. 2011;52(13):9291–7.
74. Czarny P, Kasprzak E, Wielgorski M, Udziela M, Markiewicz B, Blasiak J, Szaflik J, Szaflik JP. DNA damage and repair in Fuchs endothelial corneal dystrophy. Mol Biol Rep. 2013;40(4):2977–83.
75. Kass GE, Orrenius S. Calcium signaling and cytotoxicity. Environ Health Perspect. 1999;107 Suppl 1:25–35.
76. Sano R, Reed JC. ER stress-induced cell death mechanisms. Biochim Biophys Acta. 2013;1833(12):3460–70.

77. Engler C, Kelliher C, Spitze AR, Speck CL, Eberhart CG, Jun AS. Unfolded protein response in Fuchs endothelial corneal dystrophy: a unifying pathogenic pathway? Am J Ophthalmol. 2010;149(2):194–202.
78. Kim EC, Meng H, Jun AS. N-Acetylcysteine increases corneal endothelial cell survival in a mouse model of Fuchs endothelial corneal dystrophy. Exp Eye Res. 2014;127:20–5.
79. Kim EC, Meng H, Jun AS. Lithium treatment increases endothelial cell survival and autophagy in a mouse model of Fuchs endothelial corneal dystrophy. Br J Ophthalmol. 2013;97(8):1068–73.
80. Thastrup O, Cullen PJ, Drobak BK, Hanley MR, Dawson AP. Thapsigargin, a tumor promoter, discharges intracellular Ca2+ stores by specific inhibition of the endoplasmic reticulum Ca2+-ATPase. Proc Natl Acad Sci. 1990;87:2466–70.
81. Ziaei A, Schmedt T, Chen Y, Jurkunas U. Sulforaphane decreases endothelial cell apoptosis in Fuchs endothelial corneal dystrophy: a novel treatment. IOVS. 2013;54(10):6724–34.
82. Olson MF. Applications for ROCK kinase inhibition. Curr Opin Cell Biol. 2008;20(2):242–8.
83. Okumura N, Koizumi N, Ueno M, Sakamoto Y, Takahashi H, Tsuchiya H, Hamuro J, Kinoshita S. ROCK inhibitor converts corneal endothelial cells into a phenotype capable of regeneration in vivo endothelial tissue. Am J Pathol. 2012;181(1):268–77.
84. Okumura N, Koizumi N, Ueno M, Sakamoto Y, Takahashi H, Hirata K, Torii R, Hamuro J, Kinoshita S. Enhancement of corneal endothelium wound healing by Rho-Associated inhibitor eye drops. Br J Ophthalmol. 2011;95:1006–9.
85. Okumura N, Koizumi N, Kay EP, Ueno M, Sakamoto Y, Nakamura S, Hamuro J, Kinoshita S. The ROCK inhibitor eye drop accelerates corneal endothelium wound healing. IOVS. 2013;54(4):2493–502.

Chapter 4
Optical and Anatomic Changes in Fuchs Endothelial Dystrophy Corneas

Katrin Wacker, Jay W. McLaren, and Sanjay V. Patel

4.1 Introduction

Fuchs endothelial dystrophy (FED) is a common disease that manifests with varying degrees of severity. It is characterized by focal posterior collagenous excrescences (guttae) and progressive corneal edema, resulting in reduced corneal transparency and impaired vision [87]. In the past decade, we have improved our understanding of anatomic and optical factors that influence vision in this disease because the host cornea is retained after treatment by endothelial keratoplasty.

In 1910, Ernst Fuchs initially described the disease that has become associated with his name [24]. Although his description suggested that most of the pathologic changes in the disease were anterior in the cornea, he suggested a defective corneal endothelial layer as the underlying cause, even without the aid of a slit lamp, which was developed a year later. FED is now widely accepted to be a primary dysfunction of the corneal endothelium, but changes are apparent throughout the cornea, and are being realized early in the course of the disease. Indeed, with the advent of endothelial replacement alone in the last 15 years, it is apparent that the optical and anatomic properties of FED corneas do improve postoperatively, with significant but incomplete visual rehabilitation. Much of the renewed interest in and understanding of FED can be attributed to the pursuit of new keratoplasty techniques that enable examination of the host cornea.

K. Wacker, MD
Department of Ophthalmology, Mayo Clinic, 200 First Street SW, Rochester, MN, USA

Eye Center, Albert-Ludwigs-University of Freiburg, Killianstr. 5, 79106 Freiburg, Germany

J.W. McLaren, PhD • S.V. Patel, MD, FRCOphth (✉)
Department of Ophthalmology, Mayo Clinic, 200 First Street SW, Rochester, MN, USA
e-mail: patel.sanjay@mayo.edu

C. Cursiefen, A.S. Jun (eds.), *Current Treatment Options for Fuchs Endothelial Dystrophy*, DOI 10.1007/978-3-319-43021-8_4

To describe comprehensively and understand the optics of FED and the quality of vision in patients after treatment, it is crucial to understand the underlying structural changes in the cornea. This chapter will review the anatomic changes that can be imaged in FED in vivo and ex vivo and the optical characteristics of FED before and after corneal transplantation with relevance to visual outcomes.

4.2 Anatomic Changes

4.2.1 Anterior Cornea

Initially described as *dystrophia epithelialis corneae* by Ernst Fuchs in advanced disease with epithelial edema, anterior stromal clouding, and decreased sensitivity [24], we now know that anterior corneal changes are also present earlier in the course of the disease [3, 5, 85]. While anterior corneal changes were of little importance in the era of penetrating keratoplasty, which excised the full thickness of the host cornea, the recognition of anterior changes in the host cornea is providing a better understanding of the outcomes of endothelial keratoplasty [3, 83].

4.2.1.1 Epithelium

In advanced stages of FED, epithelial changes become obvious by slit lamp biomicroscopy. Corneas show bedewing leading to microcysts and eventually subepithelial bullae that can rupture and cause pain [11, 29]. Cysts form intra- or intercellularly [1, 73], with intracellular edema being manifested mainly in the basal epithelial cells and leading to intercellular edema as the cysts and cells rupture [1]. In FED corneas with chronic edema, map-dot-fingerprint-like modifications with folded basement membrane have been described clinically and histopathologically. These may have formed from buckling of poorly adherent epithelium and bullae or microcysts [19]. Microcysts can rupture and the cornea can recurrently erode and become infected and vascularized.

By using confocal microscopy, four different patterns of cyst formation have been described: (1) globular-shaped cystic lesions with well-defined borders and low internal reflectivity (the most frequent); (2) cystic lesions with irregular reflectivity within the cyst, surrounded by the cytoplasm of an epithelial cell; (3) tubular-shaped, elongated, and large bullae separated from other epithelial cells; and (4) abnormal epithelial cells with an increased intercellular space [29]. Image brightness in confocal microscopy indicates increased corneal backscatter (clinically termed "haze") from the epithelial basal cell layer [5, 56], a component of increased anterior corneal backscatter that has been related to outcomes of cataract surgery in FED [30]. The increased backscatter originates from the cell borders and improves quickly after endothelial keratoplasty, suggesting that intercellular edema is the source of the haze [7, 56, 83].

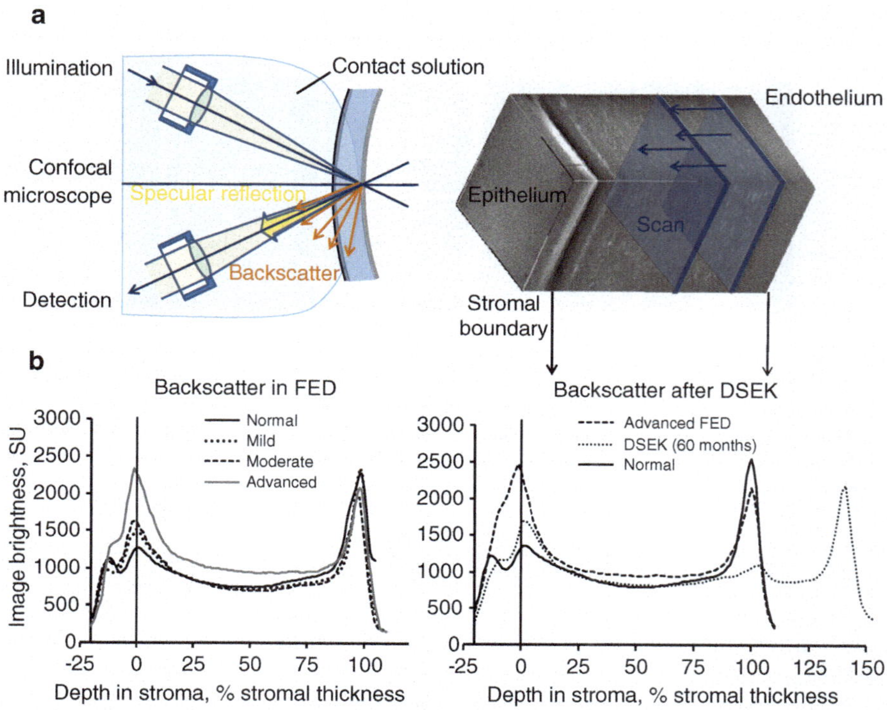

Fig. 4.1 Backscatter in Fuchs endothelial dystrophy (FED) corneas. (**a**) Confocal microscopy measures brightness of illumination at different depths of the cornea. The optical axis of the illuminator and detector are at equal angles to the normal, resulting in the detection of specular reflection (dominant) and backscatter [48]. (**b**) Corneal backscatter profiles generated from confocal images with the depth of the cornea scaled from 0% at the anterior stromal boundary to 100% at the endothelium [5]. Backscatter was standardized and measured in scatter units (SU), the concentration of a turbidity standard that produces the same image brightness. Profile of backscatter through the normal cornea and corneas with mild, moderate, and advanced FED show increasing anterior corneal backscatter with increasing severity of FED (*left*) [5]. After endothelial keratoplasty, anterior corneal backscatter that was high preoperatively in advanced FED corneas improved through 5 years, but did not return to normal (*right*) [83]

4.2.1.2 Keratocytes and Extracellular Matrix

Anterior corneal changes in FED involve cells and the extracellular matrix. In advanced disease (corneas with edema that require keratoplasty), anterior keratocytes are depleted, and a hypocellular zone develops in the anterior stroma. These changes are visible by confocal microscopy and have been confirmed by histology in tissue excised at penetrating keratoplasty [28, 56]. Confocal images of corneas with chronic edema show degenerating and depleted anterior stromal cell nuclei accompanied by subepithelial and anterior stromal fibrosis, a major contributor to increased backscattered light (Figs. 4.1 and 4.2) [54, 56]. The mechanism of subepithelial fibrosis development is unclear, but could involve epithelial or keratocyte

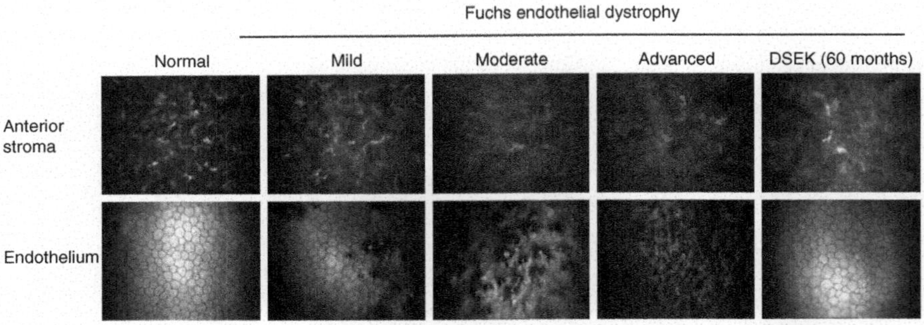

Fig. 4.2 Confocal microscopy of Fuchs endothelial dystrophy (FED) corneas. Representative confocal images of the anterior corneal stroma and the associated endothelium in a normal cornea, in mild, moderate, and advanced FED, and at 5 years after Descemet stripping endothelial keratoplasty (DSEK) for advanced FED. There is increased matrix reflectivity (backscatter) in FED associated with depletion of keratocyte nuclei. These changes persist after endothelial keratoplasty

transdifferentiation into fibroblasts [4, 28, 33, 49, 56], though the latter would require cells to traverse the Bowman layer, which is not commonly observed.

Of importance, keratocyte depletion and increased backscatter from the anterior cornea can be detected in the early stages of FED, before guttae become confluent and before edema is clinically detectable (Fig. 4.2) [5, 85]. These early anterior anatomic changes raise questions as to whether or not the primary dysfunction in FED is solely in corneal endothelial cells. They also indicate that FED is a chronic disease that has subclinical and clinical phases. After endothelial keratoplasty, keratocyte depletion persists through at least 3 years [56], and although anterior corneal backscatter improves, it does not return to normal through 5 years (Fig. 4.2) [8, 83]. Early improvement in backscatter can be attributed to resolution of corneal edema, but late persistence of elevated backscatter suggests alterations of corneal architecture in response to chronic edema before keratoplasty.

4.2.1.3 Corneal Nerves and Sensation

The nasociliary ophthalmic branch of the trigeminal nerve densely innervates the cornea to provide sensation and neurotrophic factors to the epithelium and keratocytes [3, 91]. In FED, subbasal and stromal nerves visible by confocal microscopy are tortuous, form loops, and are decreased in number early in the course of disease (Fig. 4.3) [3, 58, 66]. These changes are associated with decreased corneal sensation, even in corneas without clinically obvious anterior disease [3]; although Fuchs described decreased sensation in his original report, his patients had advanced FED with obvious anterior pathology [24]. Corneal sensitivity remains lower than normal even 2 years after endothelial keratoplasty, an indication of slow or limited repair after restoring endothelial function [3].

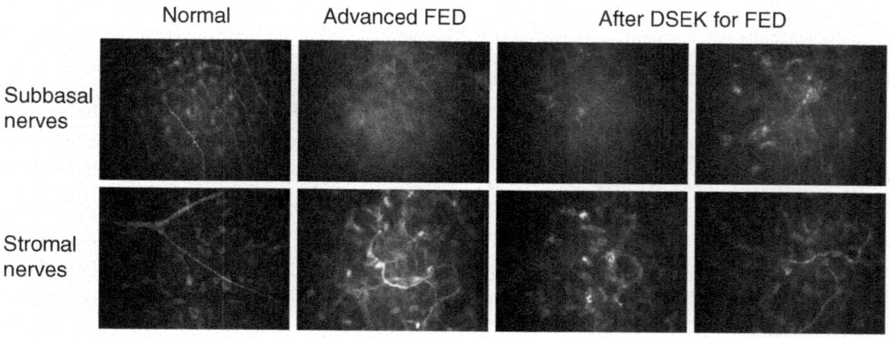

Fig. 4.3 Corneal nerves in Fuchs endothelial dystrophy (*FED*). Confocal images of subbasal and stromal nerve fiber bundles in a normal cornea and before and after Descemet stripping endothelial keratoplasty (*DSEK*) for FED. Subbasal nerve fiber bundles appear as linear bright structures between the basal epithelial cells and anterior keratocytes in normal corneas. In FED, when the subbasal nerves are visible, they typically appear finer and sparser than normal. After DSEK for FED, subbasal nerve fiber bundles typically remain fine and sparse and, occasionally, have thickened and abnormal branching patterns. Stromal nerves in normal corneas typically appear as straight brightly reflective structures with well-defined branching points. In FED, stromal nerves are often tortuous with loops and are often associated with brightly reflective keratocyte nuclei. After DSEK, the tortuosity persists, and the nerves typically appear finer than before keratoplasty, though they are still often associated with brightly reflective keratocyte nuclei

The role of corneal nerves in FED is unclear, but it is likely that they help maintain the integrity and regularity of the anterior cornea [51]. Alterations of nerve density and function might be a response to changes in the microenvironment, created by chronic edema, with reduced autocrine production of vasoactive intestinal peptide and other protective neuropeptides by the altered corneal endothelium [20]. In turn, reduced production of neurotrophic factors might affect endothelial cells and keratocytes by disinhibiting apoptosis [20]. This condition would suggest that the nerves indirectly change the anterior corneal ultrastructure, and this would affect the regularity and integrity of the anterior surface and vision [5, 85].

4.2.2 Posterior Cornea

The definitive association of posterior corneal changes with FED came after the slit lamp was introduced in 1911 by Gullstrand when Koeppe noted dimples on the endothelial surface [37]. These dimples were later termed *cornea guttata* by Vogt [82], and they remain the defining diagnostic feature of FED. Although traditionally there has been a distinction between *cornea guttata* and FED, these labels represent a spectrum of the disease and will probably be replaced by genetic definitions in the future.

4.2.2.1 Descemet Membrane

In normal corneas, Descemet membrane, the basement membrane of the endothelial cells, becomes thicker throughout life [35]. This structure has two distinct layers, a uniform anterior banded layer approximately 3 μm thick and a posterior non-banded layer that thickens from 2 μm at age 10 years to approximately 10 μm at age 80 years. In FED, Descemet membrane is thicker than normal and has an irregular contour, and the non-banded layer becomes non-uniform [35, 43]. The change in the collagen banding pattern is assumed to indicate when abnormal endothelial cell function begins. The presence of a thinner than normal non-banded posterior layer in FED suggests that endothelial dysfunction begins early in the disease; abnormal posterior banded layers then develop and account for most of the increased thickness of the membrane, and focal collagenous excrescences develop as guttae [12, 34, 92]. Guttae tend to be distributed more horizontally than vertically [1] and more inferiorly [25, 59], often appearing in the interpalpebral zone. Disease severity is usually graded based on the presence and confluence of guttae as well as the presence of clinical edema (Fig. 4.4) [40, 44].

Clinically, the Descemet membrane can appear gray and irregular in FED and is best appreciated with broad tangential illumination. With clinical confocal microscopy, Descemet membrane is not visible in normal young subjects, but occasionally becomes visible with increasing age [53]. In FED, guttae are easily visible against the endothelial cell mosaic and, when confluent, appear as voluminous ridges on the posterior corneal surface (Fig. 4.2) [56]. Abnormalities corresponding to the location of Descemet membrane in FED have been described, including a honeycombed appearance and linear structures in oblique sections, although their significance is unknown [56].

4.2.2.2 Endothelial Cells

Corneal endothelial cells form a barrier to solutes and actively transport water and electrolytes [42, 45], and this active pump keeps the normal corneal stroma dehydrated [60]. Endothelial dysfunction is thought to be the primary pathology in FED and is manifested as decreased endothelial cell density or decreased function, or both. Chronic endothelial cell dysfunction results in progressive corneal edema [14, 61], which disrupts the corneal microenvironment [15], and this could affect anterior structures. Recent evidence of anterior corneal changes early in the disease suggests that early endothelial dysfunction may also be responsible for chronic edema, assuming that the anterior corneal changes are not a primary abnormality [5, 85].

In FED, endothelial cells are disrupted by the guttae, which are often lined with a thin layer of cytoplasm, although continuity of the endothelial cell monolayer and the barrier function of the endothelium appear to remain intact until advanced stages of FED. Endothelial cells are lost, presumably by apoptosis; penetrating keratoplasty buttons express DNA fragmentation by TUNEL (terminal deoxynucleotidyl transferase-mediated dUTP nick end labeling) [9]. However, transmission electron

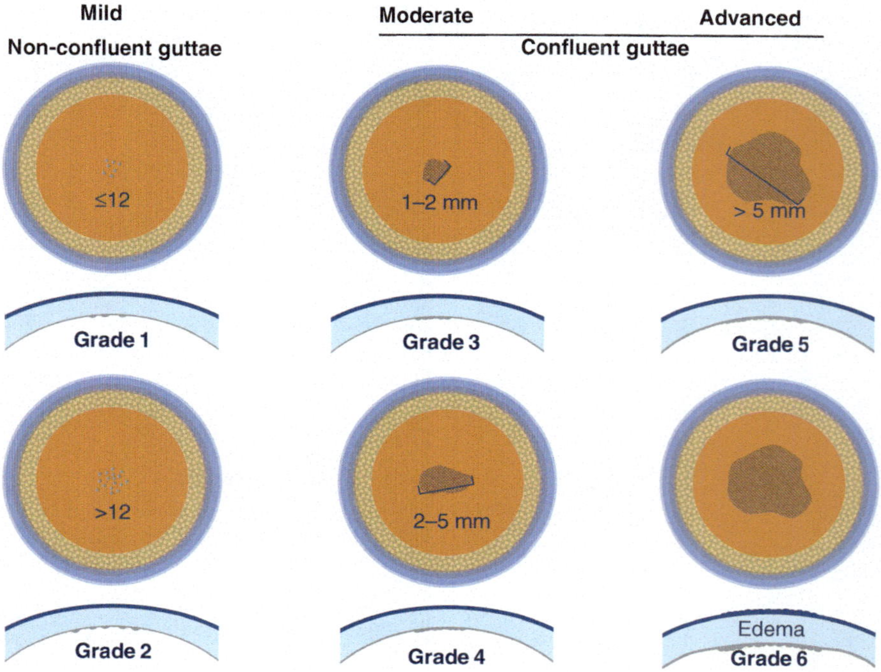

Fig. 4.4 Clinical grading of Fuchs endothelial dystrophy (FED). By using simple slit lamp retro-illumination and specular reflection, the endothelium can readily be graded in clinical practice and research settings. A modification of Krachmer's grading system is commonly used and is based on the area and confluence of guttae and the presence of edema [40, 44]. Grades 1 and 2 are corneas with 1–12 or more than 12 non-confluent central guttae, respectively (which we considered to have mild FED); grades 3 and 4 are corneas with confluent guttae of 1–2 mm or 2–5 mm in widest diameter, respectively (which we have considered to have moderate FED); grades 5 and 6 are corneas with >5-mm diameter of confluent guttae or any visible stromal or epithelial edema, respectively (which we have considered to have advanced FED)

microscopy has found little evidence of apoptosis, possibly because of cell decomposition or sampling error [34]. Endothelial cells do not reproduce significantly after trauma or in response to disease, and the endothelium is repaired by cell migration, enlargement, and redistribution [18, 81].

The endothelium in FED can be assessed macroscopically by evaluating the distribution of guttae clinically or in retro-illumination slit lamp photographs (Fig. 4.4) [26, 63]. The corneal endothelium can also be qualitatively examined by specular reflection at the slit lamp or quantitatively examined by specular or confocal microscopy. The hexagonal array of cells in normal endothelia is disrupted by guttae in FED, and these appear dark in confocal and specular images relative to the light cells. In FED, endothelial cells express polymegethism (variable cell size) and pleomorphism (variable cell shape) [10], but their density cannot be determined in the same way as in normal corneas or corneas after keratoplasty because the area of

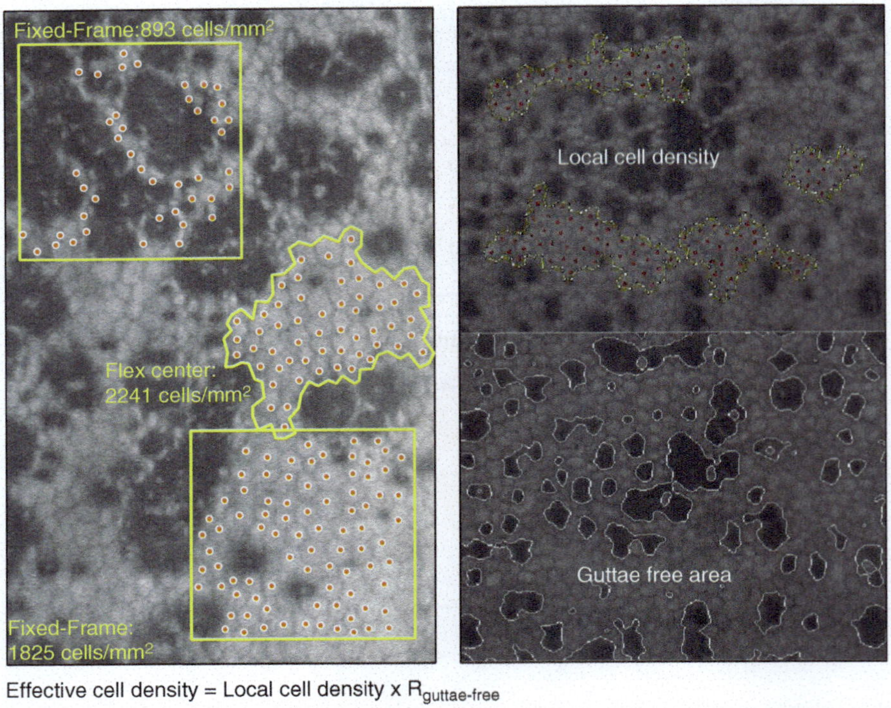

Fig. 4.5 Method of assessing endothelial cell density in Fuchs endothelial dystrophy (FED). Local endothelial cell density measurement in FED by fixed frame, variable frame, or flex center methods results in variable and imprecise estimation of cell density because of regional variation and the presence of guttae (*left*). To calculate the *effective endothelial cell density*, local cell density in several areas of contiguous cells that do not include guttae is multiplied by the ratio of the image area that is free of guttae ($R_{guttae\text{-}free}$) [46]

guttae and regional density variation would produce sampling errors [25, 46]. When considering the distribution of guttae, modified methods must be used to assess endothelial cell density. The *effective endothelial cell density* (ECD_e; Fig. 4.5) is an objective measure that estimates the overall cell density from the density of contiguous cells and the fraction of the image covered by guttae (Figs. 4.2 and 4.5). It correlates well with subjective grading of FED [46].

4.2.3 Corneal Thickness and Curvature

Central corneal thickness has been a simple and helpful measurement in clinical practice to assess corneas with edema. Corneas thicker than 640 μm are usually abnormal, and this thickness was suggested to be an indicator for combined keratoplasty and cataract extraction in the penetrating keratoplasty era [69]. Determining the presence of corneal edema when corneas are thinner than 640 μm can be a challenge when the cornea is not obviously swollen and particularly when the non-edematous (or historical) thickness is unknown. Recent evidence shows that central corneal thickness increases gradually with severity of FED, and corneas are thicker than normal even in mild disease [39, 63]. This is further evidence that corneal changes early in the disease might be the result of chronic edema.

Improvements in Scheimpflug cameras and anterior segment optical coherence tomography (AS-OCT) have enhanced our understanding of corneal curvature of the anterior and posterior surfaces, and the distribution of thickness in normal and abnormal eyes. Normal corneas are thicker vertically than horizontally, which explains against-the-rule astigmatism induced from the posterior corneal surface [74, 86]. In FED, this profile becomes abnormal with bulging of the posterior corneal surface into the anterior chamber because of central edema [13, 41]. Corneal edema in FED changes the normal ellipsoid posterior profile to a more spherical shape, effectively inducing less negative power and loss of normal posterior surface toricity [86]. Similarly, the steep anterior and posterior surface meridians, which are usually oriented vertically in normal corneas [36], are more often oblique or horizontal in FED [86]. These changes may partially explain the hyperopic shift after endothelial keratoplasty and might contribute to inaccurate refractive outcomes after cataract surgery [86].

4.3 Optical Changes

The optical quality of vision can be described in terms of the retinal point spread function, which is the image on the retina of an infinitely small point at infinity [75]. The point spread function normally has a high and narrow central peak (within the central 1° and termed small-angle domain) that decreases to a low and broad peripheral flange (beyond 1° and termed large-angle domain; Fig. 4.6) [75]. Visual acuity is determined by the shape at the center of the point spread function; the sharper the peak, the better the acuity. Abnormalities in the optical media can widen and flatten the central peak and elevate the flange. The center of the point spread function is usually degraded by optical aberrations. Low-order aberrations can be neutralized by spherocylindrical correction, and thus high-order aberrations (HOAs, traditionally thought of as irregular astigmatism) are the primary cause of optical degradation that affects visual acuity. Disability glare corresponds to the large-angle domain of the point spread function and is increased by forward light scatter (retinal straylight) that degrades the contrast of the image [75]. In eyes with spherical intraocular lens implants, changes in the shape of the point spread function can be explained by corneal pathology, and thus in pseudophakic FED patients, optical properties of the cornea can be determined from quality of vision assessed by measuring visual acuity and retinal straylight.

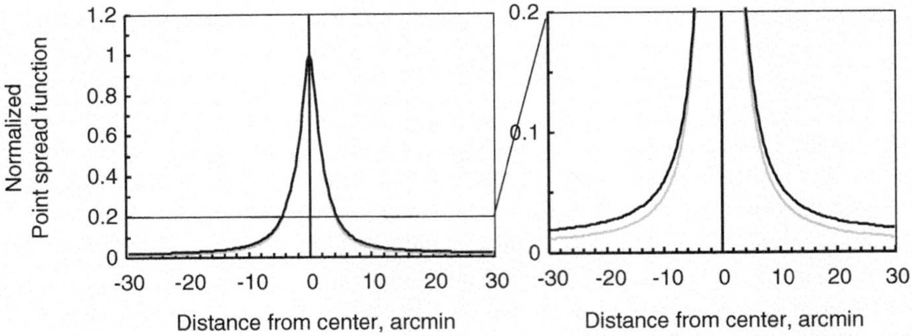

Fig. 4.6 Point spread function. The normal point spread function has a high and narrow central peak within the central 1° (small-angle domain) and a low and broad peripheral flange beyond 1° (large-angle domain). Visual acuity is determined by the shape of the center of the point spread function, which is degraded by high-order aberrations. Disability glare corresponds to the periphery of the point spread function, which is degraded by forward scatter (or straylight). The *gray line* is the point spread function under low forward scatter conditions; the *black line* is the point spread function under high forward scatter conditions. This shows that forward scatter has minimal impact on the center of the point spread function and therefore on visual acuity (Reproduced from Fig. 4.5 in McLaren et al. [47])

4.3.1 Small-Angle Domain and High-Order Aberrations

Aberrations originate from local changes in the regularity of a surface or changes in refractive index that refract and redirect a ray of light. In pseudophakic eyes with spherical intraocular lenses, high-order aberrations predominantly arise from the anterior and posterior corneal surfaces and possibly from any lamellar interface (assuming there is a change in refractive index at the interface). Aberrations create wavefront errors that can be detected by Hartman-Shack aberrometry for the whole eye. Corneal surface irregularities can be isolated and measured from elevation maps derived from videokeratoscopy or corneal tomography to generate surface-derived wavefront errors. Wavefront errors are expressed as Zernike polynomials across the optical aperture, and their amplitude is typically expressed as the root-mean-square of the total wavefront error.

Visual acuity is degraded by increased HOAs, especially those at the center of the Zernike pyramid [6]. Not all aberrations affect visual acuity equally, and different combinations of aberrations can result in variable effects on visual acuity (Fig. 4.7) [6, 47]. HOAs originating from the anterior corneal surface can be corrected with rigid contact lenses, and this was an important method of visual rehabilitation in the era of penetrating keratoplasty and still is for anterior corneal irregularity.

Understanding the role of HOAs in FED began with trying to understand incomplete visual rehabilitation after endothelial keratoplasty, for which the most common indication is FED. Few eyes achieved best-corrected Snellen acuity of 20/20 after deep lamellar endothelial keratoplasty (DLEK) [70, 71], and this was attributed

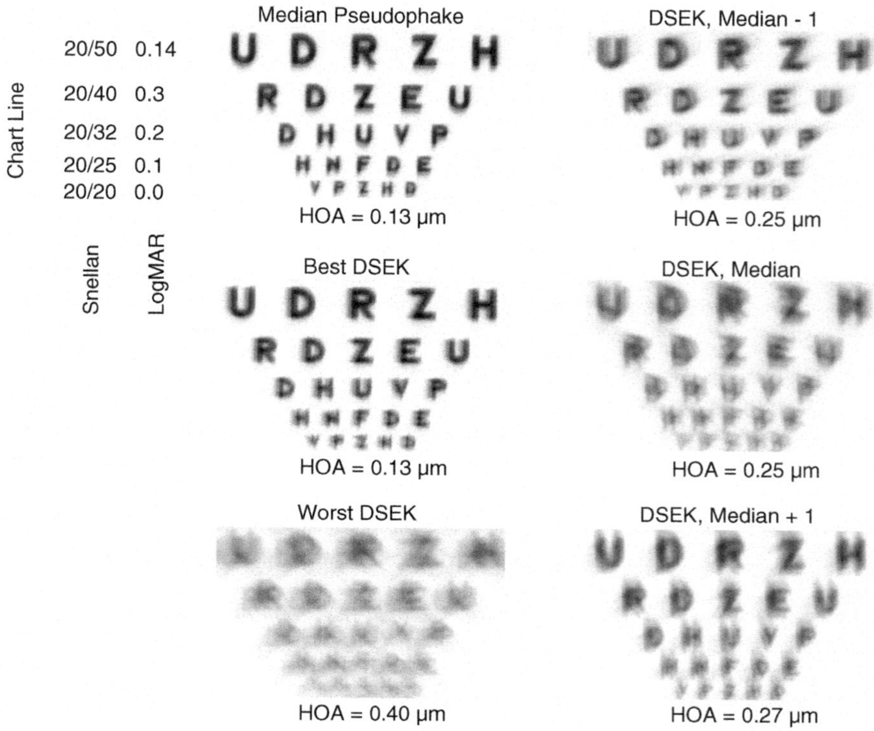

Fig. 4.7 Effect of aberrations on visual acuity. Whole eye wavefront errors were measured in pseudophakic eyes after Descemet stripping endothelial keratoplasty (*DSEK*) by Hartmann-Shack aberrometry and compared to otherwise normal pseudophakic eyes implanted with the same type of intraocular lens [47, 68]. These figures simulate the image of an eye chart on the retina in a patient with the high-order aberrations (HOA) noted. Wavefront errors were increased after DSEK compared to normal pseudophakia. The right column shows simulated eye charts in the patients with median high-order aberrations and with the next higher and next lower high-order aberrations in a study [47]. Note that similar magnitudes of wavefront error that include different combinations of aberrations can have qualitatively different effects on visual acuity because not all aberrations are equal [6] (Reproduced from Fig. 4.6 in McLaren and Patel [47]

to the donor-host lamellar interface. In DLEK, the donor and host stroma were both manually dissected. Transitioning to Descemet stripping endothelial keratoplasty (DSEK), which did not require host stromal dissection and was accompanied by microkeratome preparation of the donor, resulted in improved visual acuity outcomes, and this was attributed to a smoother lamellar interface. Because the anterior corneal surface was not surgically incised and sutures were not used, in contrast to penetrating keratoplasty, it seemed unlikely that HOAs could be a limiting factor for visual acuity after endothelial keratoplasty. This stimulated interest in assessing light scattered by the cornea as a cause of decreased visual acuity after endothelial keratoplasty (see below), especially because some eyes manifested clinical haze at the interface.

In a study that assessed quality of vision and after penetrating and endothelial keratoplasty, the center of the point spread function was significantly and similarly degraded after both procedures [67], suggesting HOAs were indeed elevated after DSEK. This was confirmed by whole eye wavefront aberrometry [68] and studies that examined both corneal surfaces after DSEK (Fig. 4.7) [38, 50, 55, 65, 88]. Apposition of irregular stromal surfaces at the lamellar interface can transmit that irregularity and the consequential aberrations to the posterior corneal surface after DLEK and to a lesser extent after DSEK. In DMEK, the posterior corneal surface should essentially be that of the posterior host stromal surface that is not disrupted during the procedure, and better visual outcomes after DMEK as compared to those after DSEK have been attributed to decreased posterior HOAs [65].

While posterior corneal HOAs are a likely explanation for decreased visual acuity after endothelial keratoplasty, decreased acuity has not been correlated with HOAs from the posterior corneal surface [65, 89] but has been correlated with HOAs from the anterior corneal surface after DSEK and DMEK [38, 55, 65, 89]. Posterior corneal HOAs are of lower magnitude than anterior corneal HOAs because of the smaller change in refractive index at the posterior corneal surface compared to anterior, and it is therefore not surprising that anterior corneal HOAs have a greater effect on visual acuity. More important might be the concept of "parallelism" (Fig. 4.8): posterior corneal HOAs reduce those from the anterior surface in corneas with "parallel" surfaces (normal corneas and penetrating grafts), but when surface "parallelism" is disrupted, such as after DLEK and DSEK (and deep anterior lamellar keratoplasty), posterior HOAs might become additive to anterior HOAs and further decrease acuity [90].

DMEK has gained popularity because of improved visual acuity outcomes compared to DSEK. While the majority of eyes have excellent visual acuity as early as 6 months after DMEK [27, 62, 64, 79], not all of them can be corrected to 20/20 [17]. Even though one would assume that the anterior and posterior corneal surfaces resume a "parallel" relationship after DMEK, the anterior corneal surface can itself be irregular and cause decreased visual acuity [55, 78]. Applying rigid contact lenses has helped improve visual acuity after DMEK, confirming this concept [80].

The irregularity of the anterior corneal surface after endothelial keratoplasty, which does not incise or suture the anterior corneal surface, was unexpected. This suggested that the underlying disease process in eyes with FED might affect the anterior surface [55, 83]. Indeed, anterior corneal aberrations are higher than normal in advanced FED, which is not unexpected in advanced disease because of epithelial or stromal edema [55]. However, even after resolution of corneal edema and at 5 years after endothelial keratoplasty, anterior corneal HOAs remained higher than normal, suggesting that the changes chronically preceded the intervention [55, 85]. Evaluation of a range of severity of FED corneas confirmed that anterior corneal HOAs are increased early in the course of disease before the epithelial surface is clinically disrupted [85], supporting the hypothesis that a chronic state of subclinical edema changes corneal structure in FED.

Posterior corneal HOAs are also increased in the early stages of FED compared to normal [85], and this is likely explained by an irregular surface from

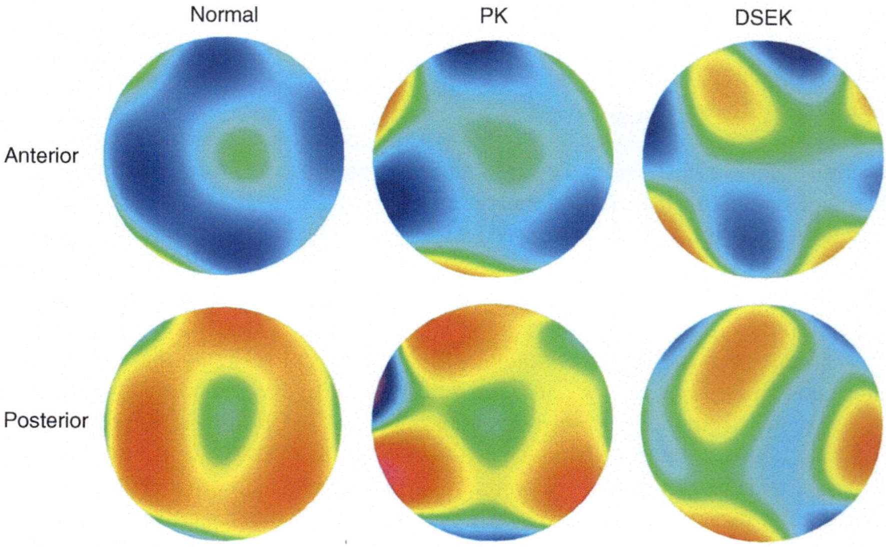

Fig. 4.8 Corneal surface "parallelism." Representative color maps of anterior and posterior corneal high-order wavefront aberrations in a normal cornea, a cornea after penetrating keratoplasty (*PK*), and a cornea after Descemet stripping endothelial keratoplasty (*DSEK*). In normal eyes and eyes after PK, color maps of the anterior surfaces show a reverse pattern with respect to those of the posterior surfaces, indicating that the two surfaces have similar shapes and that posterior aberrations normally counteract anterior aberrations (recognizing that the magnitude of aberrations is much lower from posterior than anterior). After DSEK, the same color reversal pattern is not evident indicating different shapes of the anterior and posterior surfaces and possibly resulting in more total irregularity [90]. Color map scales are not given because they are different for each example to enable illustration of the degree of parallelism in each situation (e.g., the color map scale for the normal eye has been exaggerated relative to the PK eye because the overall magnitude of wavefront error is smaller)

endothelial guttae. Of interest is that posterior corneal HOAs at 6 months after DMEK [65] are similar to those in FED prior to keratoplasty and higher than normal [85]. This raises the possibility of chronic posterior stromal changes in FED, although long-term follow-up of posterior HOAs after DMEK is required to characterize this better.

4.3.2 Large-Angle Domain and Intraocular Forward Scatter

Light scattered toward the retina is termed intraocular forward scatter and degrades retinal image quality by elevating the periphery of the point spread function and reducing image contrast [75]. Light that is scattered back toward an observer is termed backscatter and does not affect vision. Normal corneas are highly transparent [23] but are also visible at the slit lamp because of a small amount of backscattered light. When backscattered light from the cornea is higher than normal, opacities might be clinically evident and are termed "haze"; these same opacities can affect vision, i.e., the same structures that create corneal backscatter also induce forward scatter. Therefore quantifying corneal backscatter can help us understand the effects of forward scatter on vision.

Forward scatter decreases the contrast of the retinal image and is perceived as disability glare [47]. Because forward scatter has little overall effect on the center of the point spread function, it minimally affects visual acuity (Fig. 4.6) [76]. Forward scatter (or straylight) can be measured by using a "compensation comparison" technique and is very reproducible [22, 77]. Measurements of forward scatter are affected by the entire ocular media, whereas measurements of backscatter can be isolated to the cornea.

The interest in corneal light scatter was spurred from realizing that many eyes after endothelial keratoplasty could not be corrected to 20/20, and this was attributed to scatter from the donor-host lamellar interface [31]. Similarly, improvements in visual acuity outcomes from DLEK to DSEK to DMEK were attributed to smoother and anatomically more correct interfaces that would produce less scatter, even though most interfaces never develop clinically visible haze. In fact, corneal backscatter and intraocular forward scatter are correlated with visual acuity after endothelial keratoplasty [21, 54, 57]; while this association exists, causality cannot be inferred from this relationship. Based on optical principles, scattered light should have minimal effect on visual acuity, and the significant correlations between scatter and visual acuity probably indicate that common factors contribute to both scattered light and decreased visual acuity without the former necessarily causing the latter.

In a study to test the hypothesis that scattered light minimally affects visual acuity after endothelial keratoplasty, visual acuity and glare were measured in normal subjects under conditions simulating typical HOAs and excess forward scatter after DSEK [47]. Visual acuity decreased by less than 3 letters under high scatter conditions and by more than 6 letters under aberrated conditions. In another study that used adaptive optics to correct HOAs after DSEK, visual acuity improved to 20/20 [52], further confirming the optical theory that HOAs are more likely to affect visual acuity than scattered light. The role of the smoother and more anatomically correct interface, as keratoplasty has evolved from DLEK to DMEK, is probably to transmit less irregularity to the posterior corneal surface rather than produce less scattered light. Backscatter from the DSEK interface diminishes quickly after keratoplasty and is much lower than anterior corneal light scatter [7, 54, 83]. Anterior corneal scatter is therefore of more significance, improves slowly after endothelial keratoplasty, and does not return to normal even at 5 years (Fig. 4.1) [7, 83]. Because anterior corneal scatter is isolated to the host cornea, it is not the result of endothelial keratoplasty but is more likely a manifestation of the underlying disease, which in most of the cases is FED.

Increased anterior corneal scatter in FED increases disability glare compared to normal, especially in younger patients [77]. Younger patients with FED maintain better visual acuity compared to older patients, possibly because of less HOAs from lenticular changes [77]. Preoperative glare (straylight) in FED can be an indication for endothelial keratoplasty even if visual acuity appears to be minimally compromised, and preoperative straylight can predict postoperative straylight improvement after DSEK [77].

Corneas with advanced FED requiring transplantation scatter more light than normal, and this is explained in part by corneal edema. However, chronic changes in the ultrastructure of these corneas are also important because scatter does not return to normal even after resolution of edema [7]. The continued elevated anterior corneal scatter after endothelial keratoplasty might be explained by persistence of factors that increased scatter in this region in FED before keratoplasty. Increased anterior and posterior corneal backscatter has been found even in the early stages of FED, again suggesting a subclinical phase of the disease related to the presence of chronic edema (Fig. 4.1) [5, 85].

4.4 Association Between Anatomy and Optics

Early in the course of FED, both corneal surfaces can be irregular and the anterior and posterior cornea can backscatter more light than normal. Irregular surfaces and increased backscatter are associated with increased HOAs and forward scatter, respectively, which in turn decrease visual acuity and increase disability glare, respectively. The structural changes that contribute to surface irregularity and increased backscatter are probably the result of progressive and chronic subclinical corneal edema that begins early in the course of disease and persists after endothelial replacement [5, 32, 49, 83]. Posterior surface irregularity and backscatter might also be caused by guttae [85].

Corneal confocal microscopy and tomography have aided our understanding of anatomic and optical properties of FED corneas. Corneal scatter is caused in part by corneal edema (reversible component) [7], chronic anterior extracellular matrix changes [28, 33, 49], and abnormal subepithelial cells [56, 85]. The subepithelial cells probably represent fibroblasts that are responsible for subepithelial fibrosis [49], which can be present even if not clinically apparent. Increased posterior corneal backscatter in FED is caused by guttae, and their removal significantly reduces backscatter [54, 57, 85].

Anterior corneal surface irregularity occurs when epithelial and stromal edema are present but can also be present chronically prior to this [85] and after endothelial keratoplasty [55, 83]. The exact source of increased anterior aberrations is unknown in FED, but they possibly arise from a non-uniform subepithelial layer after appearance of fibroblasts and fibrosis (Fig. 4.9) [5, 56]. The epithelial stromal boundary might also become irregular from keratocyte depletion and architectural changes in the anterior cornea [28, 51, 56]. Epithelial debridement at the time of endothelial keratoplasty might improve visual outcomes [16], akin to removing basement membrane dystrophic tissue from the visual axis. Posterior surface irregularity in FED can be attributed to guttae, but it is unknown whether chronic changes in the posterior stroma might also contribute [85]. Guttae are now considered to be visually significant, but they may also influence vision by

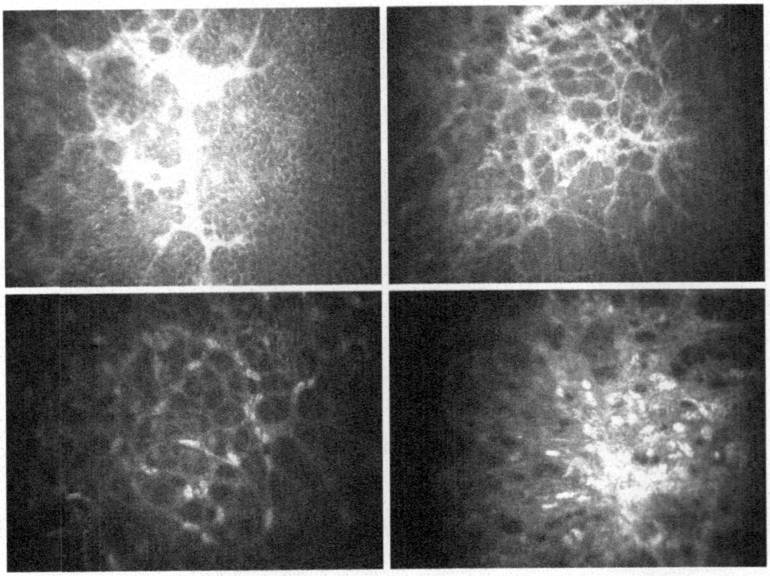

Fig. 4.9 Subepithelial cells in Fuchs endothelial dystrophy (FED). Confocal images showing subepithelial cells in FED and after endothelial keratoplasty for FED. Brightly reflective reticular networks of cells, presumably subepithelial fibroblasts, are visible deep in the basal epithelium of corneas with mild, moderate, and advanced FED. Subepithelial cells persist through at least 3 years after endothelial keratoplasty for FED, with the same reticular network of cell processes and visible oval cell nuclei. The cells are highly reflective and thus contribute to increased anterior corneal backscatter and probably to an irregular anterior corneal surface, which increases aberrations [56]

their effect on corneal edema, and separating these functions is difficult. Nevertheless, it is considered important to strip Descemet membrane during endothelial keratoplasty for FED to remove the guttae.

Graft thickness is frequently thought to influence visual outcomes after DSEK. However, there is no optical basis for this and most studies have found minimal, if any, effect of graft thickness on visual acuity [2, 72, 84]. None of the studies that claim a positive association were prospective with standardized visual acuity measurements.

4.5 Implication on Clinical Decision-Making and Prospect

As DMEK gains popularity as the treatment of choice for FED, visual acuity in eyes with healthy grafts will be determined primarily by improvement of anterior corneal irregularity, assuming central graft folds are not present. Similarly, postoperative glare will be determined by scatter from the anterior cornea. Although the course of visual outcomes might largely be determined by the chronicity of these changes in the cornea after DMEK, the optimum time to intervene in the course of FED has not been determined. At this time, even though the cornea changes subclinically early in FED, the risks of early surgery should be carefully considered, and we do not advocate intervening in the absence of FED-related symptoms. While visual outcomes are important, patient-reported outcomes are likely to become a more important measure of success in the future.

References

1. Adamis AP, Filatov V, Tripathi BJ, Tripathi RC. Fuchs' endothelial dystrophy of the cornea. Survey Ophthalmol. 1993;38:149–68.
2. Ahmed KA, McLaren JW, Baratz KH, Maguire LJ, Kittleson KM, Patel SV. Host and graft thickness after descemet stripping endothelial keratoplasty for Fuchs endothelial dystrophy. Am J Ophthalmol. 2010;150:490–7.
3. Ahuja Y, Baratz KH, McLaren JW, Bourne WM, Patel SV. Decreased corneal sensitivity and abnormal corneal nerves in Fuchs endothelial dystrophy. Cornea. 2012;31:1257–63.
4. Alomar TS, Al-Aqaba M, Gray T, Lowe J, Dua HS. Histological and confocal microscopy changes in chronic corneal edema: implications for endothelial transplantation. Investig Ophthalmol Visual Sci. 2011;52:8193–207.
5. Amin SR, Baratz KH, McLaren JW, Patel SV. Corneal abnormalities early in the course of Fuchs' endothelial dystrophy. Ophthalmology. 2014;121:2325–33.
6. Applegate RA, Sarver EJ, Khemsara V. Are all aberrations equal? J Refract Surg. 2002;18:S556–62.
7. Baratz KH, McLaren JW, Maguire LJ, Patel SV. Corneal haze determined by confocal microscopy two years after descemet stripping with endothelial keratoplasty for Fuchs corneal dystrophy. Arch Ophthalmol. 2012;130:868–74.
8. Baratz KH, Patel SV, McLaren JW, Winter EJ, Nau CB, Hodge DO, Bourne WM. Corneal haze and contrast sensitivity after deep lamellar endothelial keratoplasty versus penetrating keratoplasty. Invest Ophthalmol Vis Sci. 2006;47, Arvo E-Abstract #2372.
9. Borderie VM, Baudrimont M, Vallee A, Ereau TL, Gray F, Laroche L. Corneal endothelial cell apoptosis in patients with Fuchs' dystrophy. Invest Ophthalmol Vis Sci. 2000;41:2501–5.
10. Bourne WM. Corneal endothelium--past, present, and future. Eye Contact Lens. 2010;36:310–4.
11. Bourne WM, Hodge DO, McLaren JW. Estimation of corneal endothelial pump function in long-term contact lens wearers. Invest Ophthalmol Vis Sci. 1999;40:603–11.
12. Bourne WM, Johnson DH, Campbell RJ. The ultrastructure of Descemet's membrane. III. Fuchs' dystrophy. Arch Ophthalmol. 1982;100:1952–5.
13. Brunette I, Sherknies D, Terry MA, Chagnon M, Bourges J-L, Meunier J. 3-D characterization of the corneal shape in Fuchs dystrophy and pseudophakic keratopathy. Investig Ophthalmol Visual Sci. 2011;52:206–14.
14. Burns RR, Bourne WM, Brubaker RF. Endothelial function in patients with cornea guttata. Investig Ophthalmol Visual Sci. 1981;20:77–85.
15. Calandra A, Chwa M, Kenney MC. Characterization of stroma from Fuchs' endothelial dystrophy corneas. Cornea. 1989;8:90–7.
16. Chaurasia S, Price MO, Mckee Y, Price Jr FW. Descemet membrane endothelial keratoplasty combined with epithelial debridement and mitomycin-C application for Fuchs dystrophy with preoperative subepithelial fibrosis or anterior basement membrane dystrophy. Cornea. 2014;33:335–9.
17. Dapena I, Yeh RY, Baydoun L, Cabrerizo J, Van Dijk K, Ham L, Melles GR. Potential causes of incomplete visual rehabilitation at 6 months postoperative after descemet membrane endothelial keratoplasty. Am J Ophthalmol. 2013;156:780–8.
18. Doughman DJ, Van Horn D, Rodman WP, Byrnes P, Lindstrom RL. Human corneal endothelial layer repair during organ culture. Arch Ophthalmol. 1976;94:1791–6.
19. Eagle Jr RC, Laibson PR, Arentsen JJ. Epithelial abnormalities in chronic corneal edema: a histopathological study. Trans Am Ophthalmol Soc. 1989;87:107–19; Discussion 119–24.
20. Erie JC, Patel SV, McLaren JW, Nau CB, Hodge DO, Bourne WM. Keratocyte density in keratoconus. A confocal microscopy study(A). Am J Ophthalmol. 2002;134:689–95.

21. Espana EM, Huang B. Confocal microscopy study of donor-recipient interface after Descemet's stripping with endothelial keratoplasty. Bri J Ophthalmol. 2010;94:903–8.
22. Franssen L, Coppens JE, Van Den Berg TJTP. Compensation comparison method for assessment of retinal straylight. Investig Ophthalmol Visual Sci. 2006;47:768–76.
23. Freund DE, Mccally RL, Farrell RA, Cristol SM, L'hernault NL, Edelhauser HF. Ultrastructure in anterior and posterior stroma of perfused human and rabbit corneas. Relation to transparency. Investig Ophthalmol Visual Sci. 1995;36:1508–23.
24. Fuchs E. Dystrophia epithelialis corneae. Albrecht Von Graefes Archiv Fur Klinische Und Experimentelle Ophthalmologie. 1910;76:478–508.
25. Fujimoto H, Maeda N, Soma T, Oie Y, Koh S, Tsujikawa M, Nishida K. Quantitative regional differences in corneal endothelial abnormalities in the central and peripheral zones in Fuchs' endothelial corneal dystrophy. Investig Ophthalmol Visual Sci. 2014;55:5090–8.
26. Gottsch JD, Sundin OH, Rencs EV, Emmert DG, Stark WJ, Cheng CJ, Schmidt GW. Analysis and documentation of progression of Fuchs corneal dystrophy with retroillumination photography. Cornea. 2006;25:485–9.
27. Guerra FP, Anshu A, Price MO, Giebel AW, Price FW. Descemet's membrane endothelial keratoplasty: prospective study of 1-year visual outcomes, graft survival, and endothelial eell loss. Ophthalmology. 2011;118:2368–73.
28. Hecker LA, McLaren JW, Bachman LA, Patel SV. Anterior keratocyte depletion in Fuchs endothelial dystrophy. Arch Ophthalmol. 2011;129:555–61.
29. Hernandez-Quintela E, Mayer F, Dighiero P, Briat B, Savoldelli M, Legeais JM, Renard G. Confocal microscopy of cystic disorders of the corneal epithelium. Ophthalmology. 1998; 105:631–6.
30. Hillenaar T, Cals RHH, Eilers PHC, Wubbels RJ, Van Cleynenbreugel H, Remeijer L. Normative database for corneal backscatter analysis by in vivo confocal microscopy. Investig Ophthalmol Visual Sci. 2011;52:7274–81.
31. Hindman HB, Mccally RL, Myrowitz E, Terry MA, Stark WJ, Weinberg RS, Jun AS. Evaluation of deep lamellar endothelial keratoplasty surgery using scatterometry and wavefront analyses. Ophthalmology. 2007;114:2006–12.
32. Hsueh C-M, Lo W, Chen W-L, Hovhannisyan VA, Liu G-Y, Wang S-S, Tan H-Y, Dong C-Y. Structural characterization of edematous corneas by forward and backward second harmonic generation imaging. Biophys J. 2009;97:1198–205.
33. Iwamoto T, Devoe AG. Electron microscopic studies on Fuchs' combined dystrophy. II. Anterior portion of the cornea. Invest Ophthalmol. 1971;10:29–40.
34. Iwamoto T, Devoe AG. Electron microscopic studies on Fuchs' combined dystrophy. I. Posterior portion of the cornea. Invest Ophthalmol. 1971;10:9–28.
35. Johnson DH, Bourne WM, Campbell RJ. The ultrastructure of Descemet's membrane. I. Changes with Age in normal corneas. Arch Ophthalmol. 1982;100:1942–7.
36. Koch DD, Ali SF, Weikert MP, Shirayama M, Jenkins R, Wang L. Contribution of posterior corneal astigmatism to total corneal astigmatism. J Cataract Refractive Surg. 2012;38:2080–7.
37. Koeppe L. Klinische Beobachtungen Mit Der Nernstspaltlampe Und Dem Hornahutmikroskop. Albrecht Von Graefes Archiv Fur Klinische Und Experimentelle Ophthalmologie. 1916;91:363–79.
38. Koh S, Maeda N, Nakagawa T, Higashiura R, Saika M, Mihashi T, Fujikado T, Nishida K. Characteristic higher-order aberrations of the anterior and posterior corneal surfaces in 3 corneal transplantation techniques. Am J Ophthalmol. 2012;153:284–90.
39. Kopplin LJ, Przepyszny K, Schmotzer B, Rudo K, Babineau DC, Patel SV, Verdier DD, Jurkunas U, Iyengar SK, Lass JH, Group FTFECDGM-CS. Relationship of Fuchs endothelial corneal dystrophy severity to central corneal thickness. Arch Ophthalmol. 2012;130: 433–9.
40. Krachmer JH, Purcell Jr JJ, Young CW, Bucher KD. Corneal endothelial dystrophy. A study of 64 families. Arch Ophthalmol. 1978;96:2036–9.

41. Kwon RO, Price MO, Price Jr FW, Ambrosio Jr R, Belin MW. Pentacam characterization of corneas with Fuchs dystrophy treated with descemet membrane endothelial keratoplasty. J Refractive Surg. 2010;26:972–9.
42. Leber T. Studien Uber Den Flussigkeitswechsel Im Auge. Albrecht Von Graefes Archiv Fur Klinische Und Experimentelle Ophthalmologie. 1873;19:87–185.
43. Li JY, Terry MA, Goshe J, Shamie N, Davis-Boozer D. Graft rejection after Descemet's stripping automated endothelial keratoplasty: graft survival and endothelial cell loss. Ophthalmology. 2012;119:90–4.
44. Louttit MD, Kopplin LJ, Igo Jr RP, Fondran JR, Tagliaferri A, Bardenstein D, Aldave AJ, Croasdale CR, Price MO, Rosenwasser GO, Lass JH, Iyengar SK, Group FTFGM-CS. A multicenter study to map genes for Fuchs endothelial corneal dystrophy: baseline characteristics and heritability. Cornea. 2012;31:26–35.
45. Maurice DM. The location of the fluid pump in the cornea. J Physiol. 1972;221:43–54.
46. McLaren JW, Bachman LA, Kane KM, Patel SV. Objective assessment of the corneal endothelium in Fuchs' endothelial dystrophy. Invest Ophthalmol Vis Sci. 2014;55:1184–90.
47. McLaren JW, Patel SV. Modeling the effect of forward scatter and aberrations on visual acuity after endothelial keratoplasty. Investig Ophthalmol Visual Sci. 2012;53:5545–51.
48. McLaren JW, Wacker K, Kane KM, Patel SV. Measuring corneal haze by using scheimpflug photography and confocal microscopy. Investig Ophthalmol Visual Sci. 2015;57(1):227–35.
49. Morishige N, Yamada N, Teranishi S, Chikama T-I, Nishida T, Takahara A. Detection of subepithelial fibrosis associated with corneal stromal edema by second harmonic generation imaging microscopy. Investig Ophthalmol Visual Sci. 2009;50:3145–50.
50. Muftuoglu O, Prasher P, Bowman RW, Mcculley JP, Mootha VV. Corneal higher-order aberrations after Descemet's stripping automated endothelial keratoplasty. Ophthalmology. 2010;117:878–84.
51. Muller LJ, Pels E, Vrensen GF. The specific architecture of the anterior stroma accounts for maintenance of corneal curvature. Br J Ophthalmol. 2001;85:437–43.
52. Pantanelli SM, Sabesan R, Ching ST, Yoon G, Hindman HB. Visual performance with wave aberration correction after penetrating, deep anterior lamellar, or endothelial keratoplasty. Investig Ophthalmol Visual Sci. 2012;53(8):4797–804.
53. Patel DV, Mcghee CNJ. Contemporary in vivo confocal microscopy of the living human cornea using white light and laser scanning techniques: a major review [See comment]. Clin Exp Ophthalmol. 2007;35:71–88.
54. Patel SV, Baratz KH, Hodge DO, Maguire LJ, McLaren JW. The effect of corneal light scatter on vision after descemet stripping with endothelial keratoplasty. Arch Ophthalmol. 2009;127:153–60.
55. Patel SV, Baratz KH, Maguire LJ, Hodge DO, McLaren JW. Anterior corneal aberrations after descemet stripping endothelial keratoplasty for Fuchs endothelial dystrophy. Ophthalmology. 2012;119:1522–9.
56. Patel SV, McLaren JW. In vivo confocal microscopy of Fuchs endothelial dystrophy before and after endothelial keratoplasty. JAMA Ophthalmol. 2013;131:611–8.
57. Patel SV, McLaren JW, Hodge DO, Baratz KH. Scattered light and visual function in a randomized trial of deep lamellar endothelial keratoplasty and penetrating keratoplasty. Am J Ophthalmol. 2008;145:97–105.
58. Patel SV, McLaren JW, Kittleson KM, Bourne WM. Subbasal nerve density and corneal sensitivity after laser in situ keratomileusis: femtosecond laser Vs mechanical microkeratome. Arch Ophthalmol. 2010;128:1413–9.
59. Perez-Escudero A, Dorronsoro C, Sawides L, Remon L, Merayo-Lloves J, Marcos S. Minor influence of myopic laser in situ keratomileusis on the posterior corneal surface. Investig Ophthalmol Visual Sci. 2009;50:4146–54.
60. Polse KA, Brand R, Mandell R, Vastine D, Demartini D, Flom R. Age differences in corneal hydration control. Investig Ophthalmol Visual Sci. 1989;30:392–9.
61. Polse KA, Brand RJ, Vastine DW, Demartini DR, Sanders TL. Clinical assessment of corneal hydration control in Fuchs' dystrophy. Optometry Vision Sci. 1991;68:831–41.

62. Price MO, Giebel AW, Fairchild KM, Price FW. Descemet's membrane endothelial keratoplasty: prospective multicenter study of visual and refractive outcomes and endothelial survival. Ophthalmology. 2009;116:2361–8.
63. Repp DJ, Hodge DO, Baratz KH, McLaren JW, Patel SV. Fuchs' endothelial corneal dystrophy. Subjective grading versus objective grading based on the central-to-peripheral thickness ratio. Ophthalmology. 2013;120:687–94.
64. Rodriguez-Calvo-De-Mora M, Quilendrino R, Ham L, Liarakos VS, Van Dijk K, Baydoun L, Dapena I, Oellerich S, Melles GR. Clinical outcome of 500 consecutive cases undergoing Descemet's membrane endothelial keratoplasty. Ophthalmology. 2015;122:464–70.
65. Rudolph M, Laaser K, Bachmann BO, Cursiefen C, Epstein D, Kruse FE. Corneal higher-order aberrations after Descemet's membrane endothelial keratoplasty. Ophthalmology. 2012;119:528–35.
66. Schrems-Hoesl LM, Schrems WA, Cruzat A, Shahatit BM, Bayhan HA, Jurkunas UV, Hamrah P. Cellular and subbasal nerve alterations in early stage Fuchs' endothelial corneal dystrophy: an in vivo confocal microscopy study. Eye (Lond), Advance On Line Publication. 2012;27(1):42–9.
67. Seery LS, McLaren JW, Kittleson KM, Patel SV. Retinal point-spread function after corneal transplantation for Fuchs' dystrophy. Invest Ophthalmol Vis Sci. 2011;52:1003–8.
68. Seery LS, Nau CB, McLaren JW, Baratz KH, Patel SV. Graft thickness, graft folds, and aberrations after descemet stripping endothelial keratoplasty for Fuchs dystrophy. Am J Ophthalmol. 2011;152:910–6.
69. Seitzman GD, Gottsch JD, Stark WJ. Cataract surgery in patients with Fuchs' corneal dystrophy: expanding recommendations for cataract surgery without simultaneous keratoplasty. Ophthalmology. 2005;112:441–6.
70. Terry MA, Ousley P. Rapid visual rehabilitation after endothelial transplants with deep lamellar endothelial keratoplasty (DLEK). Cornea. 2004;23:143–53.
71. Terry MA, Ousley PJ. Deep lamellar endothelial keratoplasty visual acuity, astigmatism, and endothelial survival in a large prospective series. Ophthalmology. 2005;112:1541–8.
72. Terry MA, Straiko MD, Goshe J, Li JY, Davis-Boozer D. Descemet's stripping automated endothelial keratoplasty: the tenuous relationship between donor thickness and post-operative vision. Ophthalmology. 2012;119:1988–96.
73. Tripathi RC, Bron AJ. Cystic disorders of the corneal epithelium. II. Pathogenesis. Br J Ophthalmol. 1973;57:376–90.
74. Ueno Y, Hiraoka T, Miyazaki M, Ito M, Oshika T. Corneal thickness profile and posterior corneal astigmatism in normal corneas. Ophthalmology. 2015;122(11), e66.
75. Van Den Berg TJ, Franssen L, Coppens JE. Straylight in the human eye: testing objectivity and optical character of the psychophysical measurement. Ophthalmic Physiol Opt. 2009;29:345–50.
76. Van Den Berg TJ, Van Rijn LJ, Michael R, Heine C, Coeckelbergh T, Nischler C, Wilhelm H, Grabner G, Emesz M, Barraquer RI, Coppens JE, Franssen L. Straylight effects with aging and lens extraction. Am J Ophthalmol. 2007;144:358–63.
77. Van Der Meulen IJ, Patel SV, Lapid-Gortzak R, Nieuwendaal CP, McLaren JW, Van Den Berg TJ. Quality of vision in patients with Fuchs endothelial dystrophy and after descemet stripping endothelial keratoplasty. Arch Ophthalmol. 2011;129:1537–42.
78. Van Dijk K, Droutsas K, Hou J, Sangsari S, Liarakos VS, Melles GR. Optical quality of the cornea after descemet membrane endothelial keratoplasty. Am J Ophthalmol. 2014;158(71–79), E1.
79. Van Dijk K, Ham L, Tse WH, Liarakos VS, Quilendrino R, Yeh RY, Melles GR. Near complete visual recovery and refractive stability in modern corneal transplantation: descemet membrane endothelial keratoplasty (DMEK). Cont Lens Anterior Eye. 2013;36:13–21.
80. Van Dijk K, Parker J, Liarakos VS, Ham L, Frank LE, Melles GR. Incidence of irregular astigmatism eligible for contact lens fitting after descemet membrane endothelial keratoplasty. J Cataract Refract Surg. 2013;39:1036–46.

81. Van Horn DL, Hyndiuk RA. Endothelial wound repair in primate cornea. Exp Eye Res. 1975;21:113–24.
82. Vogt A. Weitere Ergebnisse Der Spaltlampenmikroskopie Des Vorderen Bulbusabschnittes. Arch F Ophth. 1921;106:69.
83. Wacker K, Baratz KH, Maguire LJ, McLaren JW, Patel SV. Descemet stripping endothelial keratoplasty for Fuchs' endothelial corneal dystrophy: 5-year results of a prospective study. Ophthalmology. 2015. doi:10.1016/J.Ophtha.2015.09.023.
84. Wacker K, Bourne WM, Patel SV. Effect of graft thickness on visual acuity after Descemet stripping endothelial keratoplasty: a systematic review and meta-analysis. Am J Ophthalmol. 2016;163:18–28.
85. Wacker K, McLaren JW, Amin SR, Baratz KH, Patel SV. Corneal high-order aberrations and backscatter in Fuchs endothelial corneal dystrophy. Ophthalmology. 2015;122:1645–52.
86. Wacker K, McLaren JW, Patel SV. Directional posterior corneal profile changes in Fuchs' endothelial corneal dystrophy. Invest Ophthalmol Vis Sci. 2015;56:5904–11.
87. Wilson SE, Bourne WM. Fuchs' dystrophy. Cornea. 1988;7:2–18.
88. Yamaguchi T, Negishi K, Yamaguchi K, Dogru M, Uchino Y, Shimmura S, Tsubota K. Comparison of anterior and posterior corneal surface irregularity in descemet stripping automated endothelial keratoplasty and penetrating keratoplasty. Cornea. 2010; 29:1086–90.
89. Yamaguchi T, Negishi K, Yamaguchi K, Murat D, Uchino Y, Shimmura S, Tsubota K. Effect of anterior and posterior corneal surface irregularity on vision after descemet-stripping endothelial keratoplasty. J Cataract Refract Surg. 2009;35:688–94.
90. Yamaguchi T, Ohnuma K, Tomida D, Konomi K, Satake Y, Negishi K, Tsubota K, Shimazaki J. The contribution of the posterior surface to the corneal aberrations in eyes after keratoplasty. Investig Ophthalmol Visual Sci. 2011;52:6222–9.
91. You L, Kruse FE, Volcker HE. Neurotrophic factors in the human cornea. Investig Ophthalmol Visual Sci. 2000;41:692–702.
92. Yuen HK, Rassier CE, Jardeleza MS, Green WR, De La Cruz Z, Stark WJ, Gottsch JD. A morphologic study of Fuchs dystrophy and bullous keratopathy. Cornea. 2005;24:319–27.

Chapter 5
Evolution of Posterior Lamellar Keratoplasty: PK – DLEK – DSEK/DSAEK – DMEK – DMET

Lamis Baydoun, Isabel Dapena, and Gerrit Melles

5.1 At the Start: Who Is Going to Win the Race–Lamellar or Penetrating Keratoplasty?

The idea for lamellar and penetrating replacement of corneal tissue evolved in the late eighteenth and early nineteenth century. Growing insight into transplantation biology influenced the evolution of both techniques and led to experiments with either heterologous or homologous corneal tissue transplantations.

It was in 1818 that the term "keratoplasty" was first introduced by Franz Reisinger, who conducted experiments on hetero- and homologous full-thickness transplantation [1]. However, the first successful heterograft described in 1888 was an anterior lamellar graft performed by von Hippel [2].

Still, lamellar procedures were not pursued, probably because they were perceived as technically more challenging than the penetrating technique.

5.2 After a Long Run: Penetrating Keratoplasty Takes the Lead

After numerous experiments by contemporary scientists in the past century, eventually, penetrating keratoplasty (PK) achieved its breakthrough in the early twentieth century, when Dr. Eduard Zirm performed the first successful homologous penetrating procedure in 1905 under general anesthesia and "strict" aseptic conditions [3].

L. Baydoun • I. Dapena • G. Melles, MD, PhD (✉)
Netherlands Institute for Innovative Ocular Surgery, Rotterdam, The Netherlands

Melles Cornea Clinic Rotterdam, Rotterdam, The Netherlands
e-mail: research@niios.com; baydoun@niios.com; http://www.niios.com

C. Cursiefen, A.S. Jun (eds.), *Current Treatment Options for Fuchs Endothelial Dystrophy*, DOI 10.1007/978-3-319-43021-8_5

The subsequent introduction of corticosteroids for prevention and treatment of allograft rejection and the use of microscopes and antibiotics were important contributions to make this technique popular and successful. In the following decades, amendments focused on the improvement of the surgical technique by introducing different trephines, laser-guided trephination, and suture techniques, enhancing clinical outcomes in terms of reducing postoperative unpredictable refractive errors and optimizing donor tissue preservation and preparation.

PK became the treatment of choice for a wide range of corneal disorders, affecting any corneal layer.

5.3 At the Curve: Posterior Lamellar Techniques Trying to Catch Up

From the 1950s and onward, lamellar keratoplasty techniques went through a revival phase when Dr. José Barraquer and Dr. Charles Tillett introduced the first posterior lamellar endothelial transplant underneath a manually dissected stromal flap that was secured by sutures [4–6]. The lack of adequate instruments to create thin corneal layers and limited understanding of endothelial cell physiology were probably reasons why these concepts were not further pursued. Also, these procedures were still technically more demanding than PK resulting in early complications and insufficient functional results [7]. Although a promising concept for endothelial keratoplasty was born, it took almost half a century until the first clinically successful operation was performed in 1998. Until then, namely, in the early 1990s, various scientists continued to evaluate the replacement of posterior corneal tissue underneath a sutured stromal flap in experimental animal models [8], describing a sclerocorneal approach [9] or trying to standardize flap preparation by using a microkeratome [10].

5.4 Before the Finish: Lamellar Techniques' Relay on the Fast Track – From DLEK to DSEK to DMEK

By the end of the twentieth century, PK was the standard of care for unselective treatment of all diseased corneal layers. However, the success of this surgical technique has been somewhat tempered by well-known and profound intra- and postoperative complications that could not be sufficiently solved in the past 100 years. Thus, until the late 1990s, PK as the only treatment option for endothelial diseases, such as Fuchs endothelial corneal dystrophy (FECD), was often reserved only for advanced cases with progressive corneal edema, scarring, and significant impairment of visual acuity. Still, 30–50 % of indications for PK affected solely the corneal endothelium [11], resulting in the unnecessary replacement of healthy anterior corneal tissue when treating corneal endothelial disorders.

Shortly before the turn of the millennium, within less than 10 years, a thrilling sprint in the development of endothelial keratoplasty techniques started. Each

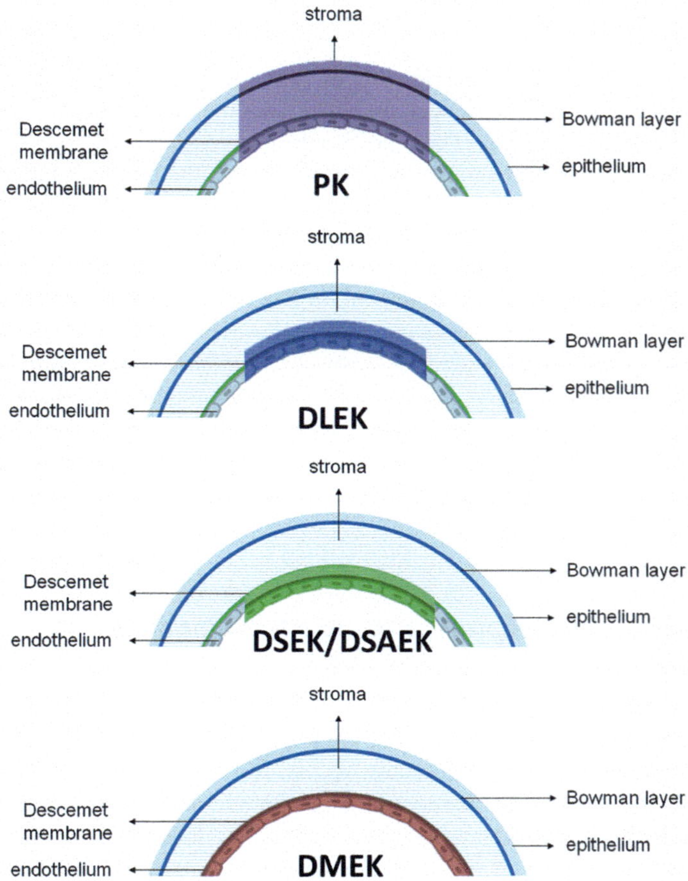

Fig. 5.1 Schematic diagram of penetrating keratoplasty and the current endothelial keratoplasty techniques (Figure had been published in modified form in Ref. [64])

refinement of the endothelial keratoplasty technique was close on the heels of the previously introduced, continuously evolving to a less invasive procedure, with thinner transplants, while extinguishing many complications associated with PK and obtaining an unexpected level of clinical outcome that, just a decade ago, could not have been thought possible (Fig. 5.1) [12].

5.4.1 Deep Lamellar Endothelial Keratoplasty (DLEK)

In 1998 Melles and colleagues introduced the first successful approach for posterior lamellar keratoplasty (PLK) in humans, in which an *unsutured* donor posterior corneal disk, consisting of posterior stroma, Descemet membrane, and endothelium, was transplanted into the anterior chamber through a limbal incision [13, 14]. In 2001, this technique was popularized as "deep lamellar endothelial keratoplasty" (DLEK) in the United States by Terry et al. [15]. In the initial PLK/DLEK technique, a posterior lamellar disk was dissected from the recipient cornea through a 9-mm sclerocorneal incision. Then, an equally sized donor disk was introduced into the recipient anterior chamber and placed against the recipient posterior cornea secured only by an air bubble, while the patient had to remain in a supine position [16]. Along with the trend of minimally invasive surgery, in the year 2000, Melles et al. improved the technique in terms of creating a smaller self-sealing 5-mm tunnel incision through which the donor (endothelium, Descemet membrane, and a layer of stroma) was inserted, while being folded like a "taco" and then unfolded inside the recipient anterior chamber [17]. The modification was popularized as "small incision" DLEK [18]. Even though this new technique soon proved to provide clinical outcomes surpassing PK and diminishing many PK-associated complications [19], [20] the technique was still challenging regarding donor and host tissue manual dissection, making it difficult to be adopted by corneal surgeons worldwide.

5.4.2 Descemet Stripping (Automated) Endothelial Keratoplasty (DSEK/DSAEK)

To simplify the concept of endothelial keratoplasty, in 2002 Melles et al. introduced a technique that facilitated selective removal ("stripping") of the host diseased corneal Descemet membrane with its endothelium using a reversed Sinskey hook. This step, known as "descemetorhexis," was followed by the insertion of a "taco-folded" posterior lamellar disk, similar to that used in PLK/DLEK, that is then positioned onto the denuded host posterior stroma [21]. This technique was later popularized as "Descemet stripping endothelial keratoplasty" (DSEK) by Price and colleagues [22, 23].

In order to facilitate donor preparation, Gorovoy and colleagues introduced an automated microkeratome that enabled standardized dissection of a donor posterior lamella from a corneoscleral button mounted on an artificial anterior chamber; to differentiate this technique from manually dissected tissue, this procedure was termed "Descemet stripping *automated* endothelial keratoplasty" (DSAEK) [24].

Facilitating donor tissue preparation by using a microkeratome enabled also eye banks to provide precut donor tissue which made this refined endothelial keratoplasty technique rapidly accessible to ophthalmic surgeons worldwide.

These reproducible novel endothelial keratoplasty techniques had evident advantages over conventional PK. Besides better functional outcomes with faster visual recovery, many PK-associated complications could be reduced: First, the intraoperative risk for bleeding or infections was considerably lessened due to the "closed" globe compared to the "open globe surgery" in PK. Second, these suture-free techniques eliminated suture-related complications, preserved the anterior corneal surface, and hereby avoided unpredictable postoperative refractive errors. Third, the lack of a large penetrating wound reduced corneal denervation and provided a tectonically stronger globe with reduced risk of angiogenetic ingrowth or traumatic wound dehiscence. Finally, and most strikingly, also the risk of allograft rejection was minimized [25, 26]. These hard facts together with the techniques' high accessibility played a key role in the remarkable increase of DSEK/DSAEK procedures in the following years and its implementation as the new "gold standard" for the treatment of endothelial pathologies.

But "where there is light, there must also be shadow" and the main "shadows," thus drawbacks of the DSEK/DSAEK techniques were that donor tissue preparation was costly, and visual acuity could vary and remain suboptimal despite technically successful surgery owing to thickness irregularities of the donor posterior stroma or stromal interface haze causing optical aberrations [27]. The visual limitation due to graft thickness irregularities was addressed by Busin et al. when introducing so-called "ultrathin DSAEK" grafts, which provided better clinical results than standard DSAEK but still required a costly microkeratome for graft preparation [28].

5.4.3 Descemet Membrane Endothelial Keratoplasty (DMEK)

In 1998, Melles and colleagues also introduced the next refinement of endothelial keratoplasty that eliminated the posterior stroma from the donor graft entirely and hereby allowed selective replacement of an autologous Descemet membrane and endothelium [29]. This modified technique was named "Descemet membrane endothelial keratoplasty" (DMEK). After the first DMEK surgeries that were performed in 2006, it soon became evident that the near anatomic restoration of the corneal anatomy provided unprecedented visual outcomes [12, 30–32] and an even lower risk of endothelial immune reaction [33, 34]. Another major advantage of DMEK over previous techniques was that, after donor preparation, the anterior corneal lamella could be used for "deep anterior lamellar keratoplasty," permitting more efficient donor tissue use [35], also known as "split cornea transplantation" [36, 37].

Despite these advances, difficulties in tissue preparation, intracameral graft unfolding, and the high incidence of postoperative graft dehiscences were perceived as the main obstacles in DMEK [38].

Soon, standardization and reproducibility of tissue preparation, provision of precut tissue, and standardization of intracameral graft unfolding aided corneal surgeons to take the first steps in DMEK or make the switch from DSEK/DSAEK to DMEK [39–43].

With increasing experience also graft detachment rates could be reduced significantly as reported by different groups worldwide [44–46].

After a decisive phase of endothelial keratoplasty innovations, posterior lamellar techniques seem to have left PK behind, when regarding the treatment of corneal endothelial disease, as in FECD, for which DMEK and DSEK/DSAEK meanwhile have become first-line choices of surgical treatment. Because of the better clinical outcomes, in particular DMEK may permit surgical intervention already at an early stage of the corneal disease.

In addition, growing experience with DMEK allowed to gain a better understanding of endothelial cell biology and physiology, as well as endothelial cell migration. For example, corneal clearance with good clinical outcomes was also observed in denuded stromal areas that were not covered by Descemet membrane and endothelium [47, 48], as observed in eyes with graft detachment or eyes that received variously shaped and sized DMEK grafts after difficult tissue preparation [49].

5.5 Modifications of Descemet Membrane Endothelial Keratoplasty

5.5.1 DMEK-S and Descemet Membrane Automated Endothelial Keratoplasty (DMAEK)

As an attempt to facilitate intraoperative handling of the thin DMEK transplant, Studeny et al. introduced DMEK-S, i.e., a manually dissected graft consisting of only Descemet membrane and endothelium in the central optical portion, supported by a peripheral stromal rim that should give the membrane stability inside the anterior chamber [50]. Da Reitz Pereira et al. [51] and McCauley et al. [52] modified the concept of DMEK-S by using a microkeratome for donor graft dissection, a technique popularized as "Descemet membrane *automated* endothelial keratoplasty" (DMAEK). In fact, DMEK-S/DMAEK provided better visual outcomes in contrast to DSEK/DSAEK and was considered to be technically less challenging than DMEK; however, a relatively high incidence of graft detachments often required air re-bubbling to achieve graft adherence [51–53].

5.5.2 Hemi-Descemet Membrane Endothelial Keratoplasty (hemi-DMEK)

Another modification of the standard DMEK technique, the so-called hemi-DMEK, was based on the idea to reduce tissue shortage.

In PK and DSEK/DSAEK, where the graft is generally thicker at the periphery than in the center, a centrally trephined graft is required for optical reasons. However in DMEK, owing to the even graft thickness of the Descemet membrane and endothe-

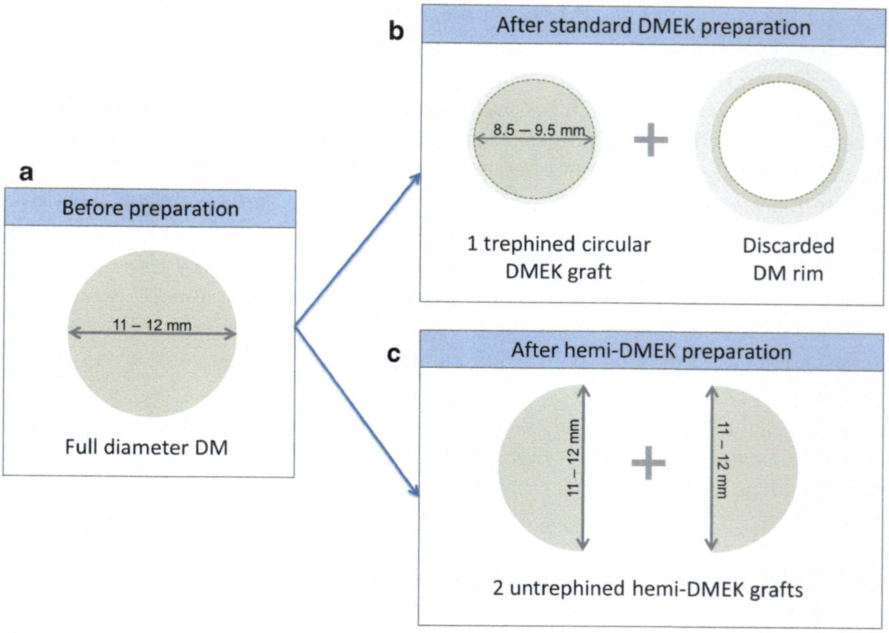

Fig. 5.2 Diagram showing graft preparation from (**a**) a full diameter (11–12 mm) corneoscleral button to achieve (**b**) one single (trephined) standard DMEK graft or (**c**) two (untrephined) semicircular hemi-DMEK grafts. Note that the overall endothelial surface area of each untrephined hemi-DMEK graft is similar to that of a trephined circular standard DMEK graft. Assuming a transplant with a homogeneous curvature, the posterior corneal curvature can be calculated using the formula for calculating the surface area of a spherical cap [63], which gives a posterior corneal surface area for a standard circular DMEK (9.0 mm) of 73 mm^2 and of 69 mm^2 for a hemi-DMEK graft (11.5 mm) (Figure has been published in Ref. [55]; reprinted with permission of Graefes Arch Clin Exp Ophthalmol)

lium throughout its whole surface area, this may no longer be necessary. In 2014 the Melles group introduced "hemi-DMEK," in which a half-moon (semicircular)-shaped Descemet membrane graft is prepared from one untrephined 11.5–12.0-mm (full) diameter donor Descemet membrane sheet and transplanted after performing a standard 9-mm descemetorhexis (Fig. 5.2). In contrast to standard DMEK graft preparation where the *trephined* central 8.5–9.5-mm circular DMEK graft is used, while the outer Descemet membrane rim is discarded, in hemi-DMEK, two semicircular grafts for two recipients may be utilized from one *untrephined* full diameter Descemet membrane sheet potentially doubling the number of endothelial grafts harvested from the same donor pool [54]. Since the total surface area of the semicircular hemi-DMEK graft is similar to the standard (circular) DMEK graft, the graft shape may be the main difference between both techniques.

In a first small case series in patients with FECD, it could be shown that visual outcomes at 6 and 12 months after hemi-DMEK may mimic those after standard DMEK [54, 55]. If further clinical trials prove that also graft survival and complication rates would be similar, hemi-DMEK could become the next step in endothelial keratoplasty for the treatment of FECD, potentially doubling the pool of endothelial graft tissue.

Despite the shape mismatch between the circular descemetorhexis and the semi-circular hemi-DMEK graft, corneal clearance was observed over the entire cornea, even over initially bare stromal areas (denuded of Descemet membrane). A similar observation was made after standard DMEK in eyes with a partially detached DMEK graft, suggesting that besides donor endothelium also host endothelial cells may be actively involved in corneal clearance after endothelial keratoplasty [56]. This new insight may have questioned the concept of performing a "keratoplasty" for corneal endothelial disorders because surgical apposition and anatomical restoration of donor endothelium may not be a requirement per se for functional recovery of the cornea [57].

Hence, endothelial keratoplasty may still not be the final innovation in the management of corneal endothelial diseases but may herald the next round for further inspiring ideas and concepts.

5.6 Will There Be a Finish Line in the Evolution of Posterior Lamellar Keratoplasty?

5.6.1 Descemet Membrane Endothelial Transfer (DMET)

Within the concept of keratoplasty, transparency and corneal deturgescence was thought to be subject to complete donor-to-host apposition. Clinical observations, however, suggested that complete donor-to-host apposition may not always be required [56, 57].

This was the starting point of a new "non-keratoplasty" concept introduced by Melles and colleagues: Descemet membrane endothelial transfer (DMET), in which after descemetorhexis, a Descemet roll is injected into the anterior chamber and secured in the main incision Fig. 5.3. While this technique would be an immense simplification of standard DMEK, corneal clearance in DMET may take up to 6 months, and endothelial cell densities may be significantly lower at 6 months postoperatively [56].

Key to DMET is a repopulation of the posterior stroma by endothelial cells either from the graft, the recipient Descemet rim, or both. If migration of the peripheral remaining host endothelial cells in eyes with FECD would potentially allow repopulation of the posterior stroma after a central descemetorhexis, that is, by eliminating the guttae which presumably are the pathological and physical barrier for cells to migrate [58], then, like DMET, also a "descemetorhexis only" could be another possible treatment approach Fig. 3. However, until now there are only anecdotal cases of corneal clearance after a descemetorhexis without graft implantation so that there is no consistent proof for its efficacy [59].

Although DMET and "descemetorhexis only" have not been implemented as "non-keratoplasty" treatment options in clinical practice, DMET may have questioned the

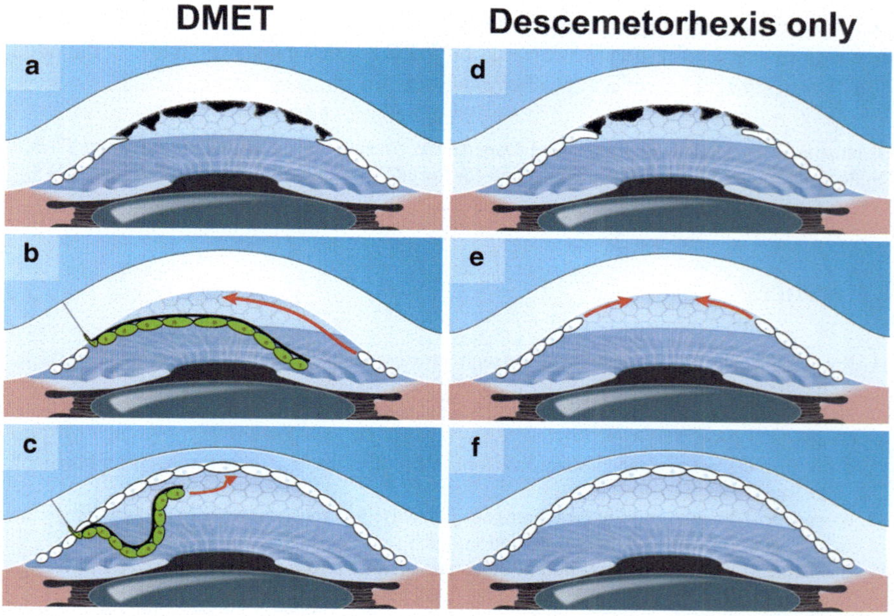

Fig. 5.3 Mechanisms behind Descemet membrane endothelial transfer (DMET) and a "descemetorhexis only" in the management of Fuchs endothelial corneal dystrophy. Regarding DMET, it is thought that the donor graft may induce recipient endothelial migration. By means of a descemetorhexis, the guttae are removed that may act as barriers to the migration of peripheral stemlike cells (**a**). When inserting a free-floating donor tissue (*green*) attached to the incision, clinical observations indicate that migration of the recipient endothelial cells is induced (**b**). Consequently, the bare stroma is covered by recipient and to some extent by donor endothelial cells that restore corneal transparency (**c**). Regarding a sole descemetorhexis, in early stages of the disease when the guttae have not progressed to the far periphery yet and there are still sufficient peripheral stemlike cells, a descemetorhexis without the insertion of donor tissue might be sufficient to induce recipient endothelial migration (**d**–**f**). Consequently, after removal physical barrier of the descemetorhexis, proliferation and migration of the peripheral of the recipient endothelial cells may be induced (**e**), resulting in a restoration of the endothelial mosaic with deturgescence of the cornea (**f**) (Figure has been published in Ref. [57]; reprinted with permission of EYE)

description of FECD as a "dystrophy" and rendered us a deeper understanding of the processes involved in endothelial cell wound healing. This insight might lead to further developments for the treatment of FECD, and it also may have opened a door to potential alternative approaches, such as cell injections or drug therapies [60–62].

5.7 Conclusion

Recent evolution in keratoplasty may not only simplify existing surgical techniques and allow for a more efficient use of donor tissue but may also provide a better understanding of the behavior of the endothelium in corneal endothelial diseases that may lead to alternative treatment options. If these newest developments would prove more successful than the current endothelial keratoplasty techniques, the need of a "keratoplasty" might need to be questioned in the near future.

Disclosure Drs Melles, Baydoun, and Dapena are consultants for DORC International/Dutch Ophthalmic, USA; Dr. Melles is a consultant for SurgiCube International.

References

1. Reisinger F. Die Keratoplastik: ein Versuch zur Erweiterung der Augenheilkunst. Bayerische Ann Chir Augenheilk. 1824;I:207–215.
2. Von Hippel A. Eine neue Methode der Hornhauttransplantation. Albrecht Von Graefes Arch Ophthalmol. 1888;34(I):108–30.
3. Zirm E. Eine erfolgreiche totale Keratoplastik. Albrecht Von Graefes Arch Ophthalmol. 1906;54:580–93.
4. Barraquer JI. Queratoplastia: Problemas que plantea la fijacion del injerto. In: Ophthalologicum Acta. London: British Medical Association; 1951. p. 999–1004.
5. Barraquer JI. Lamellar keratoplasty. (Special techniques). Ann Ophthalmol. 1972;4:437–69.
6. Tillett CW. Posterior lamellar keratoplasty. Am J Ophthalmol. 1956;41:530–3.
7. Culbertson WW. Endothelial replacement: flap approach. Ophthalmol Clin North Am. 2003;16:113–8.
8. Busin M, Monks T, Arffa RC. Endokeratoplasty in the rabbit model: a new surgical technique for endothelial transplantation. Ophthalmology. 1996;103:167.
9. Ko WW, Frueh BE, Shields CK, Costello ML, Feldman ST. Experimental posterior lamellar transplantation of the rabbit cornea. (ARVO abstract). Invest Ophthalmol Vis Sci. 1993;34:1102.
10. Jones DT, Culbertson WW. Endothelial lamellar keratoplasty (ELK). (ARVO abstract). Invest Ophthalmol Vis Sci. 1998;39:876.
11. Cursiefen C, Küchle M, Naumann GO. Changing indications for penetrating keratoplasty: histopathology of 1,250 corneal buttons. Cornea. 1998;17(5):468–70.
12. Melles GR. Posterior lamellar keratoplasty: DLEK to DSEK to DMEK. Cornea. 2006;25:879–81.
13. Melles GRJ, Eggink FAGJ, Lander F, Pels E, Rietveld FJR, Beekhuis WH, Binder PS. A surgical technique for posterior lamellar keratoplasty. Cornea. 1998;17:618–26.
14. Melles GRJ, Lander F, Beekhuis WH, Remeijer L, Binder PS. Posterior lamellar keratoplasty for a case of pseudophakic bullous keratopathy. Am J Ophthalmol. 1999;127:340–1.
15. Terry MA, Ousley PJ. Deep lamellar endothelial keratoplasty in the first United States patients: early clinical results. Cornea. 2001;20:239–43.
16. Melles GRJ, Lander F, van Dooren BTH, Pels E, Beekhuis WH. Preliminary clinical results of posterior lamellar keratoplasty through a sclerocorneal pocket incision. Ophthalmology. 2000;107:1850–7.
17. Melles GR, Lander F, Nieuwendaal C. Sutureless, posterior lamellar keratoplasty: a case report of a modified technique. Cornea. 2002;20:239–43.
18. Terry MA, Ousley PJ. Small-incision deep lamellar endothelial keratoplasty (DLEK): six-month results in the first prospective clinical study. Cornea. 2005;24:59–65.
19. Terry MA, Ousley PJ. Deep lamellar endothelial keratoplasty visual acuity, astigmatism, and endothelial survival in a large prospective series. Ophthalmology. 2005;112:1541–8.
20. Ousley PJ, Terry MA. Stability of vision, topography, and endothelial cell density from 1 year to 2 years after deep lamellar endothelial keratoplasty surgery. Ophthalmology. 2005;112: 50–7.
21. Melles GR, Wijdh RH, Nieuwendaal CP. A technique to excise the Descemet membrane from a recipient cornea (descemetorhexis). Cornea. 2004;23:286–8.

22. Gorovoy M, Price FW. New technique transforms corneal transplantation. Cataract Refract Surg Today. 2005;11:55–8.
23. Price Jr FW, Price MO. Descemet's stripping with endothelial keratoplasty in 50 eyes: a refractive neutral corneal transplant. J Refract Surg. 2005;21:339–45.
24. Gorovoy MS. Descemet-stripping automated endothelial keratoplasty. Cornea. 2006;25:886–9.
25. Chen ES, Terry MA, Shamie N, Hoar KL, Friend DJ. Precut tissue in Descemet's stripping automated endothelial keratoplasty donor characteristics and early postoperative complications. Ophthalmology. 2008;115:497–502.
26. Price MO, Gorovoy M, Benetz BA, Price Jr FW, Menegay HJ, Debanne SM, Lass JH. Descemet's stripping automated endothelial keratoplasty outcomes compared with penetrating keratoplasty from the Cornea Donor Study. Ophthalmology. 2010;117:438–44.
27. Tourtas T, Laaser K, Bachmann BO, Cursiefen C, Kruse FE. Descemet membrane endothelial keratoplasty versus Descemet stripping automated endothelial keratoplasty. Am J Ophthalmol. 2012;153(6):1082–90.
28. Busin M, Madi S, Santorum P, Scorcia V, Beltz J. Ultrathin descemet's stripping automated endothelial keratoplasty with the microkeratome double-pass technique: two-year outcomes. Ophthalmology. 2013;120(6):1186–94.
29. Melles GRJ, Rietveld FJR, Pels E, Beekhuis WH, Binder PS. Transplantation of Descemet's membrane carrying viable endothelium through a small scleral incision. Fort Lauderdale: ARVO Abstract; 1998.
30. Melles GR, Lander F, Rietveld FJ. Transplantation of Descemet's membrane carrying viable endothelium through a small scleral incision. Cornea. 2002;21:415–8.
31. Melles GR, Ong TS, Ververs B, van der Wees J. Descemet membrane endothelial keratoplasty (DMEK). Cornea. 2006;25:987–90.
32. Melles GR, Ong TS, Ververs B, van der Wees J. Preliminary clinical results of Descemet membrane endothelial keratoplasty. Am J Ophthalmol. 2008;145:222–7.
33. Dapena I, Ham L, Netuková M, van der Wees J, Melles GR. Incidence of early allograft rejection after Descemet membrane endothelial keratoplasty. Cornea. 2011;30:1341–5.
34. Anshu A, Price MO, Price Jr FW. Risk of corneal transplant rejection significantly reduced with Descemet's membrane endothelial keratoplasty. Ophthalmology. 2012;119:536–40.
35. Lie JT, Groeneveld-van Beek EA, Ham L, van der Wees J, Melles GR. More efficient use of donor corneal tissue with Descemet membrane endothelial keratoplasty (DMEK): two lamellar keratoplasty procedures with one donor cornea. Br J Ophthalmol. 2010;94(9):1265–6.
36. Heindl LM, Riss S, Laaser K, Bachmann BO, Kruse FE, Cursiefen C. Split cornea transplantation for 2 recipients—review of the first 100 consecutive patients. Am J Ophthalmol. 2011;152(4): 523–32. e2.
37. Heindl LM, Riss S, Bachmann BO, Laaser K, Kruse FE, Cursiefen C. Split cornea transplantation for 2 recipients: a new strategy to reduce corneal tissue cost and shortage. Ophthalmology. 2011;118(2):294–301.
38. Cursiefen C. Descemet membrane endothelial keratoplasty: the taming of the shrew. JAMA Ophthalmol. 2013;131(1):88–9.
39. Groeneveld EA, Lie JT, van der Wees J, Bruinsma M, Melles GR. Standardized 'no-touch' donor tissue preparation for DALK and DMEK: harvesting undamaged anterior and posterior transplants from the same donor cornea. Acta Ophthalmol. 2013;91(2):145–50.
40. Dapena I, Moutsouris K, Droutsas K, Ham L, van Dijk K, Melles GR. Standardized 'no touch' technique for Descemet membrane endothelial keratoplasty (DMEK). Arch Ophthalmol. 2011;129(1):88–94.
41. Kruse FE, Laaser K, Cursiefen C, Heindl LM, Schlötzer-Schrehardt U, Riss S, Bachmann BO. A stepwise approach to donor preparation and insertion increases safety and outcome of descemet membrane endothelial keratoplasty. Cornea. 2011;30(5):580–7.
42. Liarakos VS, Dapena I, Ham L, van Dijk K, Melles GR. Intraocular graft unfolding techniques in Descemet membrane endothelial keratoplasty. JAMA Ophthalmol. 2013;131:29–35.
43. Melles GRJ, Dapena I. How to get started with standardized 'no-touch' Descemet membrane endothelial keratoplasty (DMEK). 1st ed. Rotterdam: Netherlands Institute for Innovative Ocular Surgery; 2014.

44. Rodríguez-Calvo-de-Mora M, Quilendrino R, Ham L, Liarakos L, van Dijk K, Baydoun L, Dapena I, Oellerich S, Melles GRJ. Clinical outcome of 500 consecutive cases undergoing Descemet's membrane endothelial keratoplasty. Ophthalmology. 2015;122(3): 464–70.
45. Tourtas T, Schlomberg J, Wessel JM, Bachmann BO, Schlötzer-Schrehardt U, Kruse FE. Graft adhesion in descemet membrane endothelial keratoplasty dependent on size of removal of host's descemet membrane. JAMA Ophthalmol. 2014;132(2):155–61.
46. Price MO, Price Jr FW. Descemet's membrane endothelial keratoplasty surgery: update on the evidence and hurdles to acceptance. Curr Opin Ophthalmol. 2013;24(4):329–35.
47. Balachandran C, Ham L, Verschoor CA, Ong TS, van der Wees J, Melles GR. Spontaneous corneal clearance despite graft detachment in descemet membrane endothelial keratoplasty. Am J Ophthalmol. 2009;148(2):227–34.
48. Dirisamer M, Dapena I, Ham L, van Dijk K, Oganes O, Frank LE, van der Wees J, Melles GR. Patterns of corneal endothelialization and corneal clearance after descemet membrane endothelial keratoplasty for fuchs endothelial dystrophy. Am J Ophthalmol. 2011;152(4): 543–55.
49. Tourtas T, Heindl LM, Kopsachilis N, Bachmann BO, Kruse FE, Cursiefen C. Use of accidentally torn Descemet membrane to successfully complete Descemet membrane endothelial keratoplasty. Cornea. 2013;32:1418–22.
50. Studeny P, Farkas A, Vokrojova M, Liskova P, Jirsova K. Descemet membrane endothelial keratoplasty with a stromal rim (DMEK-S). Br J Ophthalmol. 2010;94:909–14.
51. Da Reitz Pereira C, Guerra FP, Price Jr FW, Price MO. Descemet's membrane automated endothelial keratoplasty (DMAEK): visual outcomes and visual quality. Br J Ophthalmol. 2011;95:951–4.
52. McCauley MB, Price MO, Fairchild KM, Price DA, Price Jr FW. Prospective study of visual outcomes and endothelial survival with Descemet membrane automated endothelial keratoplasty. Cornea. 2011;30:315–9.
53. Kymionis GD, Yoo SH, Diakonis VF, Grentzelos MA, Naoumidi I, Pallikaris G. Automated donor tissue preparation for Descemet membrane automated endothelial keratoplasty (DMAEK): an experimental study. Ophthalmic Surg Lasers Imaging. 2011;42:158–61.
54. Lam FC, Baydoun L, Dirisamer M, Lie J, Dapena I, Melles GR. Hemi-Descemet membrane endothelial keratoplasty transplantation: a potential method for increasing the pool of endothelial graft tissue. JAMA Ophthalmol. 2014;132(12):1469–73.
55. Lam FC, Baydoun L, Satué M, Dirisamer M, Ham L, Melles GR. One year outcome of hemi-Descemet membrane endothelial keratoplasty. Graefes Arch Clin Exp Ophthalmol. 2015;253(11):1955–8.
56. Dirisamer M, Yeh RY, van Dijk K, Ham L, Dapena I, Melles GR. Recipient endothelium may relate to corneal clearance in Descemet membrane endothelial transfer. Am J Ophthalmol. 2012;154:290–6.
57. Bruinsma M, Tong CM, Melles GRJ. What does the future hold for the treatment of Fuchs endothelial dystrophy; will 'keratoplasty' still be a valid procedure? Eye. 2013;27: 1115–22.
58. Moshirfar M, Kim G. The role of host endothelial cell proliferation in Descemet membrane endothelial transfer. Cornea. 2013;32:218–9.
59. Fernández López E, Lam FC, Bruinsma M, Baydoun L, Dapena I, Melles GRJ. Fuchs endothelial corneal dystrophy: current treatment recommendations and experimental surgical options. Expert Rev Ophthalmol. 2015;10(3):301–12.
60. Patel SV, Bachman LA, Hann CR, Bahler CK, Fautsch MP. Human corneal endothelial cell transplantation in a human ex vivo model. Invest Ophthalmol Vis Sci. 2009;50(5): 2123–31.
61. Okumura N, Koizumi N, Ueno M, Sakamoto Y, Takahashi H, Tsuchiya H, Hamuro J, Kinoshita S. ROCK inhibitor converts corneal endothelial cells into a phenotype capable of regenerating in vivo endothelial tissue. Am J Pathol. 2012;181(1):268–77.

62. Koizumi N, Okumura N, Ueno M, Kinoshita S. New therapeutic modality for corneal endothelial disease using Rho-associated kinase inhibitor eye drops. Cornea. 2014;33 Suppl 11:25–31.
63. Quilendrino R, Höhn H, Tse WH, Chi H, Dapena I, Ham L, Oellerich S, Melles GR. Do we overestimate the endothelial cell "loss" after descemet membrane endothelial keratoplasty? Curr Eye Res. 2013;38(2):260–5.
64. Van Dijk K, Baydoun L, Konder R, Melles GRJ. Contact lenses after keratoplasty. What to expect and what to look for with contact lens management in post-keratoplasty corneas. Contact Lens Spectrum. 2014;(2):36–38, 40, 42.

Chapter 6
DMEK Graft Preparation: Eye Bank Perspective and Risk Factors for Preparation Failure

Christopher G. Stoeger, Joshua D. Galloway, Zachary M. Mayko, and Christopher S. Sáles

6.1 Introduction

Historically, the initiation of a DSAEK tissue processing program required a sea change in the everyday work of eye banks. Prior to DSAEK, eye banks had existed for decades to perform one main function: to preserve corneas for the surgeon, who then prepared the tissue in the operating room as needed. DSAEK brought tissue manipulation (back) into the laboratory, which was a monumental shift for the field after more than a decade of relative stability in tissue preparation which consisted mainly of tissue preservation alone. Processing DSAEK tissue introduced a number of important considerations, many of which are pertinent to DMEK: acquisition of complex medical equipment, training technicians to use the equipment, protocols to evaluate tissue after processing, coordination of tissue processing and distribution with surgery, and the development of robust quality assurance measures. All of these activities came under increasing regulatory scrutiny by the FDA.

An organization looking to develop a DMEK program should ideally have a sound DSAEK program already in place because the latter requires infrastructure that can be shared by DMEK. In some ways, DMEK tissue processing can be easier to incorporate into an eye bank than DSAEK was during the era of PK since most of the "right things to do" are already in place at most institutes.

Although having a preexisting DSAEK program can facilitate development of a DMEK program, it cannot eliminate the unique challenges of processing DMEK tissue. Since it does not require microkeratomes, DMEK processing is in some respects less complex than DSAEK. However, this simplicity is overshadowed by

C.G. Stoeger, MBA, CEBT (✉) • J.D. Galloway, CEBT • Z.M. Mayko, MS
Lions VisionGift, Portland, OR, USA
e-mail: chris@visiongift.org

C.S. Sáles, MD, MPH
Department of Ophthalmology, Weil Cornell Medical Center, New York, NY, USA

C. Cursiefen, A.S. Jun (eds.), *Current Treatment Options for Fuchs Endothelial Dystrophy*, DOI 10.1007/978-3-319-43021-8_6

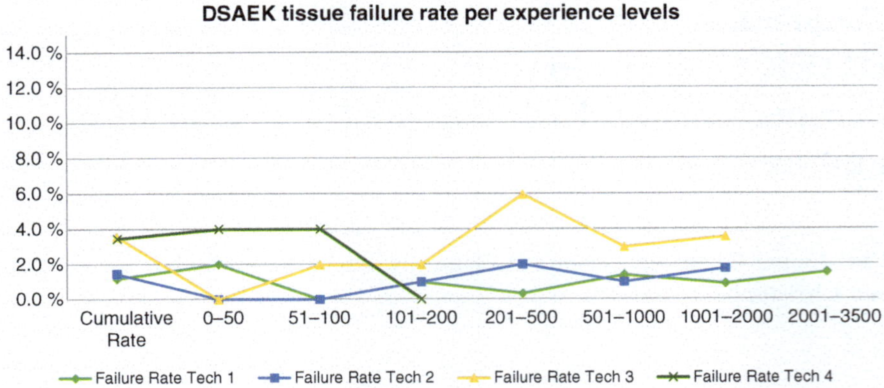

Fig. 6.1 Technician DSAEK tissue preparation failure rates are presented at different intervals of experience based on the number of processing procedures performed

the inherently delicate nature of Descemet membrane and its adherent endothelial cells (the endothelial cell-Descemet membrane complex [EDM]).

A key metric for determining the strength of any tissue processing program is the amount of tissue lost to failed preparation. Tissue failure results from a multitude of factors, which are not all related to the learning curve. Donor history, tissue selection, procedures for stripping, tissue evaluation, and training can all factor into preparation failure. Each of these factors shall be explored in greater detail in this chapter.

6.2 Learning Curve

DSAEK programs often experience higher rates of graft preparation failure early in their development [10]. In our experience, the same is true in the development of a DMEK program. Graft preparation failures that are a result of this learning curve, while most likely can never be completely avoided, can at least be minimized with careful planning and preparation.

Figures 6.1 and 6.2 are provided by Lions VisionGift to give a baseline comparison between the frequency of DSAEK and DMEK preparation failures over the course of an individual technician's learning curve. Eye banks initiating their own programs may wish to reference these data to benchmark against a known standard.

The most striking difference between the figures is a more than threefold increase in preparation failure by two of our four technicians in their first 100 DMEK preparations compared to their first 100 DSAEK preparations. What is equally impressive, however, is the progressive reduction in preparation failure achieved by technician #2 through a combination of inherent aptitude, continual feedback, and practice. The work of this technician illustrates the profound organizational impact

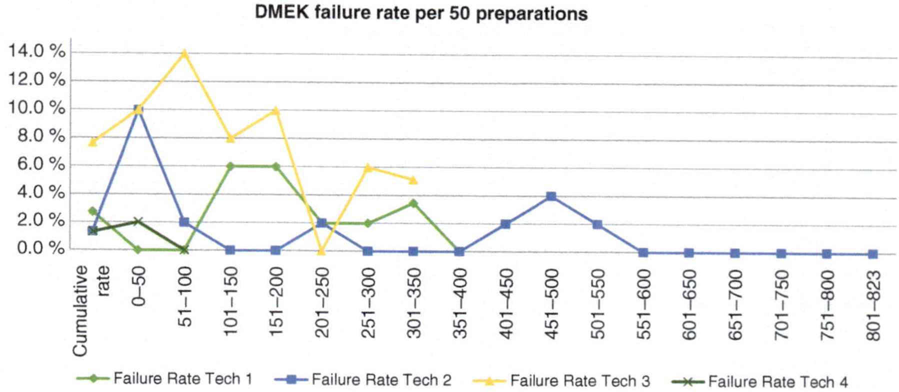

Fig. 6.2 Technician failure rates for tissue processing for Descemet membrane endothelial keratoplasty

that one individual can have on a DMEK program, if given the space and tools to improve both himself or herself and the eye bank's standard operating procedure.

6.3 Donor History and Tissue Selection

Tissue selection for DMEK preparation is different from DSAEK and previous EK preparation methods. Two main questions influence what tissue should be accepted when selecting tissue for DMEK: (1) Will the tissue satisfy surgeons' preferences? (2) Is the tissue at high risk for preparation failure when it undergoes peeling by the eye bank's technician?

6.3.1 Surgeon Preferences

Surgeons require tissue that they can successfully manipulate and transplant into recipients. Empirically, older donors provide DMEK tissue that scrolls less tightly, which can make unfurling it easier for the surgeon [1, 12]. Thickening of DM with age [2] likely imparts this desirable property.

Donors over 50 are routinely assigned to DMEK at our organization, but surgeons drive this age cutoff, and it could be lower. Many new or adopting DMEK surgeons will specifically request a lower donor age limit of 65 to decrease the chance of having to unfurl a tight scroll. To date, we do not know the lower age limit for safely and reliably peeling DMEK grafts, and our hope is that donors even younger than 50 may become acceptable for DMEK as new approaches to the procedure continue to develop.

The upper age limit for donor criteria is driven by surgeon preferences as there is limited published data available related to donor age and long-term DMEK outcomes. Mannis et al., in the landmark Cornea Donor Study (CDS), reported small but significant differences in graft failure rates for donors aged 72–75 versus younger donors. In donors aged 52–71, 74 % of corneas remained clear at 10 years. Whereas 62 % of 72–75 year old donors were clear at 10 years. These differences in graft failure rates were not apparent until after 6 years postoperatively in penetrating keratoplasty recipients [13]. As DMEK recipient outcomes are tracked for the long term, it will be important to ascertain whether older donor tissues have similar rates of graft failure to what was observed in the Cornea Donor Study.

Older donors, while easier to unfurl, are often accompanied by lower endothelial cell densities and represent a potential compromise. Our eye bank currently has a lower limit of 2000 cells/mm^2 for the endothelial cell density to be deemed suitable for EK. In practice, however, many surgeons request higher endothelial cell densities than the minimum allowed by our standard. This is a permissible practice thanks to the current donor population in the USA, but increased donor age coupled with demands for high endothelial cell densities may stress the donor pool as interest in DMEK grows.

At Lions VisionGift, we have not seen any evidence to suggest that older donors will perform inferiorly to younger donors in the long term. At our institute, the upper donor age limit is routinely set at 75. There are reports from other centers of using much older donors, especially in Europe, as reported by Schlötzer-Schrehardt et al., where the upper age of a series of 350 grafts was 95 [16]. Minimizing surgical manipulation may supplant any small long-term benefits seen in the CDS from younger donors.

6.3.2 *Identifying Donors for Successful Preparation*

Not all EDMs behave the same. Some EDMs peel readily and almost easily, whereas others are so brittle that they break into pieces with minimal force. What causes these differences? Schlötzer-Schrehardt et al. postulate that it is the ultrastructure of the membrane itself that "complicates or prevents proper DM stripping, irrespective of any surgical experience and skills." Evidence of "peg-like interlockings between DM and stroma" from electron microscopy of failed tissue preparations supports this theory [16].

Whatever the cause may be, there are corneas that eye banks should ideally exclude from the DMEK donor pool to avoid peeling EDMs that are at high risk of preparation failure. While we cannot unequivocally identify these corneas for exclusion from the donor pool, collaborative research efforts have revealed important risk factors to consider.

6.3.3 *Diabetic Donors*

In a landmark eye banking study by the University of Iowa and Iowa Lions Eye Bank, Greiner et al. recently published data showing that corneas with a history of diabetes mellitus are more difficult to peel and more likely to result in preparation

Table 6.1 Donor diabetes rating scale

Found in donor history	Point value assigned
Any history of diabetes mellitus (DM)	1
DM type 1 or 2 history of greater than or equal to 10 years in duration, DM type 2 with insulin dependence, or DM type or 1 or 2 diagnosis with related comorbidities, including: Diabetic neuropathy Diabetic nephropathy Diabetic retinopathy Peripheral vascular disease Amputation related to diabetes	2
Body mass index >30	1
Hypertension	1

Note: A cumulative score of 3 or less is considered acceptable for processing

failure. Compared to nondiabetic (1.9 %) donors, diabetic (15.3 %) donors had a startlingly higher frequency of preparation failure [8], suggesting that avoiding such donors could increase the likelihood of preparation success. Vianna et al. performed a comprehensive analysis of a large number of DMEK tissue preparations from Lions VisionGift and confirmed Greiner et al.'s findings [21]. This work also found correlates between preparation failure and the duration of diabetes, obesity, hypercholesterolemia, and hypertension.

As DMEK grows in popularity, it may be too limiting to exclude all diabetic donors from the donor pool. In light of the high prevalence of diabetes mellitus and its wide spectrum of severity in the population, we have developed a novel tool for risk-stratifying diabetic donors by the severity of their disease, as described in Table 6.1. We retrospectively applied this rating to 125 consecutive donors (only the first eye peeled was included in the analysis) and found that donors with a rating of 3 or lower on our scale were less likely to fail than those rated 4 or 5. Use of this scale has been successfully employed at Lions VisionGift since December of 2014 to help us better utilize our tissue pool.

6.3.4 *IOL Scars and Refractive Surgery*

Another important selection criterion to consider is the lens status of the donor (i.e., pseudophakic vs. phakic), especially in light of the older age demographic of DMEK donors. Recovering corneas from pseudophakic eyes is a routine practice of our eye bank, but in the setting of DMEK, the corneal incisions from cataract surgery limit the graft size by requiring the technician to peel the EDM central to scars.

We have developed a guide to aid tissue evaluation so that grafts that cannot yield an adequate graft size are excluded from the DMEK donor pool, and those that yield a marginal graft size can be avoided, when possible. This guide is illustrated in Fig. 6.3. The guide is used in conjunction with our chosen prepara-

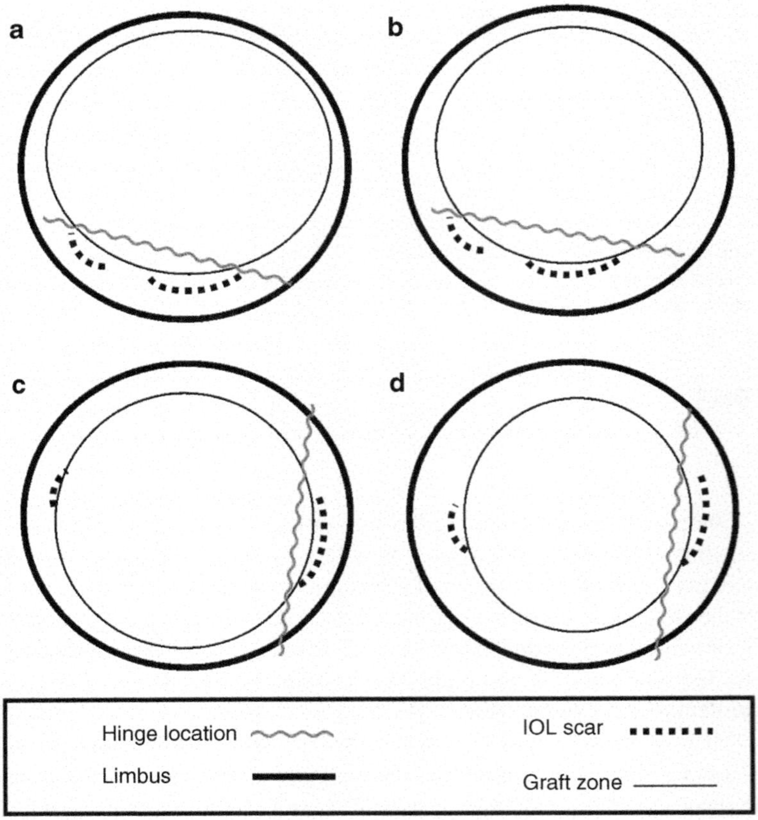

Fig. 6.3 IOL scar location can have a dramatic impact on potential graft size. Some IOL scars render the graft zone too small for practical use, while others are very close to "suitable," and still other scars pose no concerns. The hinge denotes an area of attached Descemet membrane which allows for post-preparation evaluation as well as transportation of the graft to the operating room. (**a**) Scars pose no threat to graft size. (**b**) Scars are too central to achieve a good graft size. (**c**) With careful attention to trephination placement, a suitable graft size may be obtained. (**d**) Scars are too central to obtain adequate graft size

tion technique that leaves a peripheral hinge of attached DM. This peripheral DM "hinge" keeps the graft anatomically oriented for post-preparation evaluation, transportation to the operating room, and surgical trephination. The guide is still instructive if other methods or preparation are employed but would require modification.

Laser refractive surgery such as LASIK and PRK are an exclusion for PK and ALKP [5]; however these tissues are acceptable for EK [15] so long as the endothelium is in acceptable condition. Radial keratotomy (RK) must be evaluated on a case-by-case basis due to the depth of scars associated with the procedure, but it is generally acceptable. Deep, adherent scars that raise the risk of tearing the EDM and full-thickness scars should be avoided.

6.3.5 *Mated Pairs Behave the Same*

Corneas with EDMs that are difficult to peel usually come in mated pairs. This observation reflects our own experience and has been corroborated by others [7, 18].

It is important to "listen to the tissue." If the first cornea of a mated pair proves difficult to peel or even tears and fails, it is important to understand why. When the failure is determined to be due to properties inherent in the tissue and not a processor error, do not peel the mate with the hopeful wish that the second tissue will be different. It is better to reallocate these corneas into the donor pools for penetrating keratoplasty and DSAEK, where they are unlikely to present any impediments to tissue preparation.

6.3.6 *Final Thoughts on Tissue Selection and Distribution*

Figure 6.4 illustrates our screening process, which excludes most corneas that have been recovered with the intent for transplant from the DMEK donor pool. On average, the DMEK donor pool is only 40 % of the total pool, which is a stark reality.

Reliably narrowing the donor pool down to a cohort suitable for DMEK requires a significant number of man-hours. The paired nature of DMEK failures also requires a degree of flexibility and cooperation among the staff that is unique to a DMEK program. When a tissue preparation fails, for example, it triggers a domino effect of responses across our departments to prevent a second failure and to assure that the surgeon still receives a graft as promised.

A team approach to tissue selection, preparation, and distribution is indispensable to preventing tissue loss in a DMEK program. Every department in our organization plays a critical role in implementing the donor and tissue parameters that we employ to meet surgeons' requests *and* to increase the likelihood of successful tissue processing. Table 6.2 summarizes these parameters.

6.4 Technique Selection

Choosing a technique for preparing DMEK tissue is a critical decision when starting a DMEK program. For eye banks as well as surgeons, the ultimate goal is to provide safe, healthy tissue while minimizing wastage. Whatever technique is chosen must also be easily translatable to a regulated eye bank environment. In the following section, we will explain our own chosen method of DMEK tissue preparation in detail and why we have decided to use this approach. While other eye banks may choose to invest in other methods, we will try to highlight some of the pitfalls that we experienced. Lastly, we will explain an addendum to our DMEK tissue preparation program where we have chosen to stamp our tissue with an orientation S mark (S-stamp).

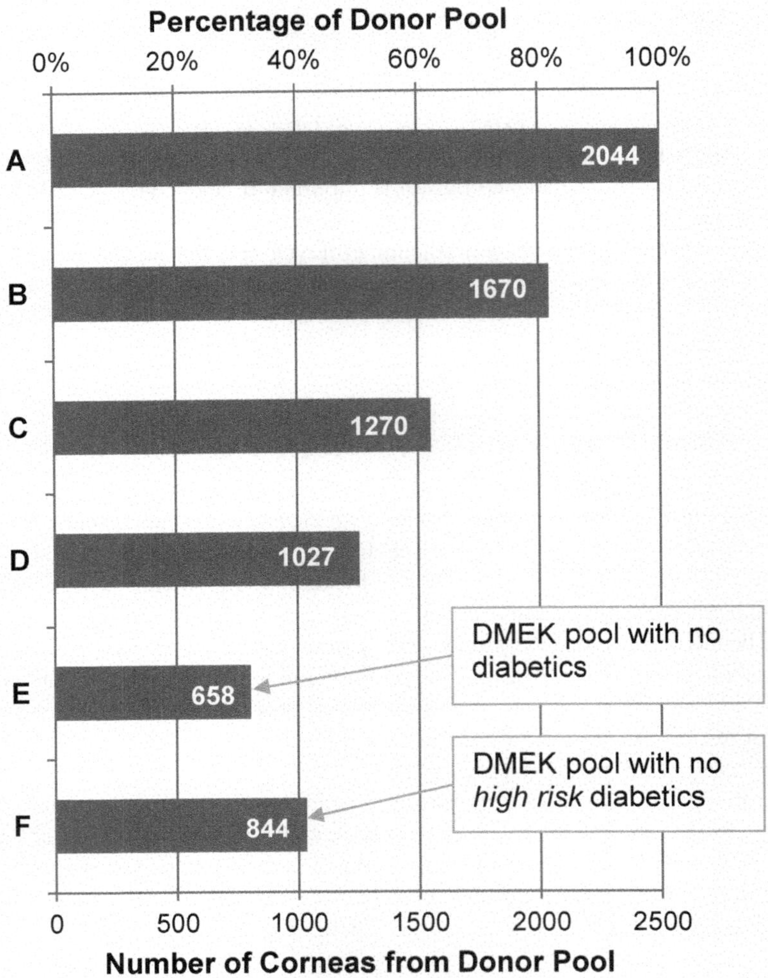

Fig. 6.4 Graphic representation of theoretic impact of diabetes rating tool based on 2014 Lions VisionGift donor and tissue data. (**a**) Corneas released for transplant. (**b**) Corneas released for transplant; ≥50 years old. (**c**) Corneas released for transplant; ≥50 years old; endothelial cell density (ECD) >2300/mm^2. (**d**) Corneas released for transplant; ≥50 years old; ECD >2300 mm^2; phakic or IOL outside of graft zone. (**e**) Corneas for transplant; ≥50 years old; ECD >2300 mm^2; phakic or IOL outside of graft zone, no diabetes mellitus (DM). (**f**) Corneas released for transplant; ≥50 years old; ECD >2300 mm^2; phakic or IOL outside of graft zone, no ≥4 DM rating

Tissue preparation techniques fall into three broad categories: big bubble, peeling, and interface sweeping. Bubbling can further be subcategorized into hydrodissection or pneumodissection. Peeling also has several iterations, including the submerged cornea using backgrounds away (SCUBA) technique and the suction block technique.

Table 6.2 Tissue selection

Parameter	Rationale
Age 40–80	Older donors are easier to peel and more desirable for surgeons due to the ease of unfurling tissue with a relatively thicker DM
IOL scars outside central 8 mm	Limitations to graft size based on placement of cataract surgery incision sites. It is impossible to peel through or around these sites. Identification of prior surgical incision sites will aid tissue selection
Diabetes risk factors are <4 on a 5-point scale	Diabetic donors are at greater risk for preparation failure. Use of a scale to risk stratify diabetic donors widens the donor pool by making low-risk diabetic donors available for DMEK
Refractive surgery acceptable	Deep radial keratotomy scars may make the EDM more difficult to peel, but otherwise refractive surgery scars are acceptable for DMEK as long as the endothelium is acceptable
Endothelial cell density >2000/mm^2	There is wide variability in individual surgeon preferences for lower ECD for DMEK. However, there is no evidence to support special requests for high ECD in order to increase the chance of a successful DMEK surgery
No excessive tearing in the mate cornea	Corneas from the same donor will exhibit similar properties

6.4.1 Peeling/SCUBA

At Lions VisionGift, we have chosen to adopt a forceps stripping or "peeling" method. This method is not without challenges, but if given the appropriate attention and practice, it is highly reproducible, has very low tissue wastage rates, and induces low amounts of cell damage.

Briefly, the technique is performed as follows: the tissue is scored peripherally with a 30 g needle, the EDM is loosened around the periphery to ensure there are no micro-adhesions, and the EDM is peeled with a set of McPherson angled tying forceps. Since it has a 5 mm platform, the angled forceps provide a large area with which to grasp the tissue. This has the effect of spreading tension exerted by the forceps over a greater area, which reduces the risk of tearing the EDM and minimizes damage to the endothelium from stress-related striae.

Our forceps stripping technique is arguably a modification to the SCUBA technique first described by Geibel, et al. [6] as a method to facilitate peeling the EDM by reducing surface tension and improving visualization. The main difference between the SCUBA technique and our forceps method is how the cornea is fixated. In the SCUBA technique, the graft is stabilized with one set of forceps, while another set of forceps is used to peel the EDM – a bimanual approach. In our technique, both hands are made available for manipulating the EDM, which is a significant ergonomic advantage for our technicians, because the tissue is stabilized with gentle suction provided by a trephine block.

6.4.2 Interface Sweeping

A commonly used interface sweeping technique is the Muraine technique and is an excellent way to prepare DMEK tissue. The rate of successful preparation with the Muraine technique is equivalent to our peeling method, and the amount of endothelial cell loss may be marginally superior [14].

The reason that we chose not to adopt the Muraine technique as our primary method of tissue preparation was the economic tradeoff, which did not outweigh its marginal benefits. The Muraine technique presents a number of additional costs per procedure compared to peeling. This includes the cost of a specialized disposable trephine and viscoelastic.

The Muraine technique is performed as follows: partial depth pre-punching of the tissue, inversion of the cornea onto an artificial anterior chamber (AAC) epithelium side-down, backing the tissue with air to inflate the cornea into a dome, coating the endothelium with viscoelastic, and carefully hydrodissecting the EDM with a LASIK cannula [14].

The primary risk of preparation failure with this approach is perforation, which can occur when the technician is sweeping the cannula in the interface between the EDM and stroma while simultaneously injecting fluid to create a hydrodissection plane. The bimanual dexterity required for this procedure, while not insurmountable, is more than required for stripping.

6.4.3 Big Bubble

The "big bubble" or pneumodissection technique is the least common technique currently used in eye banking, and we would not recommend a developing DMEK program to adopt it. The big bubble technique requires a high degree of judgment and manual dexterity as well as repeated practice to achieve consistent preparation outcomes. Careful depth control, distance, and volume of air injection are critical to obtaining a big bubble.

Briefly, the big bubble method involves precise placement of the needle prior to injection of air (or another medium) into the stroma. Care must be taken during placement of the needle to not perforate the EDM. Bubble injection follows, typically resulting in sectoral or diffuse corneal emphysema, which has the effect of thickening the tissue and allowing for further advancement of the needle into the paracentral cornea prior to Descemet separation. Success is achieved when a central bubble forms and is slowly expanded to an adequate diameter.

The main risks of this approach are accidental rupture of the EDM and failure to obtain the bubble. This can occur either because of a lack of separation or overzealous injection of media. In our experience, the skill required to reduce these risks to an acceptable level are significantly higher than other methods.

Additionally, the big bubble technique is difficult to evaluate with a slit lamp and nearly impossible to evaluate with specular microscopy. This can result in tissue being discarded unnecessarily or, conversely, tissue being transplanted that is not suitable for transplant. Alternative methods of obtaining and reporting endothelial cell density after the big bubble procedure have been proposed but have not been widely adopted.

6.4.4 Orienting DMEK Tissue

The leading cause of iatrogenic primary graft failure is inadvertent upside-down implantation of the donor tissue in the recipient. Irrespective of whose hands caused the failure, upside-down graft implantation is of great concern to our eye bank. This is because tissue loss – whether it stems from the operating room or from a breakdown in our eye bank's screening, stripping, evaluation, or distribution protocols – represents an avoidable loss of precious donor tissue.

Several methods of determining the graft's correct orientation in the anterior chamber have been developed with varying degrees of success. Slit beams, intraoperative OCT, and asymmetric notches made in the graft's periphery are among the techniques that have been published in the peer-reviewed literature [3, 11, 17].

Our eye bank developed a method of stamping the stromal side of the DMEK graft with an "S" orientation mark using a skin marker dye in which the alcohol carrier has evaporated. Although the technique was developed in conjunction with our chosen procedure for stripping the EDM, it could theoretically be employed with other preparation methods. Figure 6.5 briefly illustrates our published technique [20].

The S-stamp has eliminated iatrogenic primary graft failures caused by upside-down grafts without causing significant damage to the endothelium [19]. We have quantified the cell loss associated with the S-stamp in laboratory studies and found that on average, surgeons can expect an additional 0.6 % cell loss beyond what is caused by our standard preparation. This small incremental addition to the cell loss is aided by allowing any alcohol in the ink to evaporate prior to applying the stamp. Not all surgeons request the "S" stamp, but among those who do, the marginal amount of cell loss caused by the S-stamp is well worth the tradeoff for assured right-side-up tissue orientation.

6.5 Training

Training technicians in DMEK tissue preparation starts with the selection of staff with an aptitude for microsurgery. Although we are still refining an objective dexterity test, even in its absence, the goal of our selection process is to avoid putting technicians in a position where failure is the likely outcome through no lack of

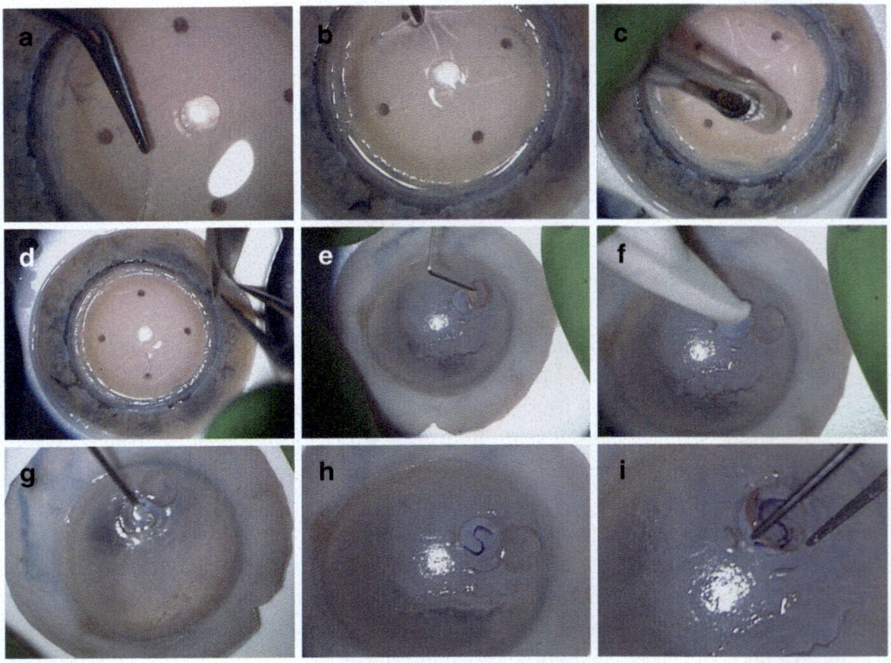

Fig. 6.5 General steps for Lions VisionGift peeling method. (**a**) Once Descemet membrane has been scored circumferentially, peeling is initiated. (**b**) Peeling is continued until 90 % of the membrane is free. (**c**) With the membrane reflected, a 2 mm punch is made through the stroma to create a window. (**d**) The membrane is now placed into its anatomical position and a wedge of sclera is resected to denote the hinge. (**e**) The cornea is placed on its scleral rim such that the stromal plug can be temporarily removed. (**f**) The window is wicked free of storage solution. (**g**) An S-stamp (Moria, Antony, France) is used to apply alcohol-free gentian violet (GV) dye, to the stromal side of Descemet membrane. GV is allowed to dry by waiting 10 s from the time the dye is applied to the stamp until it is applied to DM. (**h**) The S-stamp is clearly visible with the stromal plug reflected away. (**i**) The stromal plug is replaced just prior to placing the prepared graft into storage solution (Reproduced with permission from Wolters Kluwer. *Cornea*. 34(9):1175–8, September 2015)

training and diligence. However, manual dexterity is no guarantee of success. Extreme attention to detail, patience, and dedication to the practice required to train "muscle memory" are all important when selecting staff to undergo the rigors of training. Table 6.3 is an overview of our training procedure for new technicians.

6.5.1 Continuous Improvement

It is only with a rigid training program that tissue preparation failure can be mitigated, but even after the completion of formalized training, technicians continually receive feedback when they encounter complications. Technicians are formally evaluated annually. But since every EDM peeling procedure is recorded

Table 6.3 General rubric for training technicians

Phase	Description
1	Potential processing staff must show an interest in the procedure. Typically they circulate for the procedure a number of times prior to preparing their first graft. At a minimum, they have seen the procedure 10 times, but generally they have seen it at least 50 times
2	After an initial observation period, trainees have a preceptor walk them through the procedure a minimum of 3 times and more if the preceptor deems it necessary
3	The trainee prepares a number of practice grafts on his or her own time (without direct observation). This allows for the technician to build confidence without the pressure of a preceptor watching. Solo work could be anywhere from 10-30 practice tissues, depending on the individual
4	Once confident that the procedure is sufficiently mastered, the technician is observed for 10 preparations by the trainer, who coaches and grades the trainee. The trainee is approved to perform the procedure for transplant after 10 consecutive successful practice tissue preparations
5	After training has been completed, all preparations are recorded via a microscope camera for ongoing monitoring and feedback

and logged in our video database, even the most minor of complications are available for review by the technician and trainer. This capacity enables our eye bank to identify not only the root cause of preparation failure but also to optimize our protocols.

Being able to observe the reason for processing failures has allowed our technicians to improve and limit their failure rates tremendously. We have also found that it has fostered a culture of continual improvement and innovation among our technicians, which has proven invaluable.

6.6 Post-preparation Tissue Evaluation

A good post-preparation evaluation by the technician is an important quality control step that is difficult at best for the surgeon who prepares his or her own grafts. A well-documented evaluation of the graft aids in surgical planning and should eliminate any surprises to the surgeon related to the tissue. Although most tissue is deemed not suitable for transplant well before the post-preparation evaluation, on occasion, a thorough evaluation will reveal unacceptable endothelial cell loss that excludes prepared tissue from use.

Steps involved in tissue evaluation broadly fall into the following three categories: technician observation during peeling, post-preparation specular microscopy, and post-preparation slit lamp examination. Evaluation focuses on graft size, S-stamp quality, peripheral tears, and endothelial cell loss. Figure 6.6 demonstrates some of the evaluation steps technicians utilize to evaluate grafts prepared for DMEK. By far, the most important step in post-preparation evaluation is the slit lamp examination, which we describe in some detail.

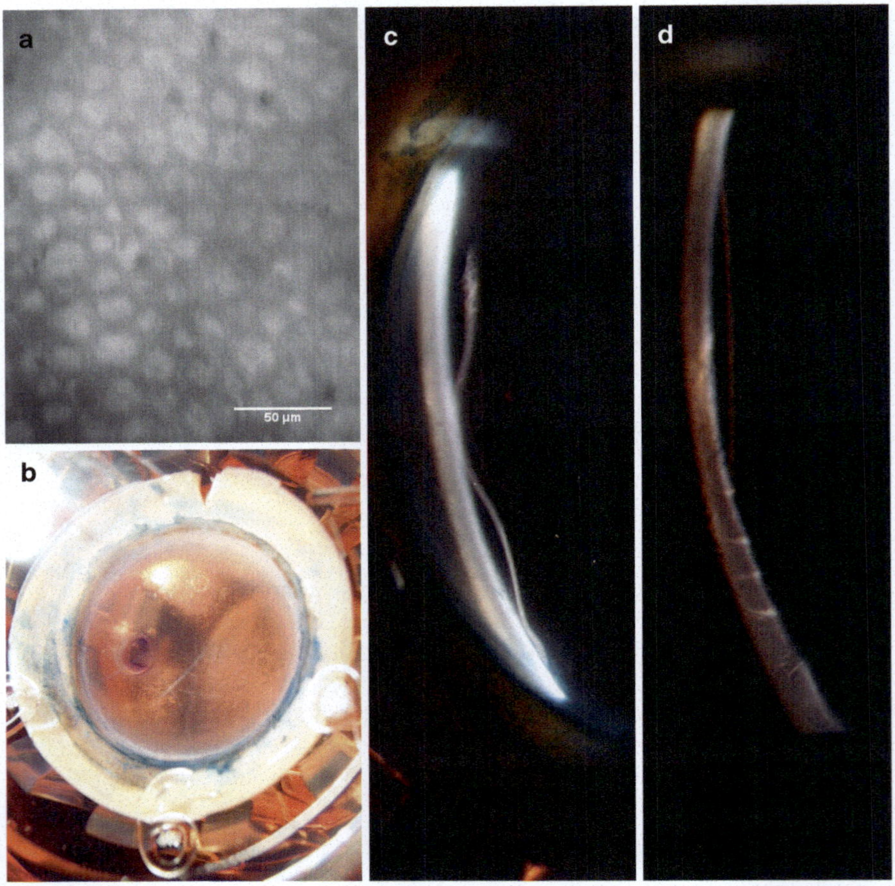

Fig. 6.6 Post DMEK preparation tissue evaluation by specular microscopy and slit lamp biomicroscopy of a single cornea. (**a**) A cropped image of endothelium with an ECD of 2703 cells/mm^2. (**b**) A 6× slit lamp image with diffuse illumination. (**c**) 10× slit lamp examination demonstrating undulating graft. (**d**) Fine slit beam at 10× as it travels across the graft and provides sharp focus to the endothelium

During the peeling of the EDM, trypan blue is used to enhance visibility of the membrane to make tissue manipulation easier. Staining has the added benefit of highlighting any areas of cell loss that may have occurred during the tissue recovery process and can focus attention to regions of interest for post-preparation slit lamp evaluation. Once prepared, the tissue is placed back in a cornea storage chamber, which facilitates evaluation with specular microscopy and slit lamp biomicroscopy.

Post-processing specular microscopy of all EK-prepared grafts is required by EBAA standards [5], but it is unwise to place much value in these cell counts because they are not as objective as they seem. Specular microscopy is limited significantly by sampling error. Post-processing cell counts can either be artificially high if large areas of cell loss have been skipped or artificially low if small areas of cell loss have been overrepresented. Specular microscopy of DMEK grafts is also inherently challenging. Obtaining a good image of the endothelium is difficult since the EDM is no longer adherent to the stroma. Should a peeling technique be employed where the center of the graft remains attached to the stroma rather than the periphery, excellent post-preparation specular microscopy may be obtained. However, in these cases, the graft is still in its native state and the post-preparation cell count has limited value to the transplant surgeon.

On the other hand, slit lamp examination is an excellent method for evaluating DMEK grafts. With a little practice by a technician already familiar with slit lamp biomicroscopy, the entire endothelium can be inspected for damage after tissue preparation. Examination begins with the use of retro-illumination, which highlights areas of endothelial stress and dropout. Care must be taken to ensure that epithelial sloughing is not confused with endothelial damage because the layers of the cornea are difficult to discern with this type of illumination. Sweeping the graft with a fine slit beam can help in this regard. The fine slit beam allows for detailed examination of the entire graft and is useful for discerning the potential trephination area.

While specular microscopy of the DMEK graft is less than ideal, its numerical result is alluring to both surgeons and eye bankers because it makes judgments about tissue viability easier. An evaluation method that yields a result with the objectivity conveyed by a number has yet to be formally adopted, but we continue to work toward this goal. One promising method is imaging the entire graft after vital dye staining with trypan blue and using a computer algorithm to estimate cell loss by quantifying the area of staining [9].

6.7 Conclusion

Eye banks have played a critical role in the advancement of endothelial keratoplasty. While DSAEK tissue preparation started as a procedure performed largely in the operating room, today most tissue is prepared in the eye bank. The same centralization of processing that has made DSAEK a "routine" procedure for the treatment of endothelial dysfunction can benefit the adoption of DMEK.

While EBAA data reveals recent growth in DMEK, it accounted for only 11 % of EK in the USA in 2014 [4], but this figure does not tell the whole story. 2014 was a watershed year for Lions VisionGift's DMEK program. DMEK supplanted DSAEK for the treatment of Fuchs dystrophy for the first time at our institution. Surgeons affiliated with Lions VisionGift who perform DMEK are now accustomed to seeing tissue as it is presented in Fig. 6.7. Undoubtedly, we will see additional "hot spots" of DMEK activity across the USA in the near future, with eye banks providing the high level of DMEK service that DSAEK has trained surgeons to expect.

Truly, we are here to honor the wish of a donor to help another see. It is through this spirit of stewardship that we share these pearls of eye banking knowledge. It is

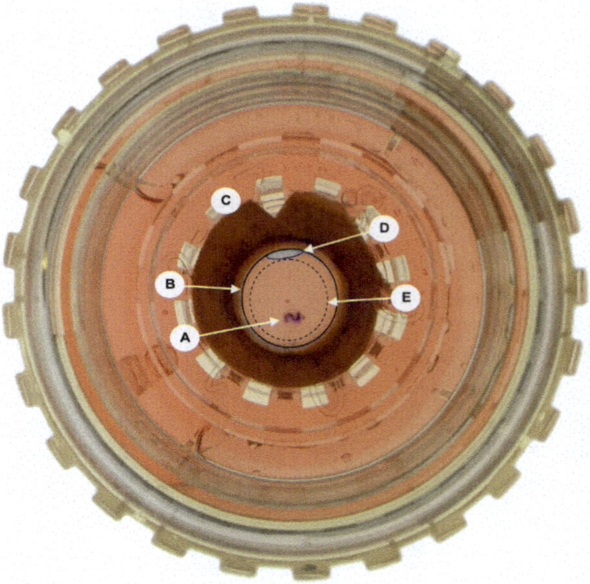

Fig. 6.7 Tissue as presented to surgeon. (**a**) A posterior view of S-stamp demonstrates orientation of the graft. (**b**) The solid line indicates the scored area of the graft. (**c**) A wedge resection of the sclera denotes the location of the hinge which assists the surgeon during the transfer of the graft from the cornea to an insertion device. (**d**) The gray oval denotes an area of the EDM that has been left intact for evaluating and shipping the tissue. This area is the "hinge" denoted by the scleral resection. (**e**) The dotted line indicates the suggested potential graft trephination zone

our hope that as new eye bank DMEK programs emerge and evolve, the information provided in this chapter will aid them in providing a high-quality graft without any undue loss of tissue.

References

1. Bennett A, Mahmoud S, Drury D, Cavanagh HD, McCulley JP, Petroll WM, Mootha VV. Impact of Donor age on corneal endothelium-descemet membrane layer scroll formation. Eye Contact Lens. 2015;41(4):236–9. doi:10.1097/icl.0000000000000108.
2. Bourne WM, Johnson DH, Campbell RJ. The ultrastructure of Descemet's membrane. III Fuchs' dystrophy. Arch Ophthalmol. 1982;100(12):1952–5.
3. Burkhart ZN, Feng MT, Price MO, Price FW. Handheld slit beam techniques to facilitate DMEK and DALK. Cornea. 2013;32(5):722–4. doi:10.1097/ICO.0b013e31827797e7.
4. Eye Bank Association of America. 2014 Eye Banking Statistical Report. Washington D.C: Eye Bank Association of America; 2015.
5. Eye Bank Association of America. Medical Standards. Washington, D.C. 2015.
6. Giebel A, Francis W, Price J. Descemet's Membrane Endothelial Keratoplasty (DMEK): The Bare Minimum. In: Francis W, Price J, Price MO, editors. DSEK: What You Need to Know About Endothelial Keratoplasty. Thorofare: Slack, Inc; 2009.

7. Gorovoy IR, Cui QN, Gorovoy MS. Donor tissue characteristics in preparation of DMEK grafts. Cornea. 2014;33(7):683–5. doi:10.1097/ico.0000000000000135.
8. Greiner MA, Rixen JJ, Wagoner MD, Schmidt GA, Stoeger CG, Straiko MD, Zimmerman MB, Kitzmann AS, Goins KM. Diabetes mellitus increases risk of unsuccessful graft preparation in Descemet membrane endothelial keratoplasty: a multicenter study. Cornea. 2014;33(11):1129–33. doi:10.1097/ico.0000000000000262.
9. Jardine GJ, Holiman JD, Stoeger CG, Chamberlain WD. Imaging and quantification of endothelial cell loss in eye bank prepared DMEK grafts using trainable segmentation software. Curr Eye Res. 2014;39(9):894–901. doi:10.3109/02713683.2014.887120.
10. Kelliher C, Engler C, Speck C, Ward D, Farazdaghi S, Jun AS. A comprehensive analysis of eye bank-prepared posterior lamellar corneal tissue for use in endothelial keratoplasty. Cornea. 2009;28(9):966–70. doi:10.1097/ICO.0b013e31819c4fcf.
11. Kruse FE, Laaser K, Cursiefen C, Heindl LM, Schlotzer-Schrehardt U, Riss S, Bachmann BO. A stepwise approach to donor preparation and insertion increases safety and outcome of Descemet membrane endothelial keratoplasty. Cornea. 2011;30(5):580–7.
12. Maier AK, Gundlach E, Schroeter J, Klamann MK, Gonnermann J, Riechardt AI, Bertelmann E, Joussen AM, Torun N. Influence of the difficulty of graft unfolding and attachment on the outcome in descemet membrane endothelial keratoplasty. Graefe's archive for clinical and experimental ophthalmology=Albrecht von Graefes Archiv fur klinische und experimentelle Ophthalmologie. 2015. doi:10.1007/s00417-015-2939-9.
13. Mannis MJ, Holland EJ, Gal RL, Dontchev M, Kollman C, Raghinaru D, Dunn SP, Schultze RL, Verdier DD, Lass JH, Raber IM, Sugar J, Gorovoy MS, Sugar A, Stulting RD, Montoya MM, Penta JG, Benetz BA, Beck RW. The effect of donor age on penetrating keratoplasty for endothelial disease: graft survival after 10 years in the Cornea Donor Study. Ophthalmology. 2013;120(12):2419–27. doi:10.1016/j.ophtha.2013.08.026.
14. Muraine M, Gueudry J, He Z, Piselli S, Lefevre S, Toubeau D. Novel technique for the preparation of corneal grafts for descemet membrane endothelial keratoplasty. Am J Ophthalmol. 2013;156(5):851–9. doi:10.1016/j.ajo.2013.05.041.
15. Phillips PM, Terry MA, Shamie N, Chen ES, Hoar KL, Stoeger C, Friend DJ, Saad HA. Descemet's stripping automated endothelial keratoplasty (DSAEK) using corneal donor tissue not acceptable for use in penetrating keratoplasty as a result of anterior stromal scars, pterygia, and previous corneal refractive surgical procedures. Cornea. 2009;28(8):871–6. doi:10.1097/ICO.0b013e318199f8d7.
16. Schlotzer-Schrehardt U, Bachmann BO, Tourtas T, Cursiefen C, Zenkel M, Rossler K, Kruse FE. Reproducibility of graft preparations in Descemet's membrane endothelial keratoplasty. Ophthalmology. 2013;120(9):1769–77. doi:10.1016/j.ophtha.2013.06.038.
17. Steven P, Le Blanc C, Velten K, Lankenau E, Krug M, Oelckers S, Heindl LM, Gehlsen U, Huttmann G, Cursiefen C. Optimizing descemet membrane endothelial keratoplasty using intraoperative optical coherence tomography. JAMA Ophthalmol. 2013;131(9):1135–42. doi:10.1001/jamaophthalmol.2013.4672.
18. Tenkman LR, Price FW, Price MO. Descemet membrane endothelial keratoplasty donor preparation: navigating challenges and improving efficiency. Cornea. 2014;33(3):319–25. doi:10.1097/ico.0000000000000045.
19. Veldman PB, Dye PK, Holiman JD, Mayko ZM, Sales CS, Straiko MD, Galloway JD, Terry MA. The S-stamp in descemet membrane endothelial keratoplasty safely eliminates upside-down graft implantation. Ophthalmology. 2015. doi:10.1016/j.ophtha.2015.08.044.
20. Veldman PB, Dye PK, Holiman JD, Mayko ZM, Sales CS, Straiko MD, Stoeger CG, Terry MA. Stamping an S on DMEK donor tissue to prevent upside-down grafts: laboratory validation and detailed preparation technique description. Cornea. 2015;34(9):1175–8. doi:10.1097/ico.0000000000000522.
21. Vianna LM, Stoeger CG, Galloway JD, Terry M, Cope L, Belfort Jr R, Jun AS. Risk factors for eye bank preparation failure of descemet membrane endothelial keratoplasty (DMEK) tissue. Am J Ophthalmol. 2015. doi:10.1016/j.ajo.2015.01.030.

Chapter 7
Donor-Tissue Splitting and Tissue Storage for DALK and DMEK Surgery

Ludwig M. Heindl and Claus Cursiefen

7.1 Donor Shortage in Corneal Transplantation

For over a century, keratoplasty ranks among the most common kinds of human tissue transplantation. In the United States alone, more than 75,000 sight-restoring corneal transplantations were performed in 2014 (2014 Eye Banking Statistical Report, available from the Eye Bank Association of America at www.restoresight.org; accessed July 28, 2015). A recent study comparing the medical cost of keratoplasty to the direct and indirect lifetime costs of the alternative – living with blindness or severe vision impairment – revealed a lifetime net benefit of nearly $6 billion per year (2013 Cost-Benefit Analysis of Corneal Transplant, available from the Eye Bank Association of America at www.restoresight.org; accessed July 28, 2015). However, in many parts of the world – including Europe and Asia – significant corneal donor shortage causes long keratoplasty waiting lists, and medically indicated corneal transplantations are being unduly postponed [1–3]. Therefore, new strategies for tackling donor shortage and reducing corneal tissue cost are needed. In other areas of transplantation surgery, split use of donor tissue has long been established to tackle donor shortage. Split-liver transplantations have been successful for several years, reducing the need for donor tissue by approximately 40 % [4, 5].

L.M. Heindl, MD (✉) • C. Cursiefen, MD, FEBO
Department of Ophthalmology, University of Cologne,
Cologne, Germany
e-mail: ludwig.heindl@uk-koeln.de; claus.cursiefen@uk-koeln.de

C. Cursiefen, A.S. Jun (eds.), *Current Treatment Options for Fuchs Endothelial Dystrophy*, DOI 10.1007/978-3-319-43021-8_7

7.2 Recent Advances in Lamellar Keratoplasty

Penetrating keratoplasty (PK), the full-thickness replacement of a diseased cornea with an allograft donor tissue, has been the standard of care for treating advanced keratoconus, anterior stromal opacity, or endothelial failure for more than 100 years [6, 7]. In the last decade, lamellar surgical techniques have been improved, allowing for selective replacement of the anterior as well as posterior pathologic corneal structures while retaining the healthy parts of the cornea [8–51].

In the surgical treatment of anterior stromal scars (e.g., advanced keratoconus, herpetic corneal scarring) or dystrophies, deep anterior lamellar keratoplasty (DALK), grafting the entire donor cornea except Descemet's membrane and the corneal endothelium, has been shown to be an effective alternative to PK [8–16]. DALK offers distinct advantages over PK, including a reduced risk of endothelial cell rejection resulting from the preservation of the recipient endothelium and a reduced rate of intraocular complications resulting from a closed-system procedure [8–16].

For the treatment of corneal endothelial disorders (e.g., Fuchs' endothelial dystrophy, pseudophakic bullous keratopathy, pseudoexfoliation syndrome keratopathy), several techniques of posterior lamellar keratoplasty have been described: deep lamellar endothelial keratoplasty (DLEK), Descemet's stripping automated endothelial keratoplasty (DSAEK), and Descemet's membrane endothelial keratoplasty (DMEK) [17–51]. In DMEK, the isolated donor endothelium-Descemet's membrane layer without any stroma is transplanted after stripping the recipient Descemet's membrane with its dysfunctional endothelium [25–51]. Compared to PK, DMEK is considered to provide faster visual rehabilitation, improved surface topography with reduction of postsurgical astigmatism, reduced risk of expulsive hemorrhage in a closed-system procedure, protection of corneal innervation for the prevention of neurotrophic keratopathy, and reduced rate of immunologic rejection against the grafted endothelium resulting from the reduced amount of foreign surface antigens on the recipient cornea and presence of the recipient's own anti-inflammatory and antiangiogenic epithelium [25–51].

The indications for keratoplasty that can be covered by either DALK or DMEK surgery comprise approximately 80 % of all indications [7]. However, DALK and DMEK currently appear to be more technically challenging for the corneal surgeon. Both novel surgical techniques have their attributes and drawbacks and are still evolving.

7.3 Split Cornea Transplantation for Two Recipients

Since in DALK the donor endothelium-Descemet's membrane layer is left over, and in DMEK the anterior part of the donor button (including the epithelium, its basement membrane, Bowman's layer, and the stroma) is left over, we have recently described a split cornea transplantation approach by combining DALK and DMEK

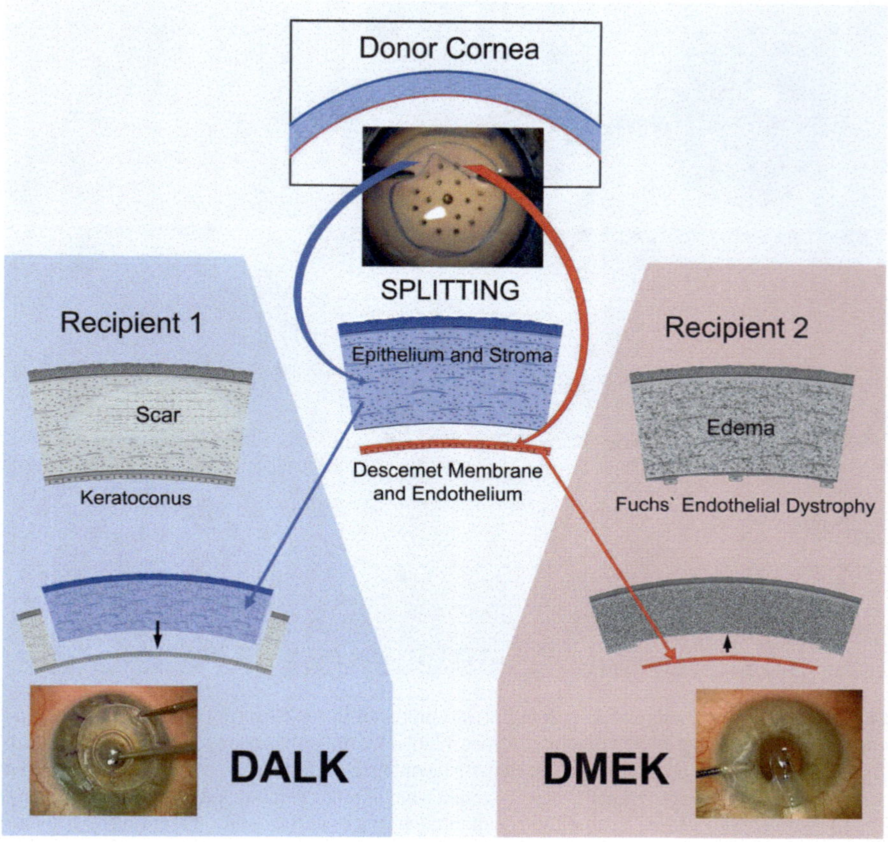

Fig. 7.1 Principle of split cornea transplantation to use one donor cornea for two recipients. A single donor cornea can be split into two parts. The anterior part (including epithelium, its basement membrane, Bowman's layer, and stroma) is transplanted using deep anterior lamellar keratoplasty (DALK) in corneal diseases affecting solely the anterior stroma and not the endothelium-Descemet's membrane layer (e.g., keratoconus). The posterior part (endothelium-Descemet's membrane layer) is grafted using Descemet's membrane endothelial keratoplasty (DMEK) in corneal endothelial diseases (e.g., Fuchs' endothelial dystrophy) without anterior stromal scarring (Modified from Refs. [52] and [53])

procedures in two recipients, in order to reduce donor shortage and cost of corneal transplantation [52–58]. That means that a full-thickness donor button is split into an anterior donor lamella for the use in a DALK procedure and into a posterior donor lamella for the use in a DMEK procedure in another patient (Fig. 7.1), so that a single donor cornea can be used for two recipients [52].

The split use of donor tissue is a relatively novel strategy in corneal transplantation. Vajpayee and coworkers described in a single case report the use of a single corneoscleral donor button in three patients by combining automated lamellar therapeutic keratoplasty for macular corneal dystrophy, DSAEK for pseudophakic

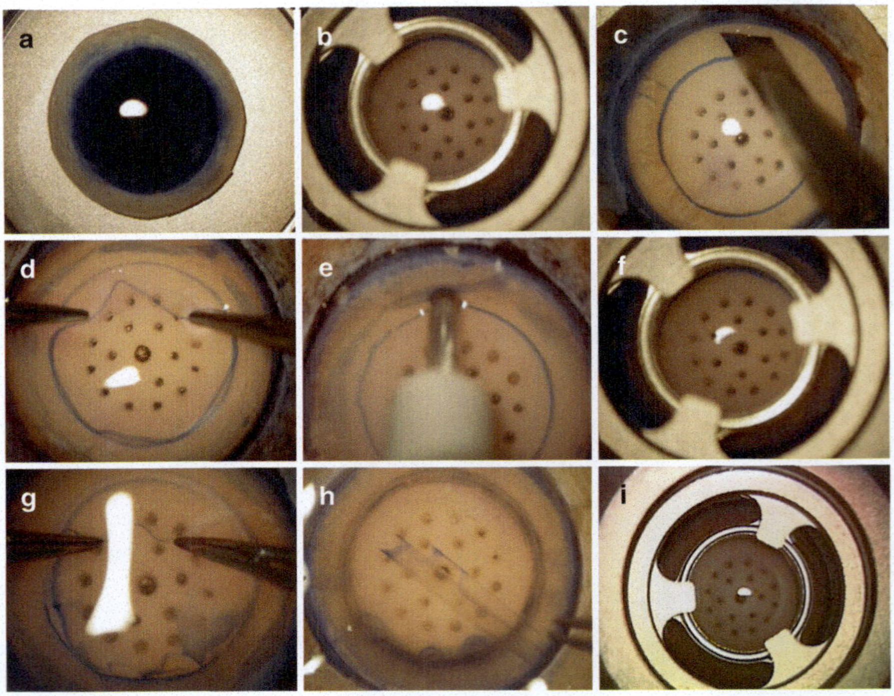

Fig. 7.2 Surgical technique of split donor cornea preparation. (**a**) Covering the corneoscleral button endothelial side up with saline and trypan blue solution. (**b**) Marking the central 8 mm by gentle trephine touch. (**c**) Incision of Descemet's membrane peripheral to the marked circle with a razor blade. (**d**) Lifting the endothelium-Descemet's membrane layer beyond the 8-mm mark using blunt anatomic forceps. (**e**) Setting three semicircular marks at the 8-mm margin using a 1-mm trephine. (**f**) Cutting through Descemet's membrane using an 8-mm trephine. (**g**) Separation of the entire endothelium-Descemet's membrane layer from the stroma underwater using blunt forceps. (**h**) Spontaneous formation of an endothelium-Descemet's membrane roll with endothelial side outward transferred into culture medium for subsequent Descemet's membrane endothelial keratoplasty (DMEK). (**i**) Circular, full-thickness trephination of the remaining anterior donor lamella using an 8.25-mm trephine for completing deep anterior lamellar keratoplasty (DALK) (Modified from Ref. [52])

bullous keratopathy, and limbal stem cell transplantation for limbal stem cell deficiency [59]. Recently, Lie and coworkers [60] as well as our group [52] reported the feasibility of split cornea transplantation by combining DALK and DMEK procedures for two recipients.

In an audit of our first 100 consecutive patients, split cornea transplantation could reduce the shortage of corneal tissue by 47 % [53]. In this initial series, a backup donor cornea was made available for every surgical intervention [53]. However, split donor cornea preparation (Fig. 7.2) could be performed successfully in all cases without inducing any significant central defects in the endothelium-Descemet's membrane layer [53]. Similarly, all DMEK surgeries stripping the recipient Descemet's membrane and inserting the endothelium-Descemet's

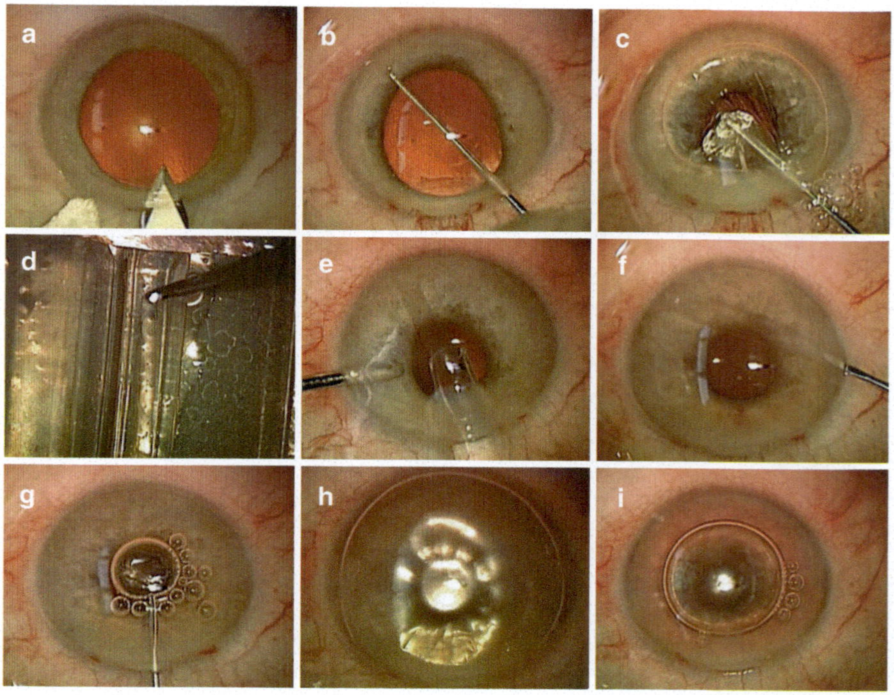

Fig. 7.3 Surgical technique of Descemet's membrane endothelial keratoplasty (DMEK). (**a**) Preparation of a 3-mm clear corneal tunnel at the 12-o'clock position. (**b**) Centripetal stripping of Descemet's membrane using a Price hook. (**c**) Complete removal of the central 9-mm Descemet's membrane. (**d**) Transfer of the donor endothelium-Descemet's membrane graft obtained from split donor cornea preparation (see Fig. 7.2) into a conventional lens injector cartridge with endothelial side outward. (**e**) Injection of the graft into the anterior chamber. (**f**) Rotation of the graft for 90°. (**g**) Unfolding of the graft by an air-bubble injection on top of the graft. (**h**) Complete filling of the anterior chamber with air pressing the graft endothelial side down against the host corneal stroma. (**i**) Reduction of the air to approximately one fifth of the anterior chamber volume or complete anterior chamber air fill is left (Modified from Refs. [51] and [52])

membrane graft (Fig. 7.3) were surgically successful [53]. In three out of the 50 eyes with anterior stromal disease (6 %), the DALK procedure (Fig. 7.4) had to be converted to PK, requiring a full-thickness corneal graft, owing to accidental macroperforation of the recipient Descemet's membrane [53]. Therefore, a backup cornea was necessary, as otherwise, the surgery for the second patient would need to be canceled, resulting in problems with general anesthesia and patient convenience [53]. The follow-up revealed good visual and refractive outcomes with low complication rates and acceptable endothelial cell loss in our first 100 consecutive patients [53].

In Lie's series, a total of 124 transplantations, i.e., 69 DMEK and 55 DALK procedures, could be performed out of a pool of 73 donor corneas, so that a total of 51 donor buttons (41 %) could be saved [60].

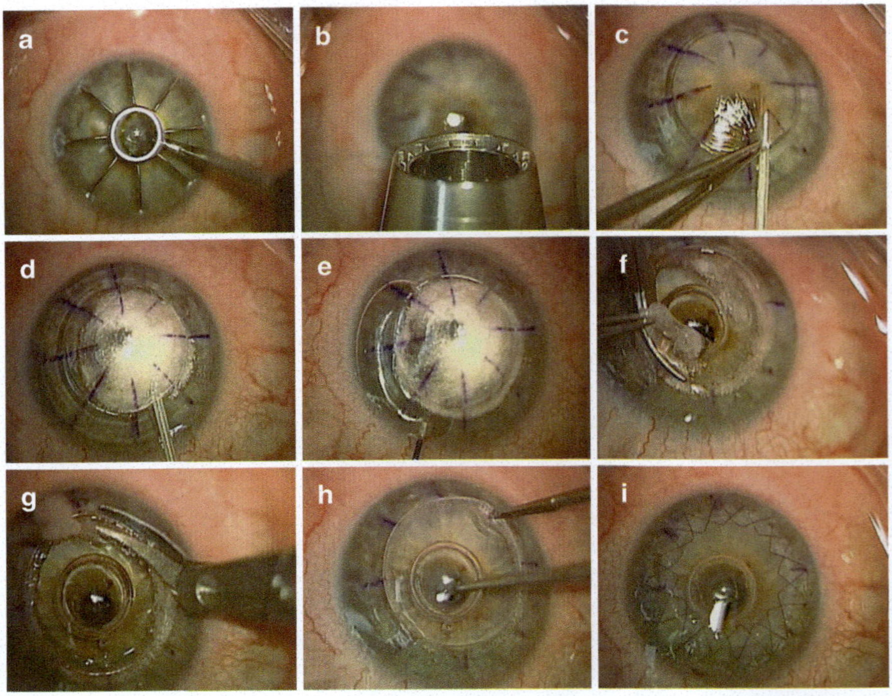

Fig. 7.4 Surgical technique of deep anterior lamellar keratoplasty (DALK). (**a**) Marking the center of the recipient corneal surface with a surgical claw. (**b**) Circular, partial-thickness trephination with an intended depth of 90 % of the preoperative pachymetry using an 8-mm trephine. (**c**) Inserting a 30-gauge needle bevel down at the peripheral trephination and advancing it centripetally just above Descemet's membrane. (**d**) Injection of a big air-bubble, resulting in a white, semiopaque disk to separate Descemet's membrane from the stroma. (**e**) Injection of a small air-bubble into the anterior chamber, becoming visible at the periphery of the big bubble formation. (**f**) Cutting out the central stromal tissue using Katzin scissors. (**g**) Evidence of bare Descemet's membrane without defects by the small air-bubble moving centrally in the anterior chamber. (**h**) Transfer of the anterior donor lamella obtained from split donor cornea preparation (see Fig. 7.2) into the recipient bed. (**i**) Fixation with a 16-bite double-running diagonal cross-stitch suture (Modified from Ref [52])

However, a recent retrospective audit of 1,141 consecutive donor corneas at our department revealed that only 15 % of corneal grafts could be performed as split cornea transplantation, resulting in 96 donor corneas being saved (8 %) [58]. The reason for this is that indications and referrals for DMEK exceed those for DALK by far (714 vs 100, respectively), at least at our department [58]. This asymmetric distribution suggests the need for scheduling DMEK and DALK recipients even more controlled.

Most recently, the Melles group published the hemi-DMEK technique splitting one endothelial graft into two half-moon-shaped grafts for two recipients [61, 62]. Since hemi-DMEK seems to provide visual outcomes similar to those in standard

DMEK [62], hemi-DMEK is a promising method for increasing the pool of endothelial graft tissue, although severe doubts remain about long-term endothelial cell counts after this approach.

In summary, due to the ongoing revolution of corneal transplantation toward lamellar keratoplasty techniques, the split use of donor corneal tissue may become a standard approach to save corneal tissue and to reduce transplantation cost in the future.

7.4 Tissue Storage for DALK and DMEK Surgery

Split cornea transplantation raises the demands on the organization and daily work in the eye banks. Firstly, microbial contamination must be avoided. Therefore, the culture media with the donor cornea tissue and its residues should be examined microbiologically before and after each surgery owing to a presumably increased risk of contamination. Secondly, sophisticated logistics of quick patient allocation is crucial. Special precautions have to be taken to precisely track the use of tissue parts, even during busy operating room days, and, in particular, to ensure that human leukocyte antigen-matched donor tissue reaches the planned recipient.

Our initial concept of performing the DMEK procedure for the patient with corneal endothelial disease immediately after completing the DALK procedure for the patient with anterior stromal disease on the same surgery day led to increasing logistical difficulties in the clinical routine. Therefore, we have changed our surgical planning concept [53, 56]. Depending on the availability of the patients, either the DALK procedure is performed first and the posterior donor lenticule is stored to complete the subsequent DMEK procedure within 7 days or the DMEK procedure is performed first and the anterior donor lenticule is stored to complete the subsequent DALK procedure within 7 days [56]. This simplifies the logistics of patient allocation and makes split cornea transplantation more feasible in the clinical routine.

Indeed, longer storage of the anterior donor lenticule without endothelium before actual use in DALK surgery could cause more edematous alterations of the graft and loss of stromal keratocytes [57] that potentially could persist and thereby degrade vision and increase complications after lamellar keratoplasty. In an experimental study using light microscopy (Fig. 7.5) and electron microscopy (Fig. 7.6), corneal epithelium and stroma revealed significantly more edematous alterations after Descemet's stripping than full-thickness corneas, with a marked increase from 1 to 3 culture weeks and marked anterior keratocyte loss within 3 culture weeks [57]. However, the 1-year outcomes (visual acuity, endothelial cell loss, central corneal thickness, and complication rate) after DALK using split donor tissue stored up to 1 week (Table 7.1) were well within the 1-year results reported by several groups for DALK using nonstored tissue [56]. Furthermore, longer storage of the posterior

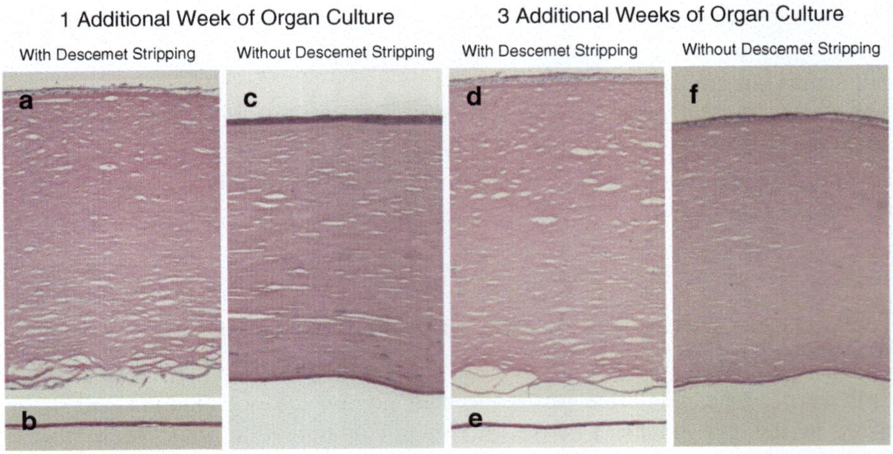

Fig. 7.5 Histopathologic graft alterations after Descemet's stripping. Histopathology of split (**a**, **b**, **d**, **e**) and full-thickness (**c**, **f**) donor corneas after one (**a**–**c**) and three (**d**–**f**) additional weeks of organ culture showing more epithelial and stromal edema after Descemet's stripping with a marked loss of keratocytes in the anterior stroma at 3 culture weeks and Descemet's membrane with intact and viable endothelium up to 3 culture weeks without significant differences between stripped and non-stripped buttons (hematoxylin-eosin, original magnification × 200) (Modified from Ref. [57])

donor lenticule before actual use in DMEK surgery could be associated with a higher endothelial cell loss [57] that potentially could persist, thereby degrading vision and increasing complications after posterior lamellar keratoplasty. An experimental study on graft alterations after Descemet's stripping revealed a linear decrease of the endothelial cell count of posterior lenticules within 4 culture weeks, showing a mean loss of 128 cells/mm^2 per week [57]. Light (Fig. 7.5) and electron microscopy (Fig. 7.6) showed an intact and viable endothelium up to 3 culture weeks in split and non-split buttons [57]. In the clinical setting, the 1-year outcomes (visual acuity, endothelial cell loss, central corneal thickness, and complication rate) after DMEK using split donor tissue stored up to 1 week (Table 7.1) were well within the 1-year results reported by several groups for DMEK using non-stored tissue [56]. Therefore, these data support the possible safety of anterior and posterior donor tissue stored in organ culture up to 1 week after splitting for the use in DALK and DMEK surgery, respectively.

In our hands, split donor cornea preparation is always performed in the operating theater. However, the tolerance of longer donor preparation-to-use times allows the implementation of a precut tissue procedure in the eye bank instead of intraoperative donor-tissue preparation for lamellar keratoplasty [63, 64].

Nevertheless, further questions concerning the ideal donor graft as well as the ideal storage conditions are still open. For DALK and DMEK surgery, we make no specific requests to the eye banks to provide tissue for split cornea transplantation with any different donor characteristics than what normally is

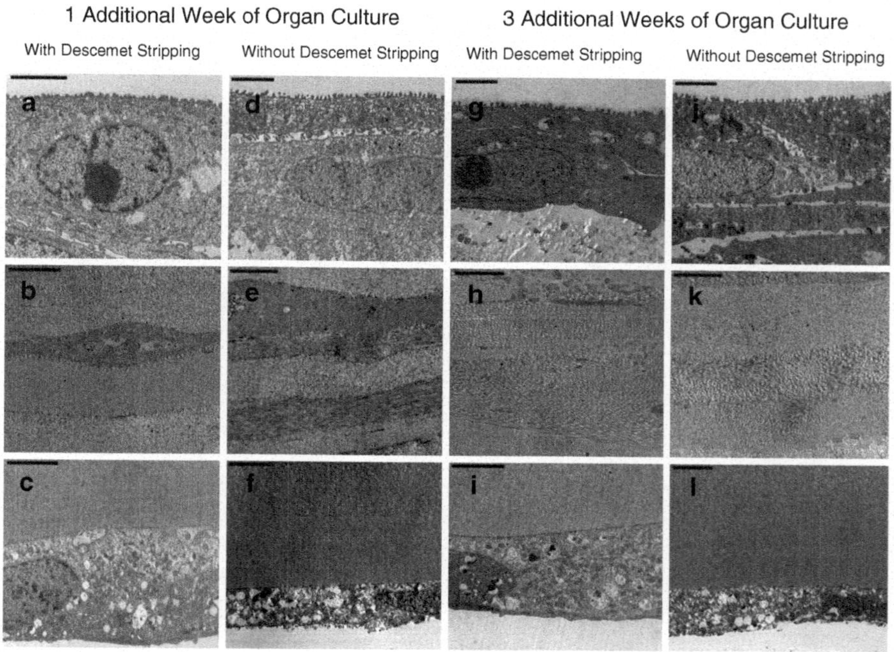

Fig. 7.6 Ultrastructural graft alterations after Descemet's stripping. Transmission electron microscopy of split (**a**–**c** and **g**–**i**) and full-thickness (**d**–**f** and **j**–**l**) donor corneas after one (**a**–**f**) and three (**g**–**l**) additional weeks of organ culture showing more epithelial (**a**, **d**, **g**, **j**) and stromal (**b**, **e**, **h**, **k**) edema after Descemet's stripping and Descemet's membrane with intact and viable endothelium (**c**, **f**, **i**, **l**) up to 3 culture weeks without significant differences between stripped and non-stripped buttons (scale bar = 2.5 μm) (Modified from Ref. [57])

requested for full-thickness PK tissue. Typically, we accept donor tissue with any donor age between 14 and 80 years; a postmortem time of up to 36 h; a donor endothelial cell density of more than 2200 cells/mm^2; in case of short-term culture, a preservation time of up to 14 days; and in case of organ culture, a preservation time of up to 34 days. All our split donor tissue is stored in Dulbecco's modified Eagle medium containing streptomycin, penicillin, and fetal calf serum at 34 °C. Further comparative studies are necessary to define better the effect of different preservation media (e.g., Optisol) and their impact on corneal tissue swelling as well as on endothelial cell loss.

Altogether, split donor corneal tissue may be stored safely for up to 1 week in organ culture before use in lamellar keratoplasty. This will revolutionize the work in the eye banks simplifying the clinical feasibility of split cornea transplantation to reduce donor shortage and cost in corneal transplantation in the future, especially in large parts of the world even more severely affected by donor-tissue shortage than in Europe.

Table 7.1 One-year outcomes after split cornea transplantation combining deep anterior lamellar keratoplasty (DALK) and Descemet's membrane endothelial keratoplasty (DMEK) in 220 eyes in dependence of the storage time after Descemet's stripping

	DALK using anterior donor lamellas with storage time after splitting				DMEK using posterior donor lamellas with storage time after splitting			
	<1 h	1–24 h	25 h–3 days	4–7 days	<1 h	1–24 h	25 h–3 days	4–7 days
	(*n*=*47*)	(*n*=*21*)	(*n*=*22*)	(*n*=*20*)	(*n*=*63*)	(*n*=*17*)	(*n*=*16*)	(*n*=*14*)
BSCVA (logMAR)	0.18±0.09	0.20±0.06	0.18±0.07	0.18±0.09	0.09±0.08	0.14±0.14	0.13±0.09	0.05±0.07
Mean±SD (range)	(0.0–0.4)	(0.1–0.4)	(0.0–0.3)	(0.0–0.4)	(–0.1–0.3)	(–0.1–0.3)	(0.0–0.3)	(–0.1–0.1)
Spherical equivalent (D)	–1.5±1.3	–2.5±1.1	–1.2±0.8	–1.1±0.9	0.8±1.3	1.1±1.3	1.3±0.9	0.4±0.6
Mean±SD (range)	(–4.5–0.0)	(–5.0––0.5)	(–3.3–0.0)	(–3.5–0.0)	(–2.8–4.5)	(–2.5–4.3)	(–0.5–3.0)	(–0.5–1.5)
Refractive astigmatism (D)	1.2±0.9	1.4±0.7	1.0±0.5	1.1±0,4	0.6±0.4	0.7±0.7	0.5±0.5	0.6±0.4
Mean±SD (range)	(0.5–3.5)	(0.5–3.0)	(0.0–2.0)	(0.5–2.0)	(0.0–1.5)	(0.0–2.5)	(0.0–1.5)	(0.0–1.5)
Endothelial cell density (cells/mm²)	1979±133	2002±61	2032±49	2007±116	1489±192	1535±238	1498±197	1543±139
Mean±SD (range)	(1734–2267)	(1784–2084)	(1969–2156)	(1700–2149)	(1007–1894)	(1002–1882)	(1187–1875)	(1352–1782)
Endothelial cell loss[a] (%)	9±4	7±3	8±3	7±3	42±9	37±11	42±10	41±7
Mean±SD (range)	(4–16)	(2–13)	(3–13)	(3–15)	(28–63)	(19–61)	(17–57)	(30–52)
Central corneal thickness (μm)	516±29	538±23	520±16	513±21	541±36	536±45	540±31	545±35
Mean±SD (range)	(480–581)	(482–572)	(495–555)	(473–559)	(437–623)	(456–600)	(488–600)	(456–597)
Complications								
Intraoperative, *n* (%)	5 (11 %)	1 (5 %)	–5 (23 %)	1 (5 %)	3 (5 %)	2 (12 %)	1 (6 %)	1 (7 %)
Postoperative, *n* (%)	9 (19 %)	2 (10 %)		4 (20 %)	38 (60 %)	12 (71 %)	7 (44 %)	11 (79 %)

Modified from Ref. [57]

BSCVA best spectacle-corrected visual acuity, *logMAR* logarithm of the minimal angle of resolution, *SD* standard deviation, *D* diopter

[a]In case of DALK, the 1-year endothelial cell density compared with the preoperative host endothelial cell density; in case of DMEK, the 1-year endothelial cell density compared with the donor endothelial cell density

References

1. Rasouli M, Caraiscos VB, Slomovic AR. Efficacy of routine notification and request on reducing corneal transplantation wait times in Canada. Can J Ophthalmol. 2009;44:31–5.
2. De By TM. Shortage in the face of plenty: improving the allocation of corneas for transplantation. Dev Ophthalmol. 2003;36:56–61.
3. Reinhard T, Böhringer D, Bogen A, Sundmacher R. The transplantation law: a chance to overcome the shortage of corneal grafts in Germany? Transplant Proc. 2002;34:1322–4.
4. Otte JB, de Ville de Goyet J, Alberti D, Balladur P, de Hemptinne B. The concept and technique of the split liver in clinical transplantation. Surgery. 1990;107:605–12.
5. Cintorino D, Spada M, Gruttadauria S, Riva S, Luca A, Volpes R, Vizzini G, Arcadipane A, Henderson K, Verzaro R, Foglieni CS, Gridelli B. In situ split liver transplantation for adult and pediatric recipients: an answer to organ shortage. Transplant Proc. 2006;38:1096–8.
6. Seitz B, Langenbucher A, Naumann GO. The penetrating keratoplasty: a 100-year success story [in German]. Ophthalmologe. 2005;102:1128–36, 1138–9.
7. Cursiefen C, Küchle M, Naumann GO. Changing indications for penetrating keratoplasty: histopathology of 1,250 corneal buttons. Cornea. 1998;17:468–70.
8. Anwar M, Teichmann KD. Big-bubble technique to bare Descemet's membrane in anterior lamellar keratoplasty. J Cataract Refract Surg. 2002;28:398–403.
9. Parthasarathy A, Por YM, Tan DT. Use of a "small-bubble technique" to increase the success of Anwar's "big-bubble technique" for deep lamellar keratoplasty with complete baring of Descemet's membrane. Br J Ophthalmol. 2007;91:1369–73.
10. Awan MA, Roberts F, Hegarty B, Ramaesh K. The outcome of deep anterior lamellar keratoplasty in herpes simplex virus-related corneal scarring, complications and graft survival. Br J Ophthalmol. 2010;94:1300–3.
11. Reinhart WJ, Musch DC, Jacobs DS, Lee WB, Kaufman SC, Shtein RM. Deep anterior lamellar keratoplasty as an alternative to penetrating keratoplasty: a report by the american academy of ophthalmology. Ophthalmology. 2011;118:209–18.
12. Braun JM, Hofmann-Rummelt C, Schlötzer-Schrehardt U, Kruse FE, Cursiefen C. Histopathological changes after deep anterior lamellar keratoplasty using the "big-bubble technique". Acta Ophthalmol. 2013;91:78–82.
13. Cursiefen C, Heindl LM. Perspectives of deep anterior lamellar keratoplasty [in German]. Ophthalmologe. 2011;108:833–9.
14. Riss S, Heindl LM, Bachmann BO, Kruse FE, Cursiefen C. Pentacam-based big bubble deep anterior lamellar keratoplasty in patients with keratoconus. Cornea. 2012;31:627–32.
15. Riss S, Heindl LM, Bachmann BO, Kruse FE, Cursiefen C. Microbubble incision as a new rescue technique for big-bubble deep anterior lamellar keratoplasty with failed bubble formation. Cornea. 2013;32:125–9.
16. Steven P, Le Blanc C, Lankenau E, Krug M, Oelckers S, Heindl LM, Gehlsen U, Huettmann G, Cursiefen C. Optimising deep anterior lamellar keratoplasty (DALK) using intraoperative online optical coherence tomography (iOCT). Br J Ophthalmol. 2014;98:900–4.
17. Price MO, Fairchild KM, Price DA, Price Jr FW. Descemet's stripping endothelial keratoplasty: five-year graft survival and endothelial cell loss. Ophthalmology. 2011;118: 725–9.
18. Price MO, Gorovoy M, Price Jr FW, Benetz BA, Menegay HJ, Lass JH. Descemet's stripping automated endothelial keratoplasty: three-year graft and endothelial cell survival compared with penetrating keratoplasty. Ophthalmology. 2013;120:246–51.
19. Terry MA, Straiko MD, Goshe JM, Li JY, Davis-Boozer D. Descemet's stripping automated endothelial keratoplasty: the tenuous relationship between donor thickness and postoperative vision. Ophthalmology. 2012;119:1988–96.
20. Li JY, Terry MA, Goshe J, Davis-Boozer D, Shamie N. Three-year visual acuity outcomes after Descemet's stripping automated endothelial keratoplasty. Ophthalmology. 2012;119: 1126–9.

21. Heindl LM, Hofmann-Rummelt C, Schlötzer-Schrehardt U, Kruse FE, Cursiefen C. Histologic analysis of descemet stripping in posterior lamellar keratoplasty. Arch Ophthalmol. 2008;126:461–4.
22. Heindl LM, Kruse FE, Cursiefen C. Complications after posterior lamellar keratoplasty (DSAEK): prevention, detection and treatment [in German]. Klin Monbl Augenheilkd. 2010;227:478–82.
23. Bucher F, Dietlein T, Hermann M, Hos D, Cursiefen C, Heindl LM. Retrocorneal membrane formation after Baerveldt shunt implantation for iridocorneal endothelial syndrome. Cornea. 2013;32:e161–3.
24. Bucher F, Roters S, Mellein A, Hos D, Heindl LM, Cursiefen C, Hermann M. "OSMO-UT-DSAEK" using THIN-C medium. Graefes Arch Clin Exp Ophthalmol. 2013;251:2181–5.
25. Melles GR, Lander F, Rietveld FJ. Transplantation of Descemet's membrane carrying viable endothelium through a small scleral incision. Cornea. 2002;21:415–8.
26. Melles GR, Ong TS, Ververs B, van der Wees J. Descemet membrane endothelial keratoplasty (DMEK). Cornea. 2006;25:987–90.
27. Rodriguez-Calvo-de-Mora M, Quilendrino R, Ham L, Liarakos VS, van Dijk K, Baydoun L, Dapena I, Oellerich S, Melles GR. Clinical outcome of 500 consecutive cases undergoing Descemet's membrane endothelial keratoplasty. Ophthalmology. 2015;122:464–70.
28. Baydoun L, van Dijk K, Dapena I, Musa FU, Liarakos VS, Ham L, Melles GR. Repeat Descemet membrane endothelial keratoplasty after complicated primary Descemet membrane endothelial keratoplasty. Ophthalmology. 2015;122:8–16.
29. Dapena I, Moutsouris K, Droutsas K, Ham L, van Dijk K, Melles GR. Standardized "no-touch" technique for descemet membrane endothelial keratoplasty. Arch Ophthalmol. 2011;129:88–94.
30. Chaurasia S, Price Jr FW, Gunderson L, Price MO. Descemet's membrane endothelial keratoplasty: clinical results of single versus triple procedures (combined with cataract surgery). Ophthalmology. 2014;121:454–8.
31. Anshu A, Price MO, Price Jr FW. Risk of corneal transplant rejection significantly reduced with Descemet's membrane endothelial keratoplasty. Ophthalmology. 2012;119:536–40.
32. Guerra FP, Anshu A, Price MO, Giebel AW, Price FW. Descemet's membrane endothelial keratoplasty: prospective study of 1-year visual outcomes, graft survival, and endothelial cell loss. Ophthalmology. 2011;118:2368–73.
33. Cursiefen C, Kruse FE. DMEK: Descemet membrane endothelial keratoplasty [in German]. Ophthalmologe. 2010;107:370–6.
34. Heindl LM, Schlötzer-Schrehardt U, Cursiefen C, Bachmann BO, Hofmann-Rummelt C, Kruse FE. Myofibroblast metaplasia after descemet membrane endothelial keratoplasty. Am J Ophthalmol. 2011;151:1019–23.
35. Kruse FE, Laaser K, Cursiefen C, Heindl LM, Schlötzer-Schrehardt U, Riss S, Bachmann BO. A stepwise approach to donor preparation and insertion increases safety and outcome of Descemet membrane endothelial keratoplasty. Cornea. 2011;30:580–7.
36. Schlötzer-Schrehardt U, Bachmann BO, Laaser K, Cursiefen C, Kruse FE. Characterization of the cleavage plane in Descemet's membrane endothelial keratoplasty. Ophthalmology. 2011;118:1950–7.
37. Rudolph M, Laaser K, Bachmann BO, Cursiefen C, Epstein D, Kruse FE. Corneal higher-order aberrations after Descemet's membrane endothelial keratoplasty. Ophthalmology. 2012;119:528–35.
38. Tourtas T, Laaser K, Bachmann BO, Cursiefen C, Kruse FE. Descemet membrane endothelial keratoplasty versus descemet stripping automated endothelial keratoplasty. Am J Ophthalmol. 2012;153:1082–90.
39. Laaser K, Bachmann BO, Horn FK, Cursiefen C, Kruse FE. Descemet membrane endothelial keratoplasty combined with phacoemulsification and intraocular lens implantation: advanced triple procedure. Am J Ophthalmol. 2012;154:47–55.
40. Steven P, Hos D, Heindl LM, Bock F, Cursiefen C. Immune reactions after DMEK, DSAEK and DALK [in German]. Klin Monbl Augenheilkd. 2013;230:494–9.

41. Cursiefen C, Steven P, Roters S, Heindl LM. Prevention and management of complications in Descemet membrane endothelial keratoplasty (DMEK) and Descemet stripping automated endothelial keratoplasty (DSAEK) [in German]. Ophthalmologe. 2013;110:614–21.
42. Steven P, Le Blanc C, Velten K, Lankenau E, Krug M, Oelckers S, Heindl LM, Gehlsen U, Hüttmann G, Cursiefen C. Optimizing descemet membrane endothelial keratoplasty using intraoperative optical coherence tomography. JAMA Ophthalmol. 2013;131:1135–42.
43. Schlötzer-Schrehardt U, Bachmann BO, Tourtas T, Cursiefen C, Zenkel M, Rössler K, Kruse FE. Reproducibility of graft preparations in Descemet's membrane endothelial keratoplasty. Ophthalmology. 2013;120:1769–77.
44. Heindl LM, Koch KR, Bucher F, Hos D, Steven P, Koch HR, Cursiefen C. Descemet membrane endothelial keratoplasty in eyes with glaucoma implants. Optom Vis Sci. 2013;90:e241–4.
45. Tourtas T, Heindl LM, Kopsachilis N, Bachmann BO, Kruse FE, Cursiefen C. Use of accidentally torn descemet membrane to successfully complete descemet membrane endothelial keratoplasty. Cornea. 2013;32:1418–22.
46. Hos D, Heindl LM, Bucher F, Cursiefen C. Evidence of donor corneal endothelial cell migration from immune reactions occurring after descemet membrane endothelial keratoplasty. Cornea. 2014;33:331–4.
47. Bucher F, Hos D, Matthaei M, Steven P, Cursiefen C, Heindl LM. Corneal nerve alterations after Descemet membrane endothelial keratoplasty: an in vivo confocal microscopy study. Cornea. 2014;33:1134–9.
48. Siggel R, Heindl LM, Cursiefen C. Descemet membrane endothelial keratoplasty (DMEK) in phakic eyes with shallow anterior chamber. Graefes Arch Clin Exp Ophthalmol. 2015;253: 817–9.
49. Bucher F, Hos D, Müller-Schwefe S, Steven P, Cursiefen C, Heindl LM. Spontaneous long-term course of persistent peripheral graft detachments after Descemet's membrane endothelial keratoplasty. Br J Ophthalmol. 2015;99:768–72.
50. Maier P, Reinhard T, Cursiefen C. Descemet stripping endothelial keratoplasty – rapid recovery of visual acuity. Dtsch Arztebl Int. 2013;110:365–71.
51. Stanzel TP, Ersoy L, Sansanayudh W, Felsch M, Dietlein T, Bachmann B, Cursiefen C. Immediate postoperative intraocular pressure changes after anterior chamber air fill in Descemet membrane endothelial keratoplasty (DMEK). Cornea. 2015;35(1):14–9.
52. Heindl LM, Riss S, Bachmann BO, Laaser K, Kruse FE, Cursiefen C. Split cornea transplantation for 2 recipients: a new strategy to reduce corneal tissue cost and shortage. Ophthalmology. 2011;118:294–301.
53. Heindl LM, Riss S, Laaser K, Bachmann BO, Kruse FE, Cursiefen C. Split cornea transplantation for 2 recipients – review of the first 100 consecutive patients. Am J Ophthalmol. 2011;152:523–32.
54. Heindl LM, Cursiefen C. Split-cornea transplantation – a novel concept to reduce corneal donor shortage [in German]. Klin Monbl Augenheilkd. 2012;229:608–14.
55. Heindl LM, Cursiefen C. One cornea, two patients: a potential new strategy for tackling donor shortage? Expert Rev Ophthalmol. 2011;6:273–6.
56. Heindl LM, Riss S, Adler W, Bucher F, Hos D, Cursiefen C. Split cornea transplantation: relationship between storage time of split donor tissue and outcome. Ophthalmology. 2013;120:899–907.
57. Heindl LM, Riss S, Adler W, Steven P, Hos D, Cursiefen C. Corneal graft alterations after Descemet stripping: implications for split cornea transplantation. JAMA Ophthalmol. 2013; 131:687–9.
58. Schaub F, Cursiefen C, Heindl LM. Retrospective appraisal of split-cornea transplantation: an audit of 1141 donor corneas. JAMA Ophthalmol. 2015;133(9):1086–7.
59. Vajpayee RB, Sharma N, Jhanji V, Titiyal JS, Tandon R. One donor cornea for 3 recipients: a new concept for corneal transplantation surgery. Arch Ophthalmol. 2007;125:552–4.
60. Lie JT, Groeneveld-van Beek EA, Ham L, van der Wees J, Melles GR. More efficient use of donor corneal tissue with Descemet membrane endothelial keratoplasty (DMEK): two lamellar keratoplasty procedures with one donor cornea. Br J Ophthalmol. 2010;94:1265–6.

61. Lam FC, Baydoun L, Dirisamer M, Lie J, Dapena I, Melles GR. Hemi-Descemet membrane endothelial keratoplasty transplantation: a potential method for increasing the pool of endothelial graft tissue. JAMA Ophthalmol. 2014;132:1469–73.
62. Lam FC, Baydoun L, Satué M, Dirisamer M, Ham L, Melles GR. One year outcome of hemi-Descemet membrane endothelial keratoplasty. Graefes Arch Clin Exp Ophthalmol. 2015;253(11):1955–8.
63. Groeneveld-van Beek EA, Lie JT, van der Wees J, Bruinsma M, Melles GR. Standardized 'no-touch' donor tissue preparation for DALK and DMEK: harvesting undamaged anterior and posterior transplants from the same donor cornea. Acta Ophthalmol. 2013;91:145–50.
64. Feng MT, Burkhart ZN, Price Jr FW, Price MO. Effect of donor preparation-to-use times on Descemet membrane endothelial keratoplasty outcomes. Cornea. 2013;32:1080–2.

Chapter 8
DSAEK and UT-DSAEK in FED: Step-by-Step Approach

Elena Albé, Vincenzo Scorcia, and Massimo Busin

The ideal keratoplasty procedure is one that takes place in a closed system and offers rapid visual rehabilitation improving visual outcomes with a low risk of complications. Descemet stripping automated endothelial keratoplasty (DSAEK) fulfills these requirements and has therefore become the gold standard for surgical treatment of endothelial decompensation [1, 2]. This "onlay" posterior lamellar keratoplasty procedure foresees the transplantation of donor Descemet membrane and endothelium attached to a layer of deep stroma. As a result, a stromal interface is created between donor tissue and recipient stroma, which has been held responsible by some authors for the suboptimal visual results obtained in a variable percentage of patients undergoing this type of surgery [3, 4].

To further improve the results of endothelial keratoplasty, a newer method was introduced by Melles [5], who named it Descemet membrane endothelial keratoplasty (DMEK), as the donor graft consisted of only Descemet membrane and endothelium. In comparison with conventional DSAEK, DMEK has shown faster visual recovery, better visual outcomes, and reduced rejection rates [6–8]. However, DMEK has not gained popularity mainly because it is technically very demanding, and complications in both during and after surgery occur much more frequently than with DSAEK [6, 7]. In addition, the surgical time required for DMEK is usually much longer than that necessary for DSAEK, and unlike DSAEK, it is not suitable for all eyes. As an example, DMEK is not a good choice

E. Albé, MD
Department of Ophthalmology, Humanitas Clinical and Research Center, Milan, Italy

V. Scorcia, MD
Department of Ophthalmology, University of "Magna Graecia", Catanzaro, Italy

M. Busin, MD (✉)
Department of Ophthalmology, Ospedale Privato "Villa Igea", Forlì, Italy

IRFO (Istituto internazionale di Ricerca e Formazione in Oftalmologia), Forlì, Italy
e-mail: mbusin@yahoo.com

C. Cursiefen, A.S. Jun (eds.), *Current Treatment Options for Fuchs Endothelial Dystrophy*, DOI 10.1007/978-3-319-43021-8_8

in cases with positive vitreous pressure or poor visibility of the anterior chamber, or when there is no barrier between anterior chamber and vitreous cavity. Finally, the learning curve of DMEK is accompanied by a high rate of tissue loss (up to 16 % in some reports), an unacceptably high detachment rate of up to 63 %, and a failure rate of up to 8 %, which is higher than that for other procedures [6, 7]. In addition, although up to about 60 % of patients undergoing DMEK in the absence of comorbidities reach 20/20 vision, still about 40 % do not, thus implying factors other than the presence of a stromal interface, as possible determinants for the final visual performance [6, 7].

In 2011, Neff et al. [4] reported post-DSAEK visual results to be better than the post-DMEK ones in patients with grafts thinner than 131 μm, thus correlating for the first-time postoperative vision to the morphologic characteristics of the DSAEK tissue transplanted. Since then, the evidence has been mounting that thinner DSAEK grafts offer a higher chance of 20/20 vision in eyes with no comorbidities. However, all these studies were retrospective in their structure. No surgical method had been standardized in order to minimize graft thickness, and a possible correlation between graft thickness and vision at a certain time after surgery was simply evaluated.

In 2009 we introduced the concept of "ultrathin" (UT) DSAEK, a simple procedure, similar to DSAEK, except that the graft is created with two microkeratome passes with the purpose of obtaining a final donor lamella thinner than 131 μm. The first passes serve to debulk and refine the donor tissue. To date, there is no doubt that the quality of microkeratome endothelial keratoplasty (EK) grafts is far superior to that of femtosecond laser EK grafts.

8.1 To Treat

DSAEK is indicated in patients with endothelial dysfunction, such as Fuchs endothelial dystrophy (FED), pseudophakic or aphakic bullous keratopathy, ICE syndrome, endothelial decompensation after penetrating keratoplasty (PK) or endothelial keratoplasty (EK), buphthalmos, and herpetic endotheliitis. Although more challenging, DSAEK can be performed in phakic eyes as well as in case of aniridia, aphakia, extensive iris trauma, anterior chamber intraocular lenses, and previous glaucoma surgery, either trabeculectomy or aqueous shunt procedures.

8.2 Not to Treat

DSAEK surgery requires the placement of an air bubble intraoperatively that is left in place a couple of hours after the surgery to support the graft in the immediate postoperative period. Therefore, conditions in which retaining a postoperative air bubble would be challenging, like aniridia, significant iris tissue defects, aphakia, anterior chamber intraocular lenses, and previous glaucoma or retinal surgery, trabeculectomy, aqueous shunt procedures, and post-vitrectomized eyes, may be considered a relative contraindication to DSAEK, being the postoperative graft attachment more complicated.

8.3 Surgical Planning

Endothelial dysfunction is assessed by the endothelial cell (EC) density measurement in the central and peripheral cornea using specular microscopy. Corneal thickness is checked by the ultrasound pachymetry or anterior segment optical coherence tomography (OCT). In phakic eyes, the lens status should be considered in the event that a concurrent cataract extraction or IOL exchange needs to be performed. If the assessment of endothelial dysfunction with central guttae and increased central corneal thickness reveals that the peripheral endothelial cell count is fairly high (at least 1800 cells/mm^2), phacoemulsification can be performed rather safely. On the contrary, when the peripheral pool of endothelial cells is low, phacoemulsification with IOL implantation should be performed just before the insertion of the donor DSAEK graft. If a modern flexible open-loop AC-IOL is well positioned and of appropriate size, it may be left in place. A sulcus-, iris-, or transscleral-fixated IOL may be placed when appropriate.

A detailed informed consent has to be provided to all patients undergoing UT-DSAEK. Preoperatively, all patients undergo a complete ophthalmological examination, including slit lamp examination, uncorrected visual acuity (UCVA) and best spectacle-corrected visual acuity (BSCVA), manifest refraction, applanation tonometry, funduscopy, and B-scan ultrasound (when required).

8.4 Surgical Technique: UT-DSAEK Graft Preparation and Transplant

8.4.1 Donor Preparation

After coating the endothelial side with a viscoelastic substance, the donor cornea is mounted on an artificial anterior chamber (AAC) of the ALTK system (Moria, Antony, France). A Moria metal reusable chamber, as well as a disposable version, can be used, which offers several advantages in the preparation of ultrathin lamellae.

Central corneal thickness (CCT) is initially measured using ultrasound pachymetry (Alcon, Fort Worth, TX). The first debulking cut is performed using a Carriazo-Barraquer (CB) microkeratome with a 300-μm head, just as one would normally create a conventional DSAEK graft. Pachymetry should be performed again following this debulking step to determine the actual thickness of the tissue.

Of all the factors that can affect the graft depth, the most important is pressure. The pressure in the system is standardized to an ideal level of 80–90 mmHg by raising the infusion bottle to a height of 120 cm above the level of the AAC and then clamping the inflation tubing at 50 cm from the entrance into the AAC.

The second cut or refinement cut is made with a 90, 110, or 130-μm microkeratome head, depending on the thickness of the residual tissue, with the goal of ultimately creating a graft approximately 100 μm or less in thickness. The bottle has to be kept still at the 120 cm height. In addition, maximal care is taken to maintain a uniform, slow movement of the hand-driven microkeratome, requiring a time between 4 and 6 s for each of the two dissections in all cases. For the second cut, the head should be oriented with the dovetail 180° away from where the first cut was initiated and the dissection performed in the opposite direction. This results in a much more planar graft. The new Moria disposable chamber has a rotating guide ring that makes it easier to move the location for initiating the second pass. In addition, the new chamber creates a larger-diameter graft. Typically, the diameter of the graft is reduced with each successive pass, but the disposable artificial chamber enables the surgeon performing the double-pass technique to create a graft that is 1–2 mm larger than the one made with the reusable chamber. The resulting tissue is very thin but it stays flat, so it behaves like a DSAEK graft and is much easier to manipulate than a DMEK graft.

The stromal side of the resulting tissue is marked to facilitate correct intraoperative orientation of the graft. The posterior donor lamella is placed on a Barron punch with the endothelial side up and cut to the desired diameter (8.5–9.0 mm).

Recently we introduced a nomogram to allow a reliable single-pass microkeratome-assisted lamellar dissection of the donor tissue with disposable heads of different sizes (Moria ALTK system; Moria SA), creating consistently thin and symmetric grafts without loss of tissue. The main graft thickness measured between 1 and 3 months postoperatively compares favorably with the results reported for double-pass microkeratome-assisted dissection of UT-DSAEK [9].

Figure 8.1 shows the OCT images of the donor tissue obtained (**a**) before debulking cut, (**b**) after debulking cut, and (**c**) after refinement cut.

8.4.2 Surgical Technique

Patients are sedated with intravenous droperidol, 3 mL (7.5 mg), immediately before the peribulbar injection of local anesthetic, which consists of a mixture of 10 mL of L-bupivacaine, 0.75 %, and 100 IU of hyaluronidase. The entire procedure is performed with the surgeon sitting at the 12 o'clock position.

A marker 9 mm in diameter can be used at the beginning of the procedure to outline the limits of the internal surface from which the endothelium is peeled off.

Then the anterior chamber is entered at the 12 o'clock position with a 25-gauge needle mounted on a 2.5-mL empty syringe.

Aqueous (approximately 0.2–0.4 mL) is aspirated and air is injected, filling the anterior chamber.

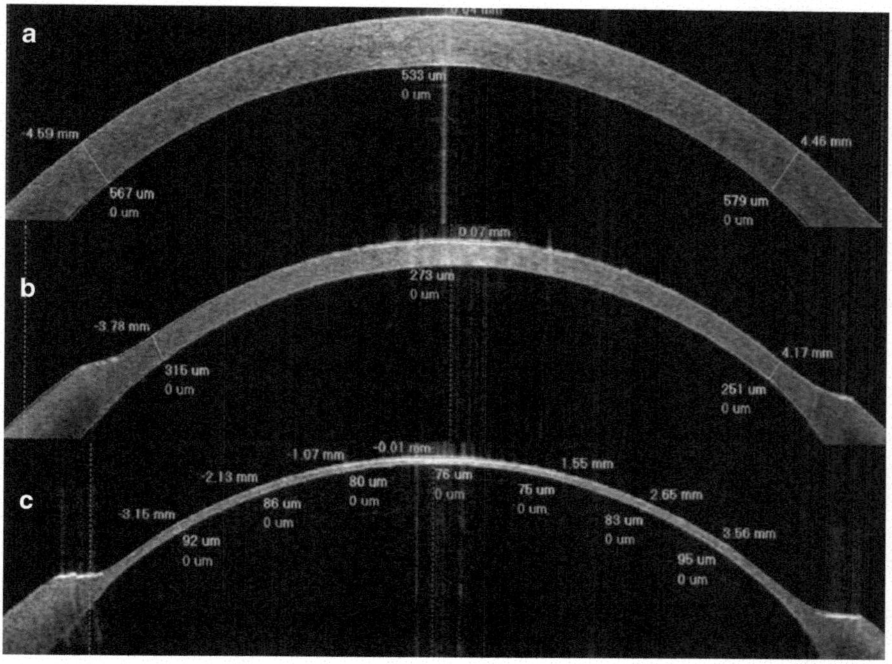

Fig. 8.1 Optical coherence tomography images of donor tissue obtained (**a**) before debulking cut, (**b**) after debulking cut, and (**c**) after refinement cut

A 25-gauge blunt cannula mounted on a syringe is introduced and used to cut through the endothelium and Descemet membrane, following the contour of the superficial mark. The cannula is therefore used to sweep away the endothelium and Descemet membrane, usually in a single piece. Whenever air is lost, the anterior chamber is reformed by injecting additional air with the syringe. Performing the entire maneuver under air enables perfect visualization of the Descemet membrane (no dye is ever used) and eliminates the need for any viscoelastic substance in the anterior chamber.

A clear cornea tunnel, 1 mm long and 3.2 mm wide, is prepared nasally.

At this point, an inferior peripheral iridectomy is performed, if not already present.

An anterior chamber maintainer is placed at the 12 o'clock position to enable continuous irrigation while performing the next surgical steps.

After punching the donor tissue to the desired size, the hollow of the punching block is filled with balanced salt solution (BSS) and the tissue left to float on the liquid cushion. The donor tissue is not folded and therefore inserted into the anterior chamber with the so-called taco technique. A corneal forceps is used to grasp the edge of the graft and drag it onto the plate of the side platform of a modified Busin glide (mini-glide or Mini Busin spatula) used to scoop the tissue, keeping the endothelial side up. As the funnel of the modified glide is smaller than the conventional

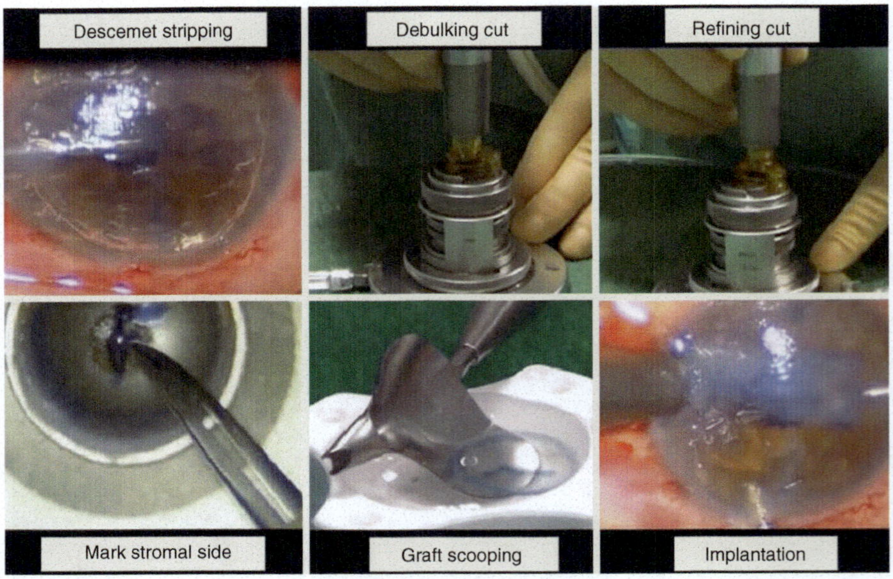

Fig. 8.2 Photographs showing the steps of the surgical technique from Descemet stripping, debulking cut, refining cut, tissue marking, graft scooping, and implantation using the pull-through technique

glide, the tip can be inserted into the wound during delivery, thus preventing squeezing of the tissue while entering the anterior chamber through the corneal incision.

The tissue is pulled into the funnel-shaped part of the Busin glide using a microincision forceps until it engages the mini-glide opening.

A side entry is created temporally.

The mini-glide is then inverted and positioned at the entrance of the nasal clear cornea tunnel. The same microincision forceps (held in the left hand when operating on the left eye and in the right hand when operating on the right eye) is inserted through the side entry and passed across the anterior chamber, exiting throughout the clear cornea tunnel to grab the graft from the mini-glide and drag it into the anterior chamber. No additional viscoelastic substance is required during insertion. The donor lamella is allowed to unfold spontaneously under continuous irrigation from the anterior chamber maintainer. When necessary, centration of the graft is achieved by gentle tapping on the corneal surface.

Figure 8.2 shows the different steps of the surgical procedure.

Both the clear cornea tunnel and the side entry are sutured watertight with interrupted 10-0 nylon sutures. The graft is attached to the posterior corneal surface by filling the anterior chamber with air injected through the temporal side entry.

Triamcinolone acetonide and gentamicin sulfate, 0.3 %, are injected subconjunctivally at the end of the procedure.

8.5 Results

In patients undergoing a triple procedure (UT-DSAEK and phacoemulsification with IOL implantation), phacoemulsification and IOL implantation are performed prior to UT-DSAEK surgery. No viscoelastics have to be used throughout the procedure; capsulorrhexis is performed using a bent needle mounted on a syringe filled with saline to maintain a closed system, while the IOL is implanted under continuous irrigation from an anterior chamber maintainer placed at the 12 o'clock position. The anterior chamber maintainer has to be inserted through a side port constructed with a 15°-disposable blade introduced in the anterior chamber under continuous irrigation delivered by the irrigation-aspiration system throughout the main port. Intracameral acetylcholine chloride is used to constrict the pupil prior to UT-DSAEK surgery.

8.6 Postoperative Care

After surgery, patients are instructed to lie supine for at least 2 h. Once this period is passed, the patients are examined about 3 h after surgery at the slit lamp to check if the graft is fully attached and in position. Some air is removed from one of the side ports using a blunt cannula if no aqueous has entered the anterior chamber from behind the iris through the inferior peripheral iridectomy.

When the graft detaches from the recipient stroma and a false chamber is seen, the graft has to be repositioned, preferably in the operating room, injecting air into the anterior chamber similarly to what is done during the primary surgery. The supine position is requested again for about 2 h.

In dubious cases, particularly when the space between the cornea and donor tissue is minimal, anterior segment optical coherence tomography (ASOCT) can be used to help diagnosing the presence of a double chamber.

Postoperatively, all patients are given topical tobramycin, 0.3 %, and dexamethasone, 0.1 %, suspension (TobraDex; Alcon, Fort Worth, Texas) combination therapy every 2 h for 2 weeks, then every 3 h for 2 additional weeks. The treatment is switched to pure steroidal eyedrops (dexamethasone 0.1 %) qid for 1 month, tid for 1 month, bid for 1 month, then finally qd to be continued indefinitely unless the patient is aphakic or steroid responder.

All sutures are removed in all cases between 4 and 6 weeks from surgery.

8.7 Complications

Primary complications associated with UT-DSAEK usually occur during the preparation of the donor tissue. Graft dislocation and primary graft failure follow in the list as more frequent complications.

Microkeratome-related complications were recorded in 7.2 % of all the dissections performed in our original work [8]. All complications occurred during the second refinement pass. Buttonholing with incomplete central dissection of the donor tissue can be handled by means of hand refinement and the tissue still used. Perforation occurred, with tissue being discarded or used anyway depending on the location of the perforation; punching the tissue eccentrically was compatible with rather peripheral sites of perforation. Improper dissection outside of the 9-mm zone, i.e., at the very end of the cut, was compatible with the normal use of the tissue. Complications during the refinement cut were more common with the use of a 50-μm microkeratome head and to a lesser extent with a 90-μm microkeratome head.

Postoperatively, graft detachment and dislocation occurred in 4.6 % of all cases. Total detachment was seen in most cases and generally successfully managed by re-bubbling (with a single or double injection). When the detachment is limited to the periphery of the graft, there is usually no interference with the vision and therefore it is not treated. Postoperative graft dislocation requiring air reinjection occurred much less often than reported after DMEK by Price et al. [6] and Guerra et al. [9] (60 %) and Laaser et al. (92 %) [10].

Primary endothelial graft failure was recorded in 2 % of the cases at 12 months follow-up and was generally successfully treated with systemic steroid treatment (1 g per kg of body weight), sub-Tenon steroid injections (Depo-Medrol every 2 weeks), and topical steroid drops. The success of the therapy depends on the delay of patient presentation to the ophthalmic care, being higher in patients presenting with initial and mild symptoms like mild loss of vision, glare, haloes, and redness.

Additional complications of the procedure include pupillary block, which is immediately treated by dilation and/or air removal at the slit lamp, persistent epithelial defect, cystoid macular edema, persistent interface haze, interface infections, and cataract formation.

Once established, Urrets-Zavalia syndrome requires surgical treatment (pupilloplasty).

Persistent epithelial defects are treated with bandage soft contact lenses and antibiotic ointment up to reepithelialization.

Cystoid macular edema is treated with systemic dorzolamide and nonsteroid anti- inflammatory medications. Intravitreal injections are seldom required.

Interface bacterial or fungal infections, which are resistant to conservative multispectrum antibiotic treatment, are surgically faced by "en bloc" removal of the recipient cornea and DSAEK graft and replaced by full-thickness keratoplasty, thus eliminating the interface infections "tout court."

The incidence of early cataract formation in phakic eyes could be significantly reduced by modifying the incision site from 3 and 9 o'clock position to 2 and 10 o'clock position delivering the graft through a clear cornea tunnel with Busin glide and pulling it with proper forceps more superiorly than the level of the pupil aperture.

8.8 UT-DSAEK Results

The prospective data from a large clinical series of 285 ultrathin DSAEK eyes by M. Busin has documented the benefits of the procedure at 2 years after surgery. This procedure offers the potential to achieve the visual results of DMEK with the ease of handling and tissue preparation of DSAEK.

The basic benefit of ultrathin DSAEK is a faster visual recovery than conventional DSAEK and an equivalent visual recovery than DMEK. The proportion of eyes achieving final acuity of 20/20 is higher than either conventional DSAEK or DMEK.

In addition, comparing UT-DSAEK to DSAEK and DMEK, all three offer an acceptable rate of cell loss.

8.8.1 Visual Outcomes

As early as 1 month postoperatively with all sutures still in place, BSCVA ≥20/20 was recorded in 11.7 % and BSCVA ≥20/40 in 63.8 %, of all eyes. BSCVA kept on improving over time, with a percentage of patients reaching 20/20 or better of 26.4 % at 6 months, 39.5 % at 1 year, and 48.8 % at 2 years after DSAEK. In particular, phakic patients younger than age 50 performed best, with 76.5 % of them reaching a BSCVA ≥20/20 as early as 6 months after UT-DSAEK.

The steep curve obtained for the UT-DSAEK values shows a continuous improvement in average logMAR BSCVA from 0.76 ± 0.49 preoperatively, to 0.35 ± 0.40 at 1 month, 0.16 ± 0.13 at 3 months, 0.12 ± 0.12 at 6 months, 0.08 ± 0.12 at 1 year, and 0.03 ± 0.09 at 2 years after UT-DSAEK, respectively.

Quite strikingly, the mean postoperative logMAR BSCVA curves of UT-DSAEK and DMEK almost overlap throughout the entire follow-up period considered, whereas the one of conventional DSAEK remains at a lower level [9, 11]. The speed of visual recovery after UT-DSAEK is somewhat slower than that recorded after DMEK, but as early as 1 year postoperatively, the percentage of eyes with BSCVA of 20/20 or better are substantially identical [9]. Based on this report, in terms of 20/20 visual recovery, UT-DSAEK performs much better than conventional DSAEK as early as 1 year in the postoperative course, with about three times as many patients achieving 20/20 or better vision.

The visual outcome recorded after UT-DSAEK indicates that the use of thin grafts allows a higher number of eyes to achieve a better visual performance in a shorter period of time than after DSAEK. However, not differently than after DMEK, the percentage of eyes without comorbidities recovering 20/20 vision after UT-DSAEK is lower than expected [6, 9, 12, 13]. This indicates that probably other factors besides the presence of a stromal interface of any type can determine the final visual result of EK. Patel et al. [14] demonstrated a small peak in corneal backscatter originating from the posterior stroma of the recipient cornea, which could be related to long-standing edema and consequent anatomical and functional changes in this part of the cornea. Recovery of normal stromal architecture might very often require a prolonged period of time, during which vision would be negatively affected. If this were true, the excellent results obtained in the eyes of younger patients undergoing phakic UT-DSAEK would be a simple consequence of a "better" recipient cornea.

Recently, Rudolph et al. [15] have reported that DSAEK increased posterior corneal high-order aberrations (HOAs), whereas DMEK displayed only minor changes in posterior corneal HOAs, possibly explaining this way to the different visual performances. Irregularity in the thickness of DSAEK grafts seems to be the main reason for this finding. Indeed it is a common experience that the microkeratome cuts deeper at the beginning than at the end of the dissection, especially if no closed-system condition is employed during the maneuver. The double-pass technique overcomes this problem by performing a second cut from the direction opposite to the one utilized for the first cut. As a result, the final thickness is similar at both ends of the dissection, and posterior corneal HOAs should be minimized.

8.8.2 *Refractive Outcomes*

The negative cylinder remained practically unchanged after UT-DSAEK (0.1 D of difference 1 year postoperatively), similarly to what was recorded after DMEK [6, 9]. Instead, a significant induced cylinder (up to 0.6 D) has been reported by several authors after DSAEK [16–19]. The most probable explanation for this is in the different size of the wound utilized for graft delivery with the different techniques. UT-DSAEK grafts can be delivered through a 3-mm wound by means of a modified mini-Busin glide, without squeezing the tissue, whereas this is less possible for thicker grafts.

After UT-DSAEK, a statistically significant ($p < 0.001$) hyperopic shift of about 0.75 D was found in the spherical equivalent (SE). After DSAEK, several authors have reported a substantially higher significant hyperopic shift (up to 1.5 D) in the SE [20–24]. The change in the posterior corneal curvature caused by the attachment of a meniscus-shaped donor graft was the main cause of the hyperopic shift recorded. However, factors other than the change of posterior corneal curvature could also play a role. Indeed, even after DMEK single procedures, Price et al. [6] and Guerra et al. [9] reported a statistically significant hyperopic shift in the SE at 3 months and to a lesser extent at 1 year postoperatively [6, 9].

Kwon et al. [25] found out that in Fuchs dystrophy, edema is usually located primarily in the central cornea, the posterior bulging of which causes the flattening of the posterior curvature with a consequent myopic shift. The mean forward displacement of the posterior surface of the cornea of DMEK eyes of this series increased postoperatively by 69 μm because of corneal deturgescence occurring as early as 1 month after surgery, thus reverting the myopic shift, or in other words, causing a hyperopic shift. This mechanism could well explain the presence of a hyperopic shift also after UT-DSAEK, despite the use of thin, "fairly plano" grafts.

8.8.3 Endothelial Cell Density

The mean endothelial cell density in the donor corneas was 2510 ± 154 (range 2100–3000). The mean endothelial cell loss at 3, 6, 12, and 24 months was 29.8 % ± 14.3 %, 33 % ± 21.1 %, 35.6 % ± 20.2 %, and 36.6 % ± 23.9 %, respectively, substantially identical to that recorded after DSAEK [16, 26–29] and DMEK [9, 30], showing that a double microkeratome pass does not affect endothelial survival. Also stabilization of cell loss is achieved as early as 1 year after UT-DSAEK, in accordance to what is seen after DSAEK. At 1 year, the endothelial cell (EC) loss was about the same as seen with DSAEK, despite the fact that the UT grafts were transplanted through a much smaller (3.0-mm) incision. In the past, a higher rate of EC loss was seen with smaller incisions because there is a typically more extensive manipulation of the tissue.

One year after UT-DSAEK, the endothelial cell loss was significantly higher in glaucoma patients overall ($p = 0.038$). Although this was reported also after DSAEK [31], the explanation for an increased cell loss remains unclear. The physical presence of a shunt in the anterior chamber may contribute to mechanical damage of the donor tissue, but normal levels of intraocular pressure controlled either by medication or by the effect of filtering surgery should be compatible with normal endothelial survival.

8.8.4 Graft Thickness (GT)

A high 98.5 % of eyes had a central thickness of the grafted lamella below 151 μm, 89 % of eyes had a central GT below 131 μm, and 69 % of eyes below 101 μm. Three months postoperatively, the mean central GT ± SD was 75.33 ± 25.9 μm, the mean peripheral 95.03 ± 36.85 μm was 92.30 ± 38.04 μm nasally, and 97.77 ± 35.66 μm temporally. The peripheral GT was significantly higher than central GT ($p < 0.0001$), but did not differ statistically between temporal and nasal side ($p = 0.0842$). The average graft thickness of DSAEK is 175 ± 38 μm. With the single-pass technique by 3 months postoperatively, 41/42 (97 %) of the grafts were of thickness ≤130 μm and 38/42 (90 %) of the grafts were of central thickness ≤100 μm [9]. Thinner grafts obtained with UT-DSAEK manifest quite ease of handling, which although not quite as easy as DSAEK, was far superior to DMEK.

8.8.5 Graft Survival

Despite 1.4 % of primary failure (the cornea not cleared by the first-month exam) and 1.4 % secondary failure (late endothelial decompensation) which required a regraft, the Kaplan-Meier graft survival probability at 1, 3, 6, 12, and 24 months was 98.6, 98.23, 97.82, 97.82, and 96.16 %, respectively [8]. All failed grafts were successfully regrafted with UT-DSAEK grafts. To date, no data is available about

DMEK graft survival probability. One-year graft survival for DSAEK in series excluding the initial learning curve of surgeons has been reported to vary between 94 and 100 % [1, 2, 16, 22, 28, 32]. Price reported recently a DSAEK graft survival rate at 5 years of 93 %, with a significantly higher value for Fuchs patients (95 %) than for patients with pseudophakic bullous keratopathy (76 %) or previous glaucoma surgery (40 %) [26].

The risk for immunologic rejection is higher in case of previous PK surgery. Rejection episodes can be reversed with corticosteroids 1 week after the onset of the rejection. The Kaplan-Meier cumulative probability of a rejection episode at 3, 6, 12, and 24 months was 0, 0.41, 2.44, and 3.27 %, respectively. From this data, it appears clearly that immunologic rejection can complicate the postoperative course of UT-DSAEK in a much lower percentage of cases than that of DSAEK [8]. Instead, the contradictory evidence in different articles of a higher rejection probability (2.44 % for UT-DSAEK versus 1 % for DMEK) but a lower rejection rate (2.8 % for UT-DSAEK versus 5.7 % for DMEK) at 1 year probably indicates a similarly low incidence of immunologic rejection with UT-DSAEK and DMEK [8].

8.9 Conclusions

Many authors claim that final visual acuity following DSAEK is suboptimal, with fewer eyes than expected achieving 20/20 vision, possibly because of the presence of a stromal interface [1–3, 17]. In comparison to most of the DSAEK series published to date, DMEK has shown a decisive improvement in terms of speed of visual recovery, percentage of patients achieving 20/20 vision, as well as rate of immunologic rejection [6–9]. However, ease of graft preparation, manipulation, delivery, and attachment, as well as feasibility of the procedure for eyes with complicated anatomy or poor intraoperative visualization, limits the use of DMEK even in the hands of an experienced corneal surgeon. Ideally, every surgeon would like to use grafts that can be manipulated as easily as DSAEK ones are, but produce the same visual results of DMEK grafts. UT-DSAEK is a technique aimed at reproducibly preparing DSAEK grafts usually thinner than 100 μm, with a double- or single microkeratome pass. In conclusion, UT-DSAEK is a procedure that shares the improved visual outcome and lower immunologic rejection rate of DMEK over DSAEK, while minimizing all types of postoperative complications. In addition, similarly to DSAEK and unlike DMEK, UT-DSAEK can be performed in all types of eyes, even in those with complicated anatomy (i.e., free communication between the anterior chamber and vitreous cavity as in aphakia, the presence of anterior chamber IOLs, etc.) or poor anterior chamber visualization [6, 9]. Finally, unlike DMEK grafts, UT-DSAEK grafts can be routinely dissected even by relatively inexperienced eye bank technicians and easily evaluated, thus reducing tissue waste and further improving the quality of tissue to be transplanted.

References

1. Lee WB, Jacobs DS, Musch DC, et al.; Ophthalmic Technology Assessment Committee Cornea and Anterior Segment Disorders Panel. Descemet's stripping endothelial keratoplasty: safety and outcomes: a report by the American Academy of Ophthalmology. Ophthalmology. 2009;116:1818–30.
2. Anshu A, Price MO, Tan DT, Price FW. Endothelial keratoplasty: a revolution in evolution. Survey Ophthalmol. 2012;57(3):236–52.
3. Letko E, Price DA, Lindoso EM, et al. Secondary graft failure and repeat endothelial keratoplasty after Descemet's stripping automated endothelial keratoplasty. Ophthalmology. 2011;118:310–4.
4. Neff KD, Biber JM, Holland EJ. Comparison of central corneal graft thickness to visual acuity outcomes in endothelial keratoplasty. Cornea. 2011;30:388–91.
5. Melles GR, Lander F, Rietveld FJ. Transplantation of Descemet's membrane carrying viable endothelium through a small scleral incision. Cornea. 2002;21:415–8.
6. Price MO, Giebel AW, Fairchild KM, Price FW. Descemet's membrane endothelial keratoplasty: prospective multicenter study of visual and refractive outcomes and endothelial survival. Ophthalmology. 2009;116:2361–8.
7. Guerra FP, Anshu A, Price MO, Giebel AW, Price FW. Descemet's membrane endothelial keratoplasty: prospective study of 1-year visual outcomes, graft survival, and endothelial cell loss. Ophthalmology. 2011;118:2368–73.
8. Busin M, Albé E. Does thickness matter: ultrathin descemet stripping automated endothelial keratoplasty. Curr Opin Ophthalmol. 2014;25(4):312–8.
9. Nahum Y, Leon P, Busin M. Postoperative graft thickness obtained with single-pass microkeratome-assisted ultrathin descemet stripping automated endothelial keratoplasty. Cornea. 2015;34(11):1362–4.
10. Laaser K, Bachmann BO, Horn FK, et al. Donor tissue culture conditions and outcome after Descemet membrane endothelial keratoplasty. Am J Ophthalmol. 2011;151:1007–18.
11. Li JY, Terry MA, Goshe J, Davis-Boozer D, Shamie N. Three-year visual acuity outcomes after descemet's stripping automated endothelial keratoplasty. Ophthalmology. 2012;119(6):1126–9.
12. Ham L, Balachandran C, Verschoor CA, et al. Visual rehabilitation rate after isolated descemet membrane transplantation: descemet membrane endothelial keratoplasty. Arch Ophthalmol. 2009;127:252–5.
13. Ham L, Dapena I, van Luijk C, et al. Descemet membrane endothelial keratoplasty (DMEK) for Fuchs endothelial dystrophy: review of the first 50 consecutive cases. Eye (Lond). 2009;23:1990–8.
14. Patel SV, Baratz KH, Hodge DO, et al. The effect of corneal light scatter on vision after descemet stripping with endothelial keratoplasty. Arch Ophthalmol. 2009;127:153–60.
15. Rudolph M, Laaser K, Bachmann BO, Cursiefen C, Epstein D, Kruse FE. Corneal higher-order aberrations after Descemet's membrane endothelial keratoplasty. Ophthalmology. 2012;119(3):528–35.
16. Busin M, Bhatt PR, Scorcia V. A modified technique for Descemet membrane stripping automated endothelial keratoplasty to minimize endothelial cell loss. Arch Ophthalmol. 2008;126(8):1133–7.
17. Price MO, Price Jr FW. Descemet's stripping with endothelial keratoplasty: comparative outcomes with microkeratome-dissected and manually dissected donor tissue. Ophthalmology. 2006;113:1936–42.
18. Gorovoy MS. Descemet-stripping automated endothelial keratoplasty. Cornea. 2006;25:886–9.
19. Terry MA, Shamie N, Chen ES, et al. Endothelial keratoplasty for Fuchs' dystrophy with cataract: complications and clinical results with the new triple procedure. Ophthalmology. 2009;116:631–9.

20. Jun B, Kuo AN, Afshari NA, et al. Refractive change after Descemet stripping automated endothelial keratoplasty surgery and its correlation with graft thickness and diameter. Cornea. 2009;28:19–23.
21. Price MO, Baig KM, Brubaker JW, Price Jr FW. Randomized, prospective comparison of precut vs surgeon-dissected grafts for Descemet stripping automated endothelial keratoplasty. Am J Ophthalmol. 2008;146:36–41.
22. Yoo SH, Kymionis GD, Deobhakta AA, et al. One-year results and anterior segment optical coherence tomography findings of Descemet stripping automated endothelial keratoplasty combined with phacoemulsification. Arch Ophthalmol. 2008;126:1052–5.
23. Koenig SB, Covert DJ, Dupps Jr WJ, Meisler DM. Visual acuity, refractive error, and endothelial cell density six months after Descemet stripping and automated endothelial keratoplasty (DSAEK). Cornea. 2007;26:670–4.
24. Koenig SB, Covert DJ. Early results of small-incision Descemet's stripping and automated endothelial keratoplasty. Ophthalmology. 2007;114:221–6.
25. Kwon RO, Price MO, Price Jr FW, et al. Pentacam characterization of corneas with Fuchs dystrophy treated with Descemet membrane endothelial keratoplasty. J Refract Surg. 2010;26:972–9.
26. Price MO, Fairchild KM, Price DA, Price FW. Descemet's stripping endothelial keratoplasty: five-year graft survival and endothelial cell loss. Ophthalmology. 2011;118:725–9.
27. Basak SK. Descemet stripping and endothelial keratoplasty in endothelial dysfunctions: three-month results in 75 eyes. Indian J Ophthalmol. 2008;56:291–6.
28. Price MO, Price Jr FW. Endothelial cell loss after Descemet stripping with endothelial keratoplasty: influencing factors and 2-year trend. Ophthalmology. 2008;115:857–65.
29. Mearza AA, Qureshi MA, Rostron CK. Experience and 12-month results of Descemet-stripping endothelial keratoplasty (DSEK) with a small-incision technique. Cornea. 2007;26:279–83.
30. Ham L, van Luijk C, Dapena I, et al. Endothelial cell density after Descemet membrane endothelial keratoplasty: 1- to 2-year follow-up. Am J Ophthalmol. 2009;148:521–7.
31. Kim P, Amiran MD, Lichtinger A, Yeng SN, Slomovic AR, Rotman DS. Outcomes of descemet stripping automated endothelial keratoplasty in patients with previous glaucoma drainage device insertion. Cornea. 2012;31(2):172–5.
32. Terry MA, Shamie N, Chen ES, et al. Endothelial keratoplasty: the influence of preoperative donor endothelial cell densities on dislocation, primary graft failure, and 1-year cell counts. Cornea. 2008;27:1131–7.

Chapter 9
DSAEK (Not Only) in Asian Eyes: What Glide to Use? Optimised Insertion Techniques

Geraint P. Williams and Donald T.H. Tan

9.1 Introduction

Dysfunction or irreparable loss of the corneal endothelium necessitates replacement with the donated corneal tissue. Historically this has been achieved by the means of a full-thickness corneal transplantation in the form of a penetrating keratoplasty (PK). More recently the advent of the selective transplantation of corneal endothelium, endothelial keratoplasty (EK), has been achieved and increasingly adopted as an alternative to PK [62].

Corneal transplantation has evolved from a full-thickness procedure (penetrating keratoplasty) to the selective use of lamellar tissue including deep anterior lamellar surgery (DALK) and Descemet stripping automated endothelial keratoplasty (DSAEK). These approaches offer advantages including maintaining the integrity of the globe, reducing the effects of suture-related irregular astigmatism, reducing the chance of corneal graft rejection and improving the speed of postoperative recovery [2, 33].

Although a method for transplanting the endothelium was described over 30 years ago, with further experimental techniques over the course of the next 10 years [14, 43, 48], a sutureless approach was first successfully undertaken by Melles nearly 20 years ago [45]. This method involving the separation of the endothelium and posterior stroma by lamellar dissection of donor tissue, the stripping of the host endothelium and the insertion of graft material has become the cornerstone of accepted current approaches.

Several different approaches have been described for the preparation of graft material including manual dissection and automation through the use of microkeratomes. The optimal means of attaching the corneal endothelial tissue to the host

G.P. Williams, PhD, FRCOphth • D.T.H. Tan, FRCSG, FRCSED, FRCOphth (✉)
Singapore National Eye Centre, Singapore, Singapore
e-mail: donald.tan.t.h@snec.com.sg

C. Cursiefen, A.S. Jun (eds.), *Current Treatment Options for Fuchs Endothelial Dystrophy*, DOI 10.1007/978-3-319-43021-8_9

stroma and minimising endothelial cell loss has evolved from the insertion of the tissue by simple folding and pulling techniques to utilising glides to support the graft through to the adoption of cartridge-based injection devises. This chapter will focus on the unique challenges presented by EK for Asian eyes and how a systematic approach to a safer and more consistent EK surgery was undertaken, a culmination in the development of an insertion device, the EndoGlide.

9.2 Disease Profile and Surgical Challenges in Southeast Asia

Singapore has a challenging mixture of patients including anatomical differences in Asian eyes such as small anterior chambers (ACs) and the presentation of advanced diseases from surrounding countries.

Anthropological studies of the anterior segment anatomy have revealed important differences between the eyes of patients from Asia compared to Caucasian patients. Much of the literature describing endothelial keratoplasty originated from European and North American centres, with higher Caucasian populations [17, 21, 45, 50, 51, 64]. It is clear that the anatomical space available to undertake the removal and insertion of corneal endothelium is less in some of the predominant ethnic groups in Southeast Asia [4, 5, 61, 69, 72]. Large-scale studies using optical coherence tomography (OCT) have demonstrated that even in open angles, the anterior chamber depth (ACD) is significantly shallower in American Chinese populations (2.77 mm ± 0.30 SD) compared to Caucasians (3.04 mm ± 0.33 SD), $p<0.0001$ [69]. Further evaluation among Singaporean Chinese, Malay and Indian ethnic groups have confirmed shallower anterior chambers but also demonstrated that although ACD is broadly similar among these populations (2.71–2.77 mm), other differences are observed. These include posterior corneal arc length (PCAL)/anterior chamber width (ACW) (which are lower in Chinese populations) and also the variability among Asian groups including anterior and posterior corneal curvature and central corneal thickness [4, 5, 61, 69, 72] and a propensity for higher vitreous pressure. These are summarised in Table 9.1. In the era of extracapsular surgery, requiring involving a large corneal or limbal wound, surgeons who are familiar with operating on Asian eyes understand appreciated the greater propensity for iris prolapse and loss of the anterior chamber due to higher vitreous pressure throughout the extracapsular procedure, and while this is somewhat can be mitigated by partial wound closure and the use of viscoelastic material in the AC, but these options are not available in EK surgery during donor insertion. These data suggest of course that the approaches to the safe removal and replacement of corneal endothelium may need modification and tailoring among populations with anatomically smaller eyes.

Historically, the principle indication for undertaking corneal transplantation for endothelial diseases in Singapore (with a predominance of Chinese (73 %) followed by Malay (12 %) and Indian patients (11 %)) over a 15-year period (1991–2006) was pseudophakic bullous keratopathy (PBK) (23 %) with only 7.1 % accounted for by Fuchs' endothelial dystrophy (FED) and 12.4 % regrafting procedures [19, 63].

Table 9.1 Anterior chamber characteristics of Asian subpopulations in Singapore and comparative American Caucasian/Chinese populations

Ethnic group	PCAL/ACW mm (SD)	ACD mm (SD)	CCT mm (SD)	ACC mm (SD)	PCC mm (SD)
Chinese	11.74 (0.42)[a]–12.92 (0.54)	2.31–2.77 (0.3)[a]	562 (32)–568 (33)	7.15 (0.34)–7.36 (0.37)	6.44 (0.36)–6.67 (0.34)
Indian	12.41 (0.51)–13.85 (0.54)	2.72 (0.37)	562 (34)	7.16 (0.4)–7.17 (0.34)	6.45 (0.35)–6.43 (0.37)
Malay	12.75 (0.51)–13.95 (0.51)	2.77 (0.34)–2.78 (0.34)	550 (37)	7.43 (0.37)–7.50 (0.42)	6.45 (0.35)–6.77 (0.36)
Caucasian	12.31 (0.44)[a]	2.48–3.04 (0.33)[a]	–	–	–

The characteristics of the anterior chamber and cornea defined by OCT are outlined. Comparative data for Chinese and Caucasian populations are presented in one series and for individual Singaporean populations in three large series [4, 5, 61, 69, 72]

PCAL posterior corneal arc length, *ACW* anterior chamber width, *PCC* posterior corneal curvature, *ACD* anterior chamber depth, *CCT* central corneal thickness, *ACC* anterior corneal curvature

[a]Direct comparison between Chinese and Caucasian populations

More recent data from the Singapore Corneal Transplant Study has indicated that the rate of PBK is proportionally even higher, up to 34 % [60].

In other countries outside of Asia, a similar high proportion of grafts were historically undertaken for PBK (25 %) in Australia with 7 % for dystrophies and 18 % regrafts [71]. These figures were mirrored from a German data from the same period with 9.5 % of grafts being undertaken for FED, 33 % for PBK and 22 % regrafts between 1996 and 2000 in Berlin [15]. Twenty-six to twenty-eight percent of keratoplasties in the Wills Eye Hospital between 1989 and 2005 were also undertaken for PBK, and 10.8–15.77 % were for FED and 17.8–22 % were regrafts [32]. A large, single centre US data also showed that PBK previously accounted for more corneal transplantation (PK) than FED (32.1 % vs. 23 %, respectively) in the Midwestern United States between 1982 and 1996 [27]. The Swedish registry revealed FED as an indication for PK in 15 % and PBK in 22 % [23]. In the United Kingdom (UK), by contrast, between 1990 and 1999 in a single, large centre study, revealed a smaller proportion of patients who underwent corneal transplantation for PBK (7.6 %), 9.3 % for FED but a remarkably higher percentage were regrafts (40.3 %) [1]. Interestingly of the high proportion of regrafts, 58.3 % were for endothelial failure or rejection. For the following decade (1999–2009), in the UK as a whole the proportion of grafts undertaken for FED continued to increase from 17.3 to 22.3 %, while the number of grafts for PBK remained stable at 14 %, while the proportion of regrafts increased from 11.9 to 16 % during the same period [35]. Similarly, the US data highlights a shift in the indication for the transplantation from PBK to FED during the last decade (as high as 80% for FED in some centres) [22, 24, 52], which is discussed further in this chapter and elsewhere (See Chap. 6).

There are other unique challenges in Asia including viral causes of endothelial failure such as cytomegalovirus (CMV) endotheliitis [20, 41]. Not only is an infectious aetiology unusual as a primary cause of endothelial failure but also presents challenges in differentiating episodes of reactivation from conventional rejection and indeed rejection as a result of reactivation of CMV.

Endothelial dysfunction has been managed historically by undertaking PK. The 5-year graft survival rates in Singapore with this procedure up to 2006 were 58.6, 50.1 and 18.3 % for FED, PBK and regrafts, respectively [63]. This represented an overall (including all indications for transplant) 5-year graft survival of 63.7 %, lower than the commensurate Australian registry data at 72 % and UK at 82 % [55, 71]. It is important to note that the success of transplantation internationally for PBK is lower, and this is reflected in the higher proportion of these cases in Asia.

The time period that these data pertain to also overlap with a paradigm shift in how corneal transplant was approached for endothelial disease. The details of the evolution from full thickness to selective endothelial transplantation are covered extensively in Chapters 6. Briefly however, the potential for undertaking a partial-thickness graft offered greater mechanical stability, a reduction in postoperative astigmatism, a theoretical reduction in antigen load and therefore a reduction in graft rejection and a faster postoperative recovery. The challenge represented by EK was on safe and reliable insertion of the graft material without a large incision. If one considers the analogy of a mechanical puzzle, the issue is akin to how one might go about the seemingly impossible task of successfully placing a model ship into a glass bottle, but without damaging it. This conundrum of course is exaggerated in the context of (i) smaller anatomical anterior chambers and (ii) a higher rate of more challenging pathology including PBK in Asia.

At the turn of the millennium, two broad approaches were conceived: the anterior 'endokeratoplasty' approach described by Busin and the posterior approach described by Melles [16, 45]. The latter gained popularity because it offered the advantage of a closed technique and evolved to become a Descemet stripping endothelial keratoplasty (DSEK), and with the assistance of a microkeratome (or latterly by femtosecond laser), a Descemet stripping automated endothelial keratoplasty (DSAEK). The term DSAEK is almost universally synonymous with endothelial keratoplasty as we understand it. Further iterations including ultrathin DSAEK, pre-Descemet's endothelial keratoplasty (PDEK) or indeed Descemet's membrane endothelial keratoplasty (DMEK) have facilitated progressively thinner grafts, and with them increasing technical challenges in the way surgeons can safely insert the corneal tissue and simultaneously maintain endothelial cell counts (ECCs). A full appraisal of these issues is beyond the scope of this chapter and is discussed elsewhere in this book.

The advent and uptake of DSAEK are reflected in a significant change in global trends in corneal transplantation generally and indeed the indications for transplantation itself. In the USA, the rate of uptake from EK rose exponentially from 3.2 to 49.7 % of all grafts between 2005 and 2014 with a corresponding drop in rates of PK from 94.9 to 41.5 % [49]. A marked shift in the indications for surgery reflected a change in the disease profile as discussed, with PBK and FED accounting for 17.8

and 47.7 %, respectively, of EK surgery by 2014. A similar increase has been observed in large series in the USA, the UK and Australia [24, 25, 33, 35, 49, 60].

These changes have also been reflected in other Asian countries, including India but with a preponderance of EKs being undertaken for bullous keratopathy (47.9 %) compared to Fuchs' endothelial corneal dystrophy (10.8 %) and regrafting (20.0 %) [47]. The high incidence of BK and the anatomical differences from Western populations already discussed highlight a particular challenge encountered in Singapore when switching from PK. This transition including the problems encountered and the steps to overcome them will be discussed in the rest of this chapter.

9.3 The Drive for Safer Donor Insertion: Adopting the Sheets Glide

EK was initiated in the Singapore National Eye Centre (SNEC) in 2006. At the time of adoption, the small-incision procedure included the use of a microkeratome-assisted preparation of the donor material (DSAEK) (Moria ALTK microkeratome, Moria) as opposed to manual preparation (DSEK) [53]. As outlined earlier in this chapter, one of the principle challenges in undertaking a small-incision keratoplasty procedure is ensuring a minimal donor endothelial cell damage for the procedure to be successful. Endothelial cell preservation is crucial as graft survival has been shown to depend on the maintenance of an adequate endothelial cell count [15]. Indeed this was one of the principle problems with penetrating keratoplasty, with gradual endothelial cell attrition and late endothelial failure accounting for a significant proportion of grafts becoming irreversibly dysfunctional (22 %) in the Singapore Corneal Transplant Study [63].

Like most centres, the initial approach to DSAEK involved 'taco'-folding the donor graft. This essentially involved bringing the endothelial side of the prepared graft into apposition and pulling the donor material into the anterior chamber through the scleral (or indeed corneal) incision, typically measuring 4–5 mm. Once inside the anterior chamber, the graft could then be opened and attached to the underlying host stromal bed with air. In order to minimise attrition, the service in SNEC employed non-compression forceps (Goosey forceps; Moria) to hold and pull the 8–8.5 mm graft.

The anatomical challenges presented by a predominantly Asian population were considerable, and in the initial phase of transition to EK, apparently insurmountable with this technique. It has subsequently become apparent from other larger series outside of Asia that the endothelial cell loss with this approach was higher compared to penetrating keratoplasty, up to 41 % at 2 years [54, 65–67]. At that time however, these data were not available, but it was apparent from the challenging case mix of small eyes in Asia combined with higher rates of PBK, late presentation and high vitreous pressure that there were significant challenges in maintaining the anterior chamber (AC) and preventing iris prolapse. This resulted in an unacceptably high endothelial cell loss (60 %), with an excessive rate of primary graft failure (25 %) from the analysis of our cohort of first 20 patients [60]. In addition to the trauma of AC instability, ECC loss was compounded by the unavoidable destruction of endothelial cells with forceps. This resulted in evident linear 'crush' injuries to the endothelium, seen on vital dye staining and confirmed with scanning electron microscopy, even with seemingly careful manipulation of the graft [44]. An alternative approach was therefore considered.

Although a direct suture 'pull-through' procedure had been described, without a means of mounting the graft on a glide, this also represented a high level of attrition with endothelial cell loss measured at up to 39.4 % at 6 months [34, 58]. The Busin glide was developed as a means of supporting the corneal donor material while opening the lip of the incision prior to pull-through with forceps from the opposite side [17]. The theoretical advantage to this approach included pulling the donor edge from the opposite corneal incision without the requirement to 'grab' the entire graft. Although this has been shown to facilitate ECC loss at less than 30 %, and despite the method appearing to have intuitive merits compared to a forceps or direct pull-through technique, the initial experience with Asian eyes in SNEC was disappointing. With the glide positioned through the wound, AC stability could not be effectively maintained resulting in immediate chamber collapse or in significant iris prolapse [60]. An alternative means of opening the corneal incision while enabling the reposition of the iris was needed and led to the adoption and modification of a Sheets glide (BD Visitec), conventionally used to insert an anterior chamber intraocular lens (IOL).

The Sheets glide offered an alternative means of avoiding forceps while maintaining the iris reposition when pulling the graft into the eye [44]. Briefly, the technique involved trimming an IOL glide, placing the prepared donor material endothelial side down on a dispersive ophthalmic viscosurgical device (OVD) and then placing the distal end of the glide through a 5-mm scleral tunnel into the anterior chamber. By employing an anterior chamber maintainer in tandem, the risk of AC collapse was avoided while preventing the problems of iris prolapse seen with forceps or indeed a pull-through technique alone. Kawai capsulorhexis forceps (model AE-4388, ASICO) were then used to grasp the edge of the donor endothelium before pulling it through into the AC while retracting the glide to stabilise the AC.

The first 20 cases undertaken at SNEC with this technique reduced the primary graft failure rate to 4.8 % [6]. In fact this was an isolated case as a series of 220 consecutive cases (0.45 %) to 2011 [60]. The evaluation of the technique following 2 years of use since inception in 2006 showed a drastic reduction in endothelial cell loss compared to the taco-folding technique at 22.4 % and manifested in graft survival at 1 year of 92 % [7]. These outcomes were encouraging when considering the burden of patients with pseudophakic bullous keratopathy in this cohort (63 %). Furthermore the visual improvement was considerable with a change from a mean best-corrected LogMAR acuity of 1.56 (0.66SD) to 0.27 (0.17SD) at 1 year.

It was apparent from an Asian patient population that the risks of taco-folding compared to the use of a Sheets glide were significant. Taco-folding conferred an odd ratio of primary graft failure of 34 % ($p<0.01$) [6]. It is interesting to note that in non-Asian populations, while the attrition from taco-folding is considerably less (34 % ECC loss at 6 months), it is still relatively high and higher than using alternative glides such as Busin's [13]. The variation in DSAEK outcomes with different insertion devices is discussed later in this chapter, but suffice it to say that different populations and surgical experience play an important role in adopting the technique that is best suited to those needs. A critical early determinant of success was comparing the Sheets glide technique against the data for penetrating keratoplasty. It is important to note that some large population studies such as the Australian graft registry have shown less favourable outcomes with DSAEK compared to PK [25]. The variation seen in SNEC with two different DSAEK donor insertion approaches highlights that a suboptimal technique can profoundly influence the outcome. To better understand therefore whether the adoption of EK offered an advantage to Singaporean patients over existing full-thickness transplantation, the outcomes were evaluated at 1 and later at 3 years following surgery.

In a cohort of patients with similar baseline characteristics, although graft survival was comparable at >92 %, endothelial cell loss was found to be significantly worse in those undergoing PK (40.9 %, $n=173$) compared to DSAEK (22.4 %, $n=68$), $p<0.001$ [7]. The Sheets glide DSAEK approach predictably also conferred less astigmatism (measured at 1.7D at 1 year) compared to PK (3.2D; $p<0.001$) and a resultant improvement in visual acuity, with the added advantage of a faster recovery [7].

Having established the safety profile and outcome of DSAEK at SNEC at a 1-year time frame, longer-term assessment was completed. At 3 years, the Sheets glide DSAEK technique maintained its advantage over conventional surgery. When comparing patients with the principal indication for DSAEK (PBK and FED), it was found that ECC loss was 39 % compared to 47 % with PK [8]. Graft survival was maintained at 87 % for DSAEK, and while comparable to PK, the latter had a higher rate of complications including wound dehiscence, infection and epitheliopathy. Reassuringly, technique-specific complications such as donor detachment occurred in only 2.6 % of cases [8]. This was substantially lower than that described in other series [59]. Overall therefore the Sheets glide technique not only offered advantages over the benchmarked procedure of PK, but also problems unique to an Asian population were circumvented.

Systematic evaluation and modification of the surgical technique is critical to optimise the outcome for patient benefits. Tailoring the approaches undertaken as outlined resulted in a significant improvement in outcome to Asian patients in terms of visual recovery, outcome and graft survival compared to conventional full-thickness grafting. Despite this success, there appeared to be room for improvement, not only in the hands of experienced EK surgeons but potentially for those learning this technique. The next section will discuss the evolution of an insertion device.

9.4 The Drive for Safer Donor Insertion: Evolution of the EndoGlide

The adoption and validation of the Sheets glide approach facilitated a wholesale change in the accepted practice in managing endothelial dysfunction in Southeast Asia. SNEC is a regional hub for many surrounding countries where keratoplasty services are less established. Patients may therefore travel considerable distances for evaluation, surgery and long-term follow-up. Access to a less invasive procedure with a relatively fast recovery represented a significant step forward in managing corneal disease in this corner of the world.

While the Sheets glide had facilitated the conversion from PK to EK, there remained an ambition to further reduce the rate of endothelial cell loss and improve AC stability, while attempting to make the procedure easier to perform consistently. While problems with iris prolapse had been largely circumvented, Sheets glide DSAEK still represented a considerable surgical challenge, in particular during the learning phase of the procedure. As DSAEK adoption has risen exponentially, the variation in practice has come into focus, in particular with variable rates seen in larger national registries such as the UK and Australia [25, 33]. It is worth noting that while the surgeon experience has been highlighted as a risk factor for graft failure, it seems that some surgeons maintain a higher failure rate despite an aggregate higher number of cases performed [25], and this may go some way to explain why centre experience in some countries appears to confer an impact on survival while individual surgeon experience does not [33]. It is therefore worth re-emphasising the point that learning the correct technique and taking appropriate measures to minimise endothelial cell trauma facilitate graft survival. In order to further control the safe passage of the donor material of different sizes and thickness into the anterior chamber, therefore, an insertion device as an alternative to the Sheets glide was conceived.

In 2008 the original Coronet EndoGlide insertion device (Network Medical Products, Ripon, UK) was created. Subsequently this has been modified for ultra-thin DSAEK to facilitate graft insertion up to 10.0 mm in diameter and up to 250 μm in thickness (Fig. 9.1). The development of the original insertion device was an iterative process considering the following parameters:

(i) Combining a glide with the pull-through technique with IOL insertion akin to a ‘USB thumbdrive’ for ease of manipulation
(ii) A means of loading the graft material into a double-coiled configuration to reduce the degree of endothelial touch
(iii) Small enough to allow insertion through a 4.5-mm scleral (or corneal) incision
(iv) Distal glide to ease passage into the anterior chamber and prevent iris prolapse
(v) Sufficient cartridge diameter to house the donor material while maintaining the incision seal, circumventing the AC collapse

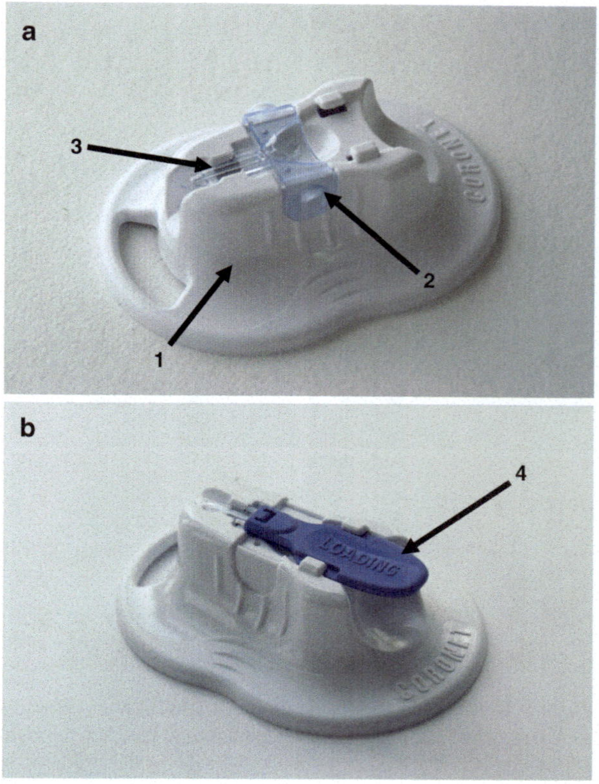

Fig. 9.1 The EndoGlide insertion device for DSAEK surgery. Colour photographs showing the components of the current Coronet 'Ultrathin' EndoGlide. Panel **a** shows the base (*1*), the saddle (*2*) and the cartridge (*3*). Once the graft has been placed on the saddle (endothelial side up) and pulled through into the introducer with Tan straight DSAEK forceps (not shown), the saddle is removed and the introducer (Panel **b**, *4*) clips into the base and cartridge. The introducer-cartridge is then removed from the base and inverted ready for transfer

(vi) Distal opening to allow safe pull-through of the graft material into the AC

The original EndoGlide was developed to allow insertion following a 4.5-mm scleral tunnel. The details of the entire procedure have been described elsewhere [38]. Briefly the precut tissue of an appropriate diameter including the anterior and posterior caps are carefully placed endothelial side up into the well of the base which together with the cartridge have been filled with balanced salt solution (BSS) (Fig. 9.2). A thin sliver of OVD is injected over the endothelium once mounted, and the BSS is drawn from the distal 'glide' end of the inserter with a sponge to help bring the graft closer to the cartridge (Fig. 9.2a). The posterior cap is pulled gently into the cartridge with straight EndoGlide forceps (Network Medical Products) from the distal opening, ensuring that the graft double coils in a straight fashion (Fig. 9.2b, c). An even coiling is essential to maintain the shape of the graft for a successful pull-through once in the AC. It is critical that an adequate but not excessive edge is revealed distally to facilitate this. The inserter is clipped into place following removal of the posterior cap and inverted so that the endothelium is facing downward.

Once loading is completed, the device is then detached from its base and introduced into a temporal scleral incision measuring 4.5 mm (Fig. 9.2). The forward-most

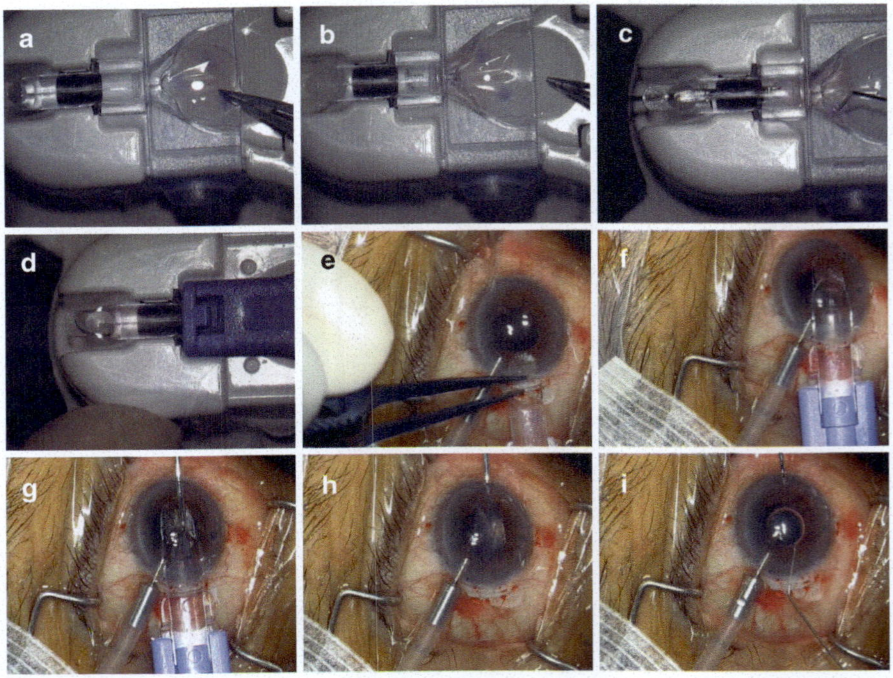

Fig. 9.2 Surgical steps in the donor preparation. Colour photographs showing the loading of corneal graft material into the EndoGlide (**a–d**) and insertion through a temporal scleral incision (**e–i**). The donor material is placed endothelial side up in the EndoGlide base and pulled into the cartridge with the assistance of forceps prior to inversion ready for insertion. The flat blade of the device is placed in the incision and advanced until a seal facilitates gentle grabbing of the graft material from the opposite nasal incision, air bubbling and removal of the EndoGlide

flat blade of the glide acts exactly like a Sheet glide to hold away the iris and prevent iris prolapse, and once the EndoGlide has been advanced to form a complete seal, the AC maintainer flow is reduced prior to the insertion of curved EndoGlide forceps (Network Medical Products) from a nasal incision (Fig. 9.2e, f). The stromal edge of the graft is grabbed carefully but firmly, and the graft material is pulled into the AC (Fig. 9.2g). Expedient but careful removal of the EndoGlide chamber is undertaken while ensuring that the donor material is still gripped, and an automatic deepening of the chamber, combined with gentle, waving side-to-side movements of the donor with the EndoGlide forceps, usually facilitates unfurling of the donor (Fig. 9.2h). Once the AC is stable, a small 1/3 air bubble is injected carefully behind the graft to maintain its position, opposed to the host corneal stroma (Fig. 9.2i). The incision is then sutured, the AC maintainer removed and a full air fill is achieved for 6-8 min, while all incisions are secured. Partial air release is undertaken before appropriate posturing. The ultrathin EndoGlide including modifications such as a removable saddle to assist coiling, a shallow base well to ease the removal of the anterior cap of the cornea (Fig. 9.1a) and a clear marking for the correct attachment

Table 9.2 Overview of insertion devices developed for DSAEK use in conventional cases

Insertion technique	Company	Type of insertion	ECC loss*
Pull-through	–	Manual retraction	39.4 %
Taco-fold	–	Manual folding	60 %
Sheets glide	BD Visitec	Glide	22 %
Busin glide	Moria	Glide	25.3 %
Rieck glide	Geuder	Glide	NA
Macaluso sealing glide	Janach	Glide	NA
Al-Ghoul injector	Enison	Glide	NA
Monarch IIB	Monarch	Cartridge injector	51.4 %
SFC-45 Visian	STAAR	Cartridge injector	NA
EndoGlide	Network Medical	Insertion device	14.9 %
Daya Endostar	Duckworth & Kent	Insertion device	NA
EndoSaver	Ocular Systems Inc.	Insertion device	28.3 %
IDEEL injector	Kaneka	Insertion device	NA
Neusidl Corneal Inserter	Fischer	Insertion device	33 %
EndoInjector	KeraMed	Insertion device	NA

Refs. [26, 29, 37, 40, 56, 68]
Summary table of insertion techniques and devices. Common/currently available devices are highlighted in bold
*ECC = Endothelial Cell Count
NA data not available from a human series

and insertion of the graft has facilitated an enhanced safety and ease of use (Fig. 9.1b) [3].

At the time of its development, there were no commercially available insertion devices, but subsequently a number of other 'platform inserters' have been introduced, including the Daya Endostar (Duckworth & Kent), Rieck glide (Geuder), Al-Ghoul injector (Ension, PA, USA), Macaluso sealing glide (Janach) and the EndoInjector, formerly Endoshield (KeraMed, California), but many have not made it to clinical use, with the exception of the EndoSerter (Ocular Systems Inc., Winston-Salem, North Carolina) and the Neusidl Corneal Inserter (Fischer Surgical, Imperial, Montana) devices, both platform inserters [3]. It is important to consider that the insertion of biological graft material is not the same as a synthetic IOL with coiling and injecting potentially causing endothelial cell damage. This was exemplified in a study that assessed a bifold folding technique compared with the employment of a Monarch IIB injection cartridge in a cohort of 179 patients. The bifold technique resulted the ECC loss at 12 months was 42.5 %, and with the cartridge 51.4 % [70]. Another cartridge-based device SFC-45 Visian implantable Collamer lens cartridge (STAAR Surgical, California) was compared in a cadaveric series following the microkeratome-prepared donor tissue [42]. While the immediate endothelial cell loss was significantly better than the forceps delivery, this was not substantiated in a patient series. An isolated case report however demonstrated an endothelial cell loss of 21 % at 5 months.

A published literature is available for the Neusidl corneal inserter [26, 40, 68] and EndoSerter [29, 37, 56], both FDA-approved devices (Table 9.2). The Neusidl inserter has been employed in a larger series of patients in the USA and small series of Asian patients from Japan. Terry's group initially published a series of cadaveric eyes ($n = 10$) and compared them to their conventional forceps approach. In the preliminary cadaveric series, it was found that endothelial cell loss was comparable in both groups [26]. When a randomised control trial ($n = 100$ eyes) was undertaken, however, there was found to be a higher percentage (33 %) of endothelial cell loss with the Neusidl injector compared to the forceps [68]. The only evidence from an Asian population came from a small series in Japan ($n = 6$) which showed a mean endothelial cell loss of 31.4 % at 12 months [40]. An alternative device, the EndoSerter which facilitates insertion through a 4-mm incision, was first evaluated in a large, non-randomised study ($n = 175$) and compared to forceps insertion, and revealed that despite respectable visual outcomes to an early 6-month time point, endothelial cell loss, while lower than forceps (44.1 %), was relatively high at 28.3 % [29]. Although ECC was measured at 2997 ± 231 cells/mm^2 at 6 months, the percentage loss data was not available [37]. Additionally, a small cadaveric study demonstrated no difference from the Sheets glide technique with the EndoSerter, but no patient data was available to support this [56].

The EndoGlide was approved for use in Europe with CE marking and as a class 1 medical device by the US Food and Drug Administration (FDA) in 2009 and the EndoGlide Ultrathin in 2012. The outcomes of the ongoing evaluation will be discussed in the following section.

9.5 Surgical Outcomes with the EndoGlide

Having developed the EndoGlide, a device designed to circumvent the difficulty of donor endothelium insertion into anatomically smaller eyes, SNEC surgeons were able to confirm the feasibility of the insertion device. Previously adopted techniques resulted in an unacceptable attrition to endothelial cell counts, which in turn drastically impaired graft survival. To validate its early adoption, the outcomes of the first 25 eyes in Asian patients who underwent EndoGlide-assisted DSAEK at SNEC were analysed [38]. The majority had with PBK ($n = 12$) or FED ($n = 9$) and an average graft diameter of 8.75 mm. The endothelial cell loss was measured at 13.1 % at 6 months ($n = 20$) and 15.6 % at 12 months ($n = 11$), representing a mean ECC of 2,575 cells/mm^2. This translated into a visual outcome of 6/12 or better in 57 % of eyes and the remainder between 6/12 and 6/48, all due to pre-existing visual pathology and with non-losing vision.

Encouraged by the early outcomes from the EndoGlide, an evaluation of a larger series ($n = 100$) of patients with PBK ($n = 59$) or FED demonstrated similar outcomes [36]. With no immediate insertion problems encountered, a mean visual acuity of 6/12 was achieved and in all patients free of coexisting visual impairment such as retinal or optic nerve disease. The mean endothelial cell loss again was encouraging at 14.9 % at 12 months, with no significant difference between PBK and FED. In order to confirm this reduction, a comparative analysis at 3 years with the Sheets glide showed an endothelial cell loss of 29.7 % at 3 years compared to 38.5 % ($p < 0.05$) [9]. Subgroup analysis in patients with FED revealed a significant difference between the EndoGlide and Sheets glide approaches.

Other groups have also compared DSAEK outcome against other approaches such as the Busin glide and the EndoSerter injector [28, 30]. A comparative clinical trial conducted in the UK showed that at 6 months, the visual outcomes in a series of patients undergoing DSAEK by EndoGlide ($n = 22$) and Busin glide ($n = 30$) were found to be similar [30]. The rate of endothelial cell loss however was significantly higher in the Busin glide group (47.5 % vs. 25.8 %, $p < 0.0001$). It is worth noting that the approach to Busin glide insertion, while comparable to the preferred EndoGlide temporal approach, is contrary to the original description by Busin and has been argued to be the cause for the higher loss due to excessive manipulation and AC collapse by pulling the graft from a temporal incision [18]. Comparison between the EndoGlide and EndoSerter in a separate study from Canada revealed comparable results at 12 months (41.2 % vs. 31.4 %, $p = 0.45$) [28]; however in both, the endothelial cell loss was comparatively high compared to other studies, but explained by a higher re-bubbling rate [9, 28, 29, 36, 38].

The initial series evaluating the EndoGlide inserter found a good safety profile with no detachments and no primary graft failures in the first 6 months [38]. Loading events were made challenging in the learning phase as a result of pulling the graft into the cartridge too rapidly, inadequately lubricating the chamber or in very thin grafts. These resulted in a W configuration as opposed to a double coil and could be avoided with a careful pull-through, using a Sinskey hook to massage the stromal side of the graft upward on the insertion or using a second pair of forceps at the proximal end of the graft to unfurl a W configuration [38]. Complications were reported including the AC collapse during insertion, a non-healing epithelial defect and the presence of vitreous in phaco-DSAEK case. All made a full recovery by 6 months including visual outcomes of 6/21 or better and ECC loss <22 %. In the larger series at 1 year, one graft developed a primary graft failure due to incorrect 'upside-down' insertion, and two grafts required re-bubbling (both successful) [36]. A clearer picture of late complications was also appreciated. The rate of rejection remained low at 2.6 %, while 1.3 % failed [36]. These figures are comparable or lower than other larger series [59]. The EndoGlide therefore remains the standard of care for DSAEK in SNEC among other centres.

9.6 Special Circumstances

Although PBK represents a comparative challenge, the outcomes compared to FED have been shown to be favourable with the EndoGlide. Other scenarios however pose additional challenges, and complex situations include the presence of glaucoma tubes in the AC, combining the DSAEK with glaucoma, cataract surgery, undertaking surgery with AC-IOLs, following failed corneal transplantation such as previous PK and secondary to infective causes of endothelial failure such as cytomegalovirus (CMV) endotheliitis.

A retrospective assessment of 45 complex cases in Asian eyes at SNEC demonstrated a higher rate of endothelial cell loss of 27 % at 12 months [39]. This cohort however included the eyes with single or multiple risk factors including previous surgery such as trabeculectomy, penetrating keratoplasty, vitrectomy, glaucoma tubes and aphakia [11, 12, 46]. Ten percent had a combined phaco-DSAEK including a combination of risk factors. Complications predictably increased including three that required a re-bubble procedure and one graft that had primary failure. Maintaining an adequate air fill presented a particular problem in an aphakic, vitrectomised eye and highlights the extreme end of surgical difficulty in DSAEK. Though higher than 'routine' cases, the outcomes including complications were comparable to other insertion approaches despite the anticipated risks in these eyes [34, 58]. Furthermore the ability to undertake EK in eyes with existing failed PK offers a potential avenue to visually rehabilitate the eyes where further full-thickness transplantation would be precluded because of the risk of rejection associated with an increased antigen load. EK graft size has been implicated in EK survival [6, 57], and the deliberate selection of larger grafts (9.0 mm) may have boosted the overall cell count and circumvented problems of cell loss in complex eyes where preventing contact between the endothelium and surrounding structures in the AC is more difficult.

Although uncommon outside of Asia-Pacific, CMV endotheliitis is a devastating albeit potentially reversible viral inflammatory condition which is causing endothelial cell loss [20, 31, 41]. While it is particularly important to recognise that graft CMV endotheliitis may masquerade as a graft rejection and/or failure, paradoxically once medical management with valganciclovir has been commenced and tapered to control inflammation, DSAEK may actually offer a route to replace the host endothelium or CMV-induced failed graft [10].

9.7 The Asian Experience in Non-Asian Eyes

The ability to undertake selective removal and transplantation of 50-200 um of tissue without complication is challenging, and the UK data shows that some surgeons consistently perform less well than peers manifest in centre-related discrepancies in the UK [33]. As discussed, the importance of optimised training and surgical approaches in facilitating a safe procedure are paramount if 'flattening the surgical learning curve' is to be achieved. To date the few studies undertaken have demonstrated a favourable outcome when utilising the EndoGlide insertion device for DSAEK. This approach has not only improved outcomes locally, but has been adopted worldwide in populations outside of Asia including the UK [30].

9.8 Conclusions

EK has represented a significant change in how the management of corneal endothelial disease is managed. The learning curve for modern DSAEK is significant, and in certain populations, seemingly tried and tested techniques may have unacceptable safety profiles. In this chapter, we have outlined some of the approaches in undertaking DSAEK and how these were modified and developed for an Asian population. The advent of the Sheets glide and latterly the EndoGlide insertion device have facilitated the advent of a consistent and safe DSAEK for an Asian population, even in complex situations which may have otherwise have precluded the adoption of EK.

References

1. Al-Yousuf N, Mavrikakis I, Mavrikakis E, Daya SM. Penetrating keratoplasty: indications over a 10-year period. Br J Ophthalmol. 2004;88:998–1001.
2. Allan BD, Terry MA, Price Jr FW, Price MO, Griffin NB, Claesson M. Corneal transplant rejection rate and severity after endothelial keratoplasty. Cornea. 2007;26:1039–42.
3. Ang AY, Liu YC, Tan DT, Mehta JS. Descemet stripping automated endothelial keratoplasty with the EndoGlide Ultrathin graft insertion device. Expert Rev Med Devices. 2014;11:573–9.
4. Ang M, Chong W, Huang H, Wong TY, He MG, Aung T, Mehta JS. Determinants of posterior corneal biometric measurements in a multi-ethnic Asian population. PLoS One. 2014;9, e101483.
5. Ang M, Chong W, Tay WT, Yuen L, Wong TY, He MG, Saw SM, Aung T, Mehta JS. Anterior segment optical coherence tomography study of the cornea and anterior segment in adult ethnic South Asian Indian eyes. Invest Ophthalmol Vis Sci. 2012;53:120–5.
6. Ang M, Htoon HM, Cajucom-UY HY, Tan D, Mehta JS. Donor and surgical risk factors for primary graft failure following Descemet's stripping automated endothelial keratoplasty in Asian eyes. Clin Ophthalmol. 2011;5:1503–8.
7. Ang M, Mehta JS, Anshu A, Wong HK, Htoon HM, Tan D. Endothelial cell counts after Descemet's stripping automated endothelial keratoplasty versus penetrating keratoplasty in Asian eyes. Clin Ophthalmol. 2012;6:537–44.
8. Ang M, Mehta JS, Lim F, Bose S, Htoon HM, Tan D. Endothelial cell loss and graft survival after Descemet's stripping automated endothelial keratoplasty and penetrating keratoplasty. Ophthalmology. 2012;119:2239–44.
9. Ang M, Saroj L, Htoon HM, Kiew S, Mehta JS, Tan D. Comparison of a donor insertion device to sheets glide in Descemet stripping endothelial keratoplasty: 3-year outcomes. Am J Ophthalmol. 2014;157(1163–1169), e3.
10. Anshu A, Chee SP, Mehta JS, Tan DT. Cytomegalovirus endotheliitis in Descemet's stripping endothelial keratoplasty. Ophthalmology. 2009;116:624–30.
11. Anshu A, Price MO, Price FW. Descemet's stripping endothelial keratoplasty: long-term graft survival and risk factors for failure in eyes with preexisting glaucoma. Ophthalmology. 2012;119:1982–7.
12. Anshu A, Price MO, Price Jr FW. Descemet's stripping endothelial keratoplasty under failed penetrating keratoplasty: visual rehabilitation and graft survival rate. Ophthalmology. 2011;118:2155–60.

13. Bahar I, Kaiserman I, Sansanayudh W, Levinger E, Rootman DS. Busin guide vs forceps for the insertion of the donor lenticule in descemet stripping automated endothelial keratoplasty. Am J Ophthalmol. 2009;147(220–226), e1.
14. Barraquer JN, Rutllan JN. Microsurgery of the cornea: an atlas and textbook. Scriba: Barcelona; 1984.
15. Bertelmann E, Pleyer U, Rieck P. Risk factors for endothelial cell loss post-keratoplasty. Acta Ophthalmol Scand. 2006;84:766–70.
16. Busin M, Arffa RC, Sebastiani A. Endokeratoplasty as an alternative to penetrating keratoplasty for the surgical treatment of diseased endothelium: initial results. Ophthalmology. 2000;107:2077–82.
17. Busin M, Bhatt PR, Scorcia V. A modified technique for descemet membrane stripping automated endothelial keratoplasty to minimize endothelial cell loss. Arch Ophthalmol. 2008;126:1133–7.
18. Busin M, Scorcia V. A prospective study comparing EndoGlide and Busin glide insertion techniques in descemet stripping endothelial keratoplasty. Am J Ophthalmol. 2012;154:416–7; author reply 417.
19. Chan CM, Wong TY, Yeong SM, Lim TH, Tan DT. Penetrating keratoplasty in the Singapore National Eye Centre and donor cornea acquisition in the Singapore Eye Bank. Ann Acad Med Singapore. 1997;26:395–400.
20. Chee SP, Bacsal K, Jap A, Se-Thoe SY, Cheng CL, Tan BH. Corneal endotheliitis associated with evidence of cytomegalovirus infection. Ophthalmology. 2007;114:798–803.
21. Chen ES, Shamie N, Terry MA. Descemet-stripping endothelial keratoplasty: improvement in vision following replacement of a healthy endothelial graft. J Cataract Refract Surg. 2008;34:1044–6.
22. Chen ES, Terry MA, Shamie N, Hoar KL, Phillips PM, Friend DJ. Endothelial keratoplasty: vision, endothelial survival, and complications in a comparative case series of fellows vs attending surgeons. Am J Ophthalmol. 2009;148(26–31), e2.
23. Claesson M, Armitage WJ, Fagerholm P, Stenevi U. Visual outcome in corneal grafts: a preliminary analysis of the Swedish Corneal Transplant Register. Br J Ophthalmol. 2002;86:174–80.
24. Cornea Donor Study Investigator G, Gal RL, Dontchev M, Beck RW, Mannis MJ, Holland EJ, Kollman C, Dunn SP, Heck EL, Lass JH, Montoya MM, Schultze RL, Stulting RD, Sugar A, Sugar J, Tennant B, Verdier DD. The effect of donor age on corneal transplantation outcome results of the cornea donor study. Ophthalmology. 2008;115:620–6 e6.
25. Coster DJ, Lowe MT, Keane MC, Williams KA, Australian Corneal Graft Registry C. A comparison of lamellar and penetrating keratoplasty outcomes: a registry study. Ophthalmology. 2014;121:979–87.
26. Davis-Boozer D, Terry MA, Greiner MA, Holiman J, Saad HA, Alqudah AA, Li JY. In vitro evaluation of endothelial cell loss using the Neusidl Corneal Inserter. Cornea. 2013;32:479–82.
27. Dobbins KR, Price Jr FW, Whitson WE. Trends in the indications for penetrating keratoplasty in the midwestern United States. Cornea. 2000;19:813–6.
28. Elbaz U, Yeung SN, Lichtinger A, Zauberman NA, Goldich Y, Ziai S, Chan CC, Rootman DS, Slomovic AR. EndoGlide versus EndoSerter for the insertion of donor graft in descemet stripping automated endothelial keratoplasty. Am J Ophthalmol. 2014;158(257–262), e1.
29. Foster JB, Swan KR, Vasan RA, Greven MA, Walter KA. Small-incision Descemet stripping automated endothelial keratoplasty: a comparison of small-incision tissue injector and forceps techniques. Cornea. 2012;31:42–7.
30. Gangwani V, Obi A, Hollick EJ. A prospective study comparing EndoGlide and Busin glide insertion techniques in descemet stripping endothelial keratoplasty. Am J Ophthalmol. 2012;153(38–43), e1.
31. Ghauri AJ, Williams GP, Shah S, Murray PI, Rauz S. Post-phacoemulsification cytomegalovirus corneal endotheliitis diagnosis and management. JRSM Short Rep. 2012;3:42.

32. Ghosheh FR, Cremona FA, Rapuano CJ, Cohen EJ, Ayres BD, Hammersmith KM, Raber IM, Laibson PR. Trends in penetrating keratoplasty in the United States 1980-2005. Int Ophthalmol. 2008;28:147–53.
33. Greenrod EB, Jones MN, Kaye S, Larkin DF, National Health Service B, Transplant Ocular Tissue Advisory G, Contributing O. Center and surgeon effect on outcomes of endothelial keratoplasty versus penetrating keratoplasty in the United Kingdom. Am J Ophthalmol. 2014;158:957–66.
34. Kaiserman I, Bahar I, Mcallum P, Slomovic AR, Rootman DS. Suture-assisted vs forceps-assisted insertion of the donor lenticula during Descemet stripping automated endothelial keratoplasty. Am J Ophthalmol. 2008;145:986–90.
35. Keenan TD, Jones MN, Rushton S, Carley FM, National Health Service B, Transplant Ocular Tissue Advisory G, Contributing O. Trends in the indications for corneal graft surgery in the United Kingdom: 1999 through 2009. Arch Ophthalmol. 2012;130:621–8.
36. Khor WB, Han SB, Mehta JS, Tan DT. Descemet stripping automated endothelial keratoplasty with a donor insertion device: clinical results and complications in 100 eyes. Am J Ophthalmol. 2013;156:773–9.
37. Khor WB, Kim T. Descemet-stripping automated endothelial keratoplasty with a donor tissue injector. J Cataract Refract Surg. 2014;40:1768–72.
38. Khor WB, Mehta JS, Tan DT. Descemet stripping automated endothelial keratoplasty with a graft insertion device: surgical technique and early clinical results. Am J Ophthalmol. 2011;151(223–32), e2.
39. Khor WB, Teo KY, Mehta JS, Tan DT. Descemet stripping automated endothelial keratoplasty in complex eyes: results with a donor insertion device. Cornea. 2013;32:1063–8.
40. Kobayashi A, Yokogawa H, Sugiyama K. Clinical results of the Neusidl Corneal Inserter((R)), a new donor inserter for Descemet's stripping automated endothelial keratoplasty, for small Asian eyes. Ophthalmic Surg Lasers Imaging. 2012;43:311–8.
41. Koizumi N, Suzuki T, Uno T, Chihara H, Shiraishi A, Hara Y, Inatomi T, Sotozono C, Kawasaki S, Yamasaki K, Mochida C, Ohashi Y, Kinoshita S. Cytomegalovirus as an etiologic factor in corneal endotheliitis. Ophthalmology. 2008;115(292–297), e3.
42. Kuo AN, Harvey TM, Afshari NA. Novel delivery method to reduce endothelial injury in descemet stripping automated endothelial keratoplasty. Am J Ophthalmol. 2008;145:91–6.
43. Mcculley JP, Maurice DM, Schwartz BD. Corneal endothelial transplantation. Ophthalmology. 1980;87:194–201.
44. Mehta JS, Por YM, Beuerman RW, Tan DT. Glide insertion technique for donor cornea lenticule during Descemet's stripping automated endothelial keratoplasty. J Cataract Refract Surg. 2007;33:1846–50.
45. Melles GR, Eggink FA, Lander F, Pels E, Rietveld FJ, Beekhuis WH, Binder PS. A surgical technique for posterior lamellar keratoplasty. Cornea. 1998;17:618–26.
46. Mitry D, Bhogal M, Patel AK, Lee BS, Chai SM, Price MO, Price Jr FW, Jun AS, Aldave AJ, Mehta JS, Busin M, Allan BD. Descemet stripping automated endothelial keratoplasty after failed penetrating keratoplasty: survival, rejection risk, and visual outcome. JAMA Ophthalmol. 2014;132:742–9.
47. Mohamed A, Chaurasia S, Murthy SI, Ramappa M, Vaddavalli PK, Taneja M, GARG P, Chinta S, Basu S, Rathi VM, Sangwan VS. Endothelial keratoplasty: a review of indications at a tertiary eye care Centre in South India. Asia Pac J Ophthalmol (Phila). 2014;3:207–10.
48. Mohay J, Lange TM, Soltau JB, Wood TO, Mclaughlin BJ. Transplantation of corneal endothelial cells using a cell carrier device. Cornea. 1994;13:173–82.
49. Park CY, Lee JK, Gore PK, Lim CY, Chuck RS. Keratoplasty in the United States: a 10-year review from 2005 through 2014. Ophthalmology. 2015;122(12):2432–42.
50. Price Jr FW, Price MO. Descemet's stripping with endothelial keratoplasty in 50 eyes: a refractive neutral corneal transplant. J Refract Surg. 2005;21:339–45.
51. Price Jr FW, Price MO. Descemet's stripping with endothelial keratoplasty in 200 eyes: early challenges and techniques to enhance donor adherence. J Cataract Refract Surg. 2006;32:411–8.

52. Price MO, Gorovoy M, Price Jr FW, Benetz BA, Menegay HJ, Lass JH. Descemet's stripping automated endothelial keratoplasty: three-year graft and endothelial cell survival compared with penetrating keratoplasty. Ophthalmology. 2013;120:246–51.
53. Price MO, Price Jr FW. Descemet's stripping with endothelial keratoplasty: comparative outcomes with microkeratome-dissected and manually dissected donor tissue. Ophthalmology. 2006;113:1936–42.
54. Price MO, Price Jr FW. Endothelial cell loss after descemet stripping with endothelial keratoplasty influencing factors and 2-year trend. Ophthalmology. 2008;115:857–65.
55. Rahman I, Carley F, Hillarby C, Brahma A, Tullo AB. Penetrating keratoplasty: indications, outcomes, and complications. Eye (Lond). 2009;23:1288–94.
56. Riaz KM, Grewal DS, Cervantes P, Basti S. Endothelial damage with two DSAEK insertion techniques performed by a novice corneal surgeon in residency training: a comparative analysis. Cornea. 2014;33:91–5.
57. Romano V, Tey A, Hill NM, Ahmad S, Britten C, Batterbury M, Willoughby C, Kaye SB. Influence of graft size on graft survival following Descemet stripping automated endothelial keratoplasty. Br J Ophthalmol. 2015;99:784–8.
58. Sarnicola V, Toro P. Descemet-stripping automated endothelial keratoplasty by using suture for donor insertion. Cornea. 2008;27:825–9.
59. Suh LH, Yoo SH, Deobhakta A, Donaldson KE, Alfonso EC, Culbertson WW, O'brien TP. Complications of Descemet's stripping with automated endothelial keratoplasty: survey of 118 eyes at One Institute. Ophthalmology. 2008;115:1517–24.
60. Tan, D., Ang, M., Arundhati, A., Khor, W-B. 2015. Development Of Selective Lamellar Keratoplasty Within An Asian Corneal Transplant Program: The Singapore Corneal Transplant Study. American Ophthalmological Society. 2015;113:T101–23
61. Tan DK, Chong W, Tay WT, Yuen LH, He M, Aung T, Tan DT, Wong TY, Mehta JS. Anterior chamber dimensions and posterior corneal arc length in Malay eyes: an anterior segment optical coherence tomography study. Invest Ophthalmol Vis Sci. 2012;53:4860–7.
62. Tan DT, Dart JK, Holland EJ, Kinoshita S. Corneal transplantation. Lancet. 2012;379:1749–61.
63. Tan DT, Janardhanan P, Zhou H, Chan YH, Htoon HM, Ang LP, Lim LS. Penetrating keratoplasty in Asian eyes: the Singapore Corneal Transplant Study. Ophthalmology. 2008;115(975–982), e1.
64. Terry MA. Endothelial keratoplasty: clinical outcomes in the two years following deep lamellar endothelial keratoplasty (an American Ophthalmological Society thesis). Trans Am Ophthalmol Soc. 2007;105:530–63.
65. Terry MA. Endothelial keratoplasty: a comparison of complication rates and endothelial survival between precut tissue and surgeon-cut tissue by a single DSAEK surgeon. Trans Am Ophthalmol Soc. 2009;107:184–91.
66. Terry MA, Chen ES, Shamie N, Hoar KL, Friend DJ. Endothelial cell loss after Descemet's stripping endothelial keratoplasty in a large prospective series. Ophthalmology. 2008;115(488–496), e3.
67. Terry MA, Shamie N, Chen ES, Phillips PM, Shah AK, Hoar KL, Friend DJ. Endothelial keratoplasty for Fuchs' dystrophy with cataract: complications and clinical results with the new triple procedure. Ophthalmology. 2009;116:631–9.
68. Terry MA, Straiko MD, Goshe JM, Shamie N, Shah A, Alqudah AA, Davis-Boozer D. Endothelial keratoplasty: prospective, randomized, masked clinical trial comparing an injector with forceps for tissue insertion. Am J Ophthalmol. 2013;156(61–68), e3.
69. Wang YE, Li Y, Wang D, He M, Lin S. Comparison of factors associated with occludable angle between american Caucasians and ethnic Chinese. Invest Ophthalmol Vis Sci. 2013;54:7717–23.
70. Wendel LJ, Goins KM, Sutphin JE, Wagoner MD. Comparison of bifold forceps and cartridge injector suture pull-through insertion techniques for Descemet stripping automated endothelial keratoplasty. Cornea. 2011;30:273–6.

71. Williams KA, Muehlberg SM, Lewis RF, Coster DJ. How successful is corneal transplantation? A report from the Australian Corneal Graft Register. Eye (Lond). 1995;9(Pt 2):219–27.
72. Yuen LH, He M, Aung T, Htoon HM, Tan DT, Mehta JS. Biometry of the cornea and anterior chamber in Chinese eyes: an anterior segment optical coherence tomography study. Invest Ophthalmol Vis Sci. 2010;51:3433–40.

Chapter 10
Intra- and Postoperative Complications and Their Management in DMEK (Including Re-DMEK)

Bjoern Bachmann and Claus Cursiefen

10.1 Preoperative Considerations

Preoperative considerations and planning of DMEK surgery are essential for the surgical success and start with correct *donor recipient matching*. When planning the surgery, the recipient's anterior chamber depth has to be taken into account. Total control of the anterior chamber depth after implantation of the DMEK roll is essential for uncomplicated unfolding of the graft [1]. In small hyperopic eyes, the corneal diameter tends to be smaller and the anterior chamber can be extremely shallow. A high vitreous pressure during surgery will further impair surgical manoeuvres for intracameral unfolding of the DMEK graft. This can complicate, e.g. the correct placement of an air bubble inside the Descemet's membrane (DM) roll, and the reduced amount of anterior chamber volume can hamper the mobility of the graft. In such cases grafts of smaller diameter are favourable for intracameral manipulations and unfolding of the graft. If the patient in addition is younger and remains phakic, the anterior chamber may be even smaller. In these hyperopic phakic eyes, an anterior chamber maintainer may become necessary to be able to implant the graft [2]. Care has to be taken not to flush out the donor role. DMEK in phakic and hyperopic eyes even with anterior chambers below 2.5 mm is possible and leads to excellent visual results, but the endothelial cell loss is significantly higher [2].

In addition to the graft diameter, unfolding of the graft can actively be influenced by choosing grafts from older donors. Compared to younger donors, DM from older donors, meaning donors above 60 years of age, has less rolling tendency. These grafts are favourable in patients with a very deep anterior chamber, e.g. after vitrectomy or high myopic eyes where almost no vitreous pressure can be expected. Active shallowing of the anterior chamber during DMEK by the release of fluid via

B. Bachmann (✉) • C. Cursiefen
Department of Ophthalmology, University of Cologne, Cologne, Germany
e-mail: bjoern.bachmann@uk-koeln.de

C. Cursiefen, A.S. Jun (eds.), *Current Treatment Options for Fuchs Endothelial Dystrophy*, DOI 10.1007/978-3-319-43021-8_10

a paracentesis is important to keep grafts with a strong rolling tendency unfolded. By choosing DM from older donors, unfolding in these patients is much simpler and needs less manipulation after implantation as long as the correct orientation of the graft is kept from the beginning of the implantation process.

These factors, donor age and graft diameter can also be used for the adjustment of the graft's intracameral behaviour in patients with marked changes of the anterior segment anatomy like excessive anterior synechia, aphakia, anterior chamber lens or intracameral tubes after implantation of glaucoma drainage devices. If pronounced changes of the anterior segment exist, depending on the surgeons experience, Descemet's Stripping (Automated) Endothelial Keratoplasty (DS(A)EK) or even perforating corneal transplantation (PK) should be considered as an alternative approach.

In terms of graft diameter, an individualised approach should be taken, using much larger diameters for recipient eyes with larger corneal diameter and deep anterior chamber, e.g. in buphthalmos. In some of these eyes diameters up to 11 mm can be used safely, whereas routinely in "normal" eyes smaller diameters like 8 mm are a safe option.

10.2 Complications During Graft Preparation

Technically, graft preparation can be performed hours or days before surgery [3]. Since there is a chance of losing the graft during preparation due to tearing, increasing the interval between graft preparation and transplantation improves the predictability and reliability whether the surgery will take place or not. Moreover, graft preparation outside the operation theatre saves costs and staff time. This approach has already been successfully adopted in some eye clinics in the United States and in Europe [4]. However, in most countries eye banks do not offer precut grafts for DMEK. If DMEK precut grafts are not available and if the grafts are available just the day when the DMEK is supposed to take place, a safe, reliable and reproducible technique for graft preparation with a high success rate of the stripping procedure is essential. Many variations in graft preparation have been described for the separation of DM from the corneal stroma [1, 5, 6]. There are techniques utilising the injection of air or fluid in deep stromal layers which can either lead the pure separation of DM from the corneal stroma or result in DM separation with a small layer of corneal stroma attached (Dua's layer) [7, 8]. The classic technique for DM stripping uses forceps for pulling DM from the posterior corneal stroma which results in a very high success rate of 98 % [1, 6, 9]. Pulling can either be started from the outest periphery at the border of DM to the trabecular meshwork or after scraping away a peripheral ring of DM giving access to a circular edge of the remaining DM. With either technique tearing of DM can occur. To avoid larger DM tears into the centre of the graft, thorough evaluation of the DM's edge for smaller tears before stripping is essential. In particular, grafts originating from donors with a history of cataract surgery or other anterior segment surgery frequently have scars with firm adhesions around the inner corneal entrance of the corneal incisions. DM from this area is generally firmly attached and cannot be stripped which results in tearing of the

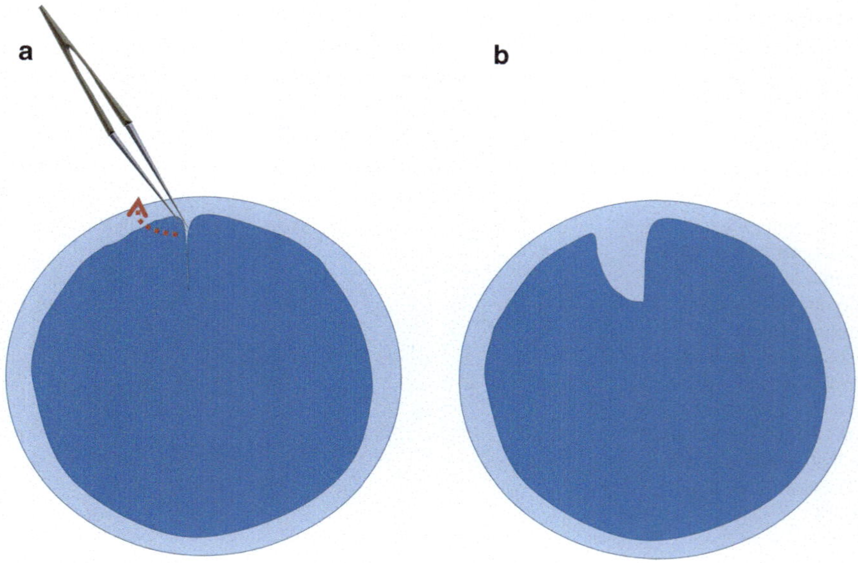

Fig. 10.1 (**a**) Peripheral tears can be removed by radial pulling of Descemet's membrane to the periphery (*red dotted arrow*) on one side of the tear. (**b**) This will turn the tip of the tear into a rounded edge

graft. If such tears can be identified, further enlargement of the tear can be avoided by two techniques: the tear can be removed by radial pulling of DM to the periphery on one side of the tear (Fig. 10.1a). This will turn the tear into a rounded edge of DM (Fig. 10.1b). This technique resembles the rescue manoeuvres for managing a radial tear during continuous curvilinear capsulorhexis. However, some DM will be lost and this manoeuvre should therefore preferably be performed in smaller peripheral tears only. In larger tears directed towards the centre of the graft, DM from both sides of the graft can be grasped with two forceps and evenly pulled towards the centre (Fig. 10.2) [1]. The advantage of the two forceps technique is that no additional loss of DM results. However, the synchronised use of two forceps for DM stripping needs training and if not performed very even offers the risk of further tear enlargement. A third approach is stripping DM from the opposite site of larger peripheral tears without any further manipulation of the tissue around the affected area. This technique can be applied if adhesions of DM are limited to one or two quadrants of the graft.

In general stripping close to the tear needs intense observation. Further enlargement of the tear during pulling has to be excluded. Tangential pulling will enlarge the tear and must be avoided.

Even grafts which have been completely torn into two pieces can be used for transplantation as long as a certain amount of donor endothelial cells is preserved [10]. However, torn DMs are by far more difficult to graft and overlapping of DM from the same tissue can occur reducing the total number of viable grafted corneal endothelial cells.

Peripheral tears barely cause problems once the different techniques how to approach these tears have been adopted. Central tears are more challenging to manage

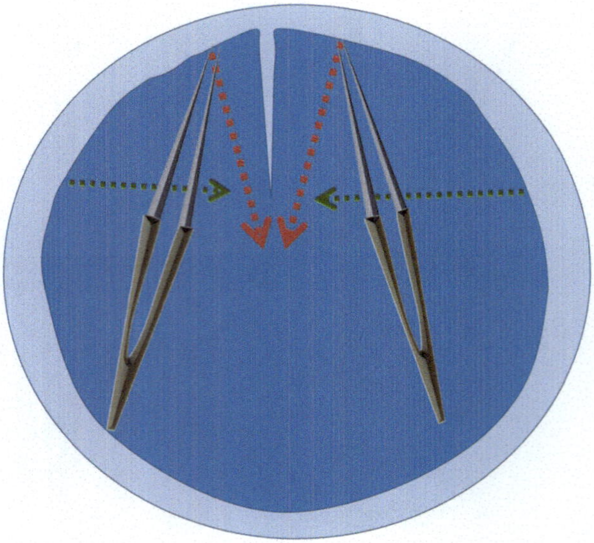

Fig. 10.2 In larger radially directed tears, two forceps can be used to pull Descemet's membrane from both sides of the tear in parallel (*red dotted arrow*) without further tear enlargement. Before approaching the tear, Descemet's membrane should be stripped close to the tip of the tear by pulling almost orthogonally to the tear direction (*green dotted arrow*). The advantage of the two forceps technique is that no additional loss of Descemet's membrane will result

since one has to avoid further damage of this central tissue which will result in endothelial cell damage right in the centre of the optical zone. To strip DM with central adhesions, stripping has to be stopped as soon as tearing is recognised. Stripping should then be proceeded from the two sites orthogonal to the initial stripping direction. When approaching the adhesive zone, DM still attached to the corneal stroma has to be grasped with a forceps to avoid further enlarging of the tear. Technically, implantation and unfolding of grafts with central tears do not differ from intact grafts. However, the graft should be placed with the defect as peripheral as possible preferable towards the 12 o'clock position. Depending on the graft preparation technique, DM becomes trephined before stripping is completed. Trephination can be performed eccentrical to shift the central tear towards the periphery of the graft (Fig. 10.3).

10.3 Intraoperative Complications

A smooth course of DMEK surgery can be hindered by factors of which many of them can be identified preoperatively already. Small, hyperopic eyes with high vitreous pressure offer only little space for unfolding manoeuvres after graft implantation. A cornea appearing cloudy at the slit lamp is in general even less transparent under the surgery microscope. Anterior segment abnormalities, e.g. in patients with a history of glaucoma drainage device implantation, in aphakic eyes or in eyes with larger iris defects or anterior synechia increase the risk of having difficulties to unfold and place the graft correctly.

These factors should be taken into account when planning the surgery. The first decision to be made is whether the risk of complications outperforms the benefits of DMEK instead of DS(A)EK. Frequently patients with complex anterior segment

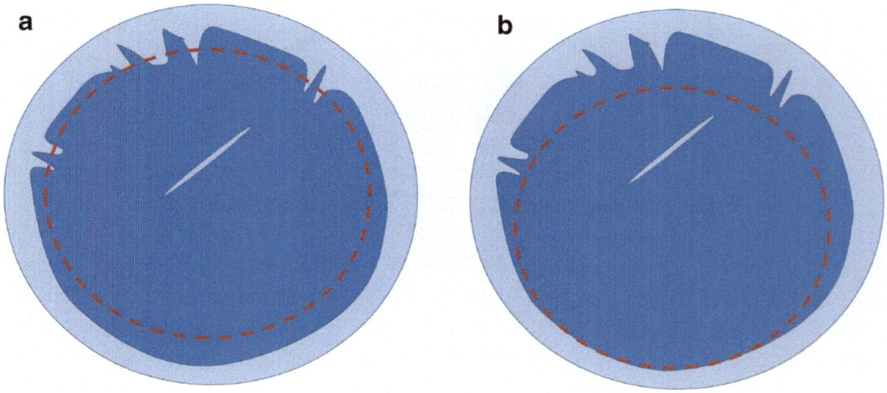

Fig. 10.3 (**a**) If a high number of tears approaching the trephination line (*red dotted circle*) or centrally located tears occur, eccentrical trephination (**b**; *red dotted circle*) results in a sharp outline of the graft without tears in the peripheral edge and can also shift a central tear towards the periphery of the graft

disorders are on a higher risk for graft rejections which are barely seen after DMEK (1 % within 2 years) but occur more frequently after DS(A)EK (15-fold higher) [11]. Moreover, the functional results and the healing process are more favourable making DMEK the method of choice in most patients [12]. However, surgeries on higher risk for intraoperative complications are more likely to result in higher endothelial cell loss due to mechanical stress and are thus on a higher risk of (primary) graft failures. With careful planning of the surgery and with growing experience of the surgeon, even corneal endothelial diseases in the face of complex anterior segment disorders can be successfully treated with DMEK.

When high vitreous pressure is expected, the following measures should be considered:

- Oculopression before surgery
- Administration of drugs with lowering effect on vitreous pressure (acetazolamide, mannitol)
- Low systolic and mean arterial blood pressure during surgery
- Cataract surgery in combination with DMEK (Triple-DMEK) in phakic eyes [2]

Eyes with a small corneal diameter and a shallow anterior chamber give little space for unfolding the graft. Therefore, adapting the graft size to the anterior chamber depth and the corneal white-to-white distance facilitates the unfolding process. To the authors' experience, graft diameters of as little as 7 mm can be helpful for DMEK in very small eyes. Intracameral unfolding of the DMEK graft can also be hampered by anterior synechia or by intracameral tubes from drainage devices [13]. In such cases the mechanical barrier should be removed by lysis of the anterior synechia or surgical shortening of the intracameral tube.

Not only small eyes but also very large eyes or eyes after vitrectomy with a deep anterior chamber without vitreous pressure can make unfolding of the DMEK graft difficult. Once the graft is partially unfolded by external manoeuvres or by an

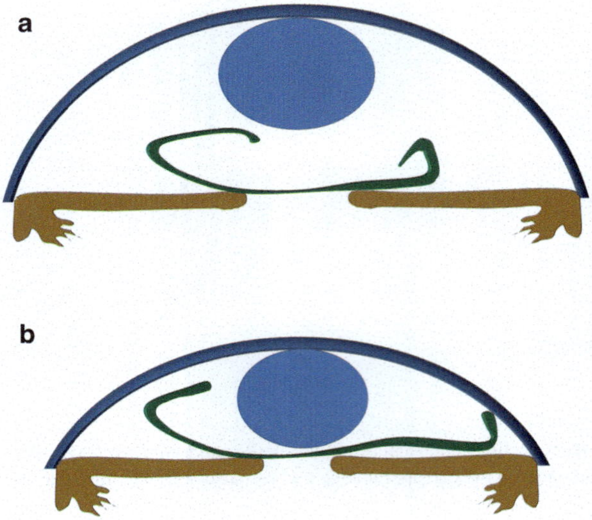

Fig. 10.4 (**a**) Very large eyes or eyes after vitrectomy with a deep anterior chamber without vitreous pressure can make unfolding of the DMEK graft difficult. After partial unfolding of the graft (e.g. by an intracameral air bubble), the graft will almost always spontaneously form a roll again. (**b**) In normal-sized eyes with normal vitreous pressure, anterior chamber depth can be adjusted and flattened by fluid release. Thus, the peripheral parts of an unfolded graft can be trapped between the iris and the cornea which keeps the graft unfolded and prevents it from spontaneous rolling

intracameral air bubble, the graft will spontaneously form a roll again in case the anterior chamber is very deep (Fig. 10.4a). In an eye where the anterior chamber depth can be adjusted and flattened by fluid release, the peripheral parts of an unfolded graft are trapped between iris and cornea which keeps the graft unfolded and prevents it from spontaneous rolling (Fig. 10.4b). In eyes after vitrectomy or large eyes with very deep anterior chambers, the donor size should be enlarged (depending on the recipient's diameter of the cornea), and again, corneas from an older donor should be used since the rolling behaviour in these grafts is much less pronounced.

If during DMEK surgery, unexpected rolling behaviours are noted in pseudophakic eyes which have been operated on before elsewhere, care should be taken to rule out vitreous prolapse and such prolapse should be removed to avoid incarceration between the recipients' cornea and the DMEK role.

Correct unfolding and positioning of the graft is substantially influenced by the transparency of the recipient's cornea. Graft orientation during unfolding in eyes with cloudy corneas can easily be lost. Certain techniques have been described to confirm the orientation of the unfolding process.

Orientation marks are an easy measure to confirm the orientation not only during the surgery but also thereafter during the postoperative course [14]. Three marks can be set at the margin of the graft using a 1-mm trephine during graft preparation of which two of them are set close together and the third one is placed with little distance.

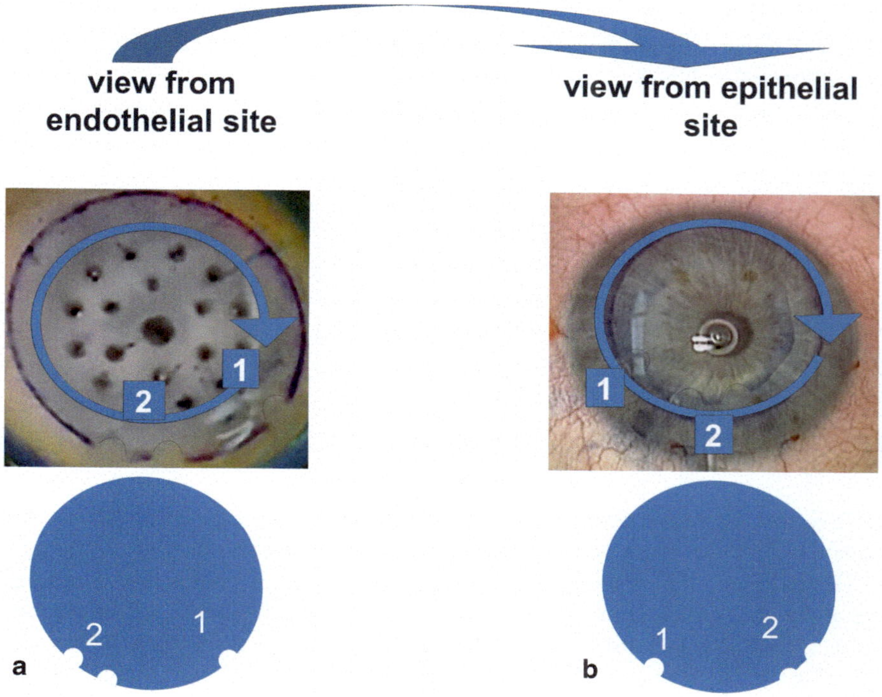

Fig. 10.5 Orientation marks set by small trephinations of the edge of Descemet's membrane help to identify the graft orientation. (**a**) Two marks are set close together and the third one is placed with little distance. This results in a clockwise order of the marks of 1–2 when the graft is seen from the endothelial site. (**b**) The order changes if the unfolded graft is directed correctly inside the anterior chamber when it is seen from the epithelial site. Here the clockwise order of the marks is 2–1, meaning that one mark is placed with little distance to the other two marks which sit closer together (Reproduced with the kind permission of Elsevier Inc. from Ref. [14])

This results in a clockwise order of the marks of 1–2 when the graft is seen from the endothelial site. The order changes when the graft is turned which is the case if the graft is placed correctly at the backsite of the corneal stroma, and it is seen from the epithelial site. Here the clockwise order of the marks is 2–1, meaning that one mark is placed with little distance to the other two marks which sit closer together (Fig 10.5).

To confirm the correct orientation of a partially unfolded graft with curled edges, the tip of a cannula can be placed between graft and recipient's cornea. When the cannula is moved from the centre of graft into the peripheral roll, one can recognise the blue shimmer of the stained graft. In contrast, when the graft orientation is false, the tip of the cannula cannot be placed inside the roll when starting the movement from the centre since the roll opens downwards (Moutsouris sign) [15]. A (hand-held) slit beam is another option to visualise the graft orientation by identifying the direction towards the rolled graft edges directed [16].

Novel microscopes offer online OCT imaging during surgery. Hereby, all steps of preparation and implantation can be visualised even in very cloudy recipient corneas

[17]. These devices not only help to identify orientation and localisation of the graft but also help to visualise the remaining amount of fluid after gas tamponade.

Intraoperative bleeding after iridectomy during DMEK is a rare but possibly serious complication which can lead to early termination of the surgery. An iridectomy should therefore always be performed before the recipient's DM stripping. Otherwise, massive corneal edema will be the result in case the surgery has to be finished after stripping and before correct graft placement. To avoid intraoperative bleeding, an iridotomy with a Nd:YAG laser can be placed (at 6 o'clock position) before surgery. Even if the iridotomy is too small at the beginning of the surgery, widening of the opening by blunt spreading with a microscissor offers a reduced and only minimal risk of bleeding.

10.4 Postoperative Complications

DMEK-specific early postoperative complications comprise a *rise in intraocular pressure* (IOP) due to gas tamponade, graft detachment and primary graft failure.

Depending on the surgeon's choice, the amount of gas fill of the anterior chamber at the end of the surgery can vary and can be adjusted to 100 % of the anterior chamber volume. In most patients where a sufficient iridotomy or iridectomy is placed at 6 o'clock position, the pupillary block caused by the anterior chamber gas fill will not result in a raise of IOP. If the surgeon chooses a 100 % gas fill of the anterior chamber, opening of the iridotomy should be supported by topical administration of pilocarpine during the first postoperative days. The duration of pilocarpine administration depends on the type of gas used for tamponade (slower resorption of SF6 20 % compared with room air) [18]. However, postoperative blood or fibrin plugs in the opening of the iridotomy can cause an increase of IOP. In such cases reopening of the iridotomy can be achieved by additional Nd:YAG laser application.

After DMEK the patients are usually asked to keep a supine position to support graft attachment during the first postoperative days. However, in supine position even peripheral iridotomies can be covered and plugged by the gas tamponade. In such cases, sitting position can lead to reopening of the iridotomy and will thus lower the IOP within minutes. In addition local and systemic IOP-lowering drug administration can help to overcome the pupillary block situation.

If the rise in IOP is very high and a full iris bombe configuration with peripheral touch between the iris and the cornea persists, release of intracameral air might be necessary. This can be performed after local administration of anaesthetics and antiseptics in a sitting position at the slit lamp by the opening of a paracentesis at 3 or 9 o'clock position with a blunt instrument (e.g. spatula or forceps). Thus, only air to the level of the paracentesis will be released leaving an intracameral air bubble above that level for further support of the graft but allowing for fluid transfer through the pupil again. This usually results in an immediate deepening of the anterior chamber. Even without symptomatic angle closure, pressure values of up to 40 mmHg can be measured in the first postoperative hours. Care should be taken especially in glaucoma patients to monitor IOP closely in the early postoperative period [18].

An IOP increase can also be related to local steroid administration. Such steroid-related IOP peaks are seen in around 20 % of all patients after DMEK [19]. Since graft rejection barely occurs after DMEK, local steroids should be tapered fast or changed to substances with a decreased impact on IOP (e.g. loteprednol etabonate) in patients with a steroid-associated elevation of IOP.

A common complication after DMEK is *partial graft detachment*. Smaller peripheral detachments of the graft are seen in up to 50 % of patients and more. Most detachments will resolve by themselves with spontaneous reattachment over time but the patient's visual acuity can be reduced during that time [20]. Moreover, if the graft tends to roll, a fold can develop. Smaller peripheral folds usually do not influence the final visual acuity. However, myofibroblastic transformation of the endothelial cells can occur which increases the folds or increases the detached area. Therefore, larger graft dehiscence should either be treated by an additional intracameral gas tamponade (rebubbling) or should at least be observed tightly. In case larger peripheral fold formation is observed, rebubbling should be performed immediately before myofibroblastic transformation of the endothelial cells cause wrinkling of the graft which can promote graft dehiscence [21]. It seems that in areas of overlapping between the graft's and the recipient's DM, graft detachment is more likely to occur [22]. Therefore, the stripped area of the recipient's posterior corneal surface should be larger than the graft. When the graft is centred correctly, this will avoid such areas of overlapping. Rebubbling should preferably be performed from a site where DMEK tissue is attached to avoid the risk of further enlarging the detachment by injecting air between the graft and the recipient's corneal stroma.

Another common postoperative complication after DMEK with or without cataract surgery (Triple-DMEK) is the formation of *cystoid macular edema* (CME) occurring in about 12 % of all patients [23, 24]. The overall prognosis of CME is good. However, a prolonged course of the disease with significant visual impairment can occur. High-frequency postoperative treatment with prednisolone acetate eye drops 1 % hourly the first week after DMEK significantly reduces the development of CME after (Triple-) DMEK [24].

Primary graft failure is very rare and most commonly associated with intraoperative complications. Postoperatively wrong graft orientation can be identified by the rolling behaviour of the detached DM or by markings of the graft [14]. These can be identified during slit lamp examination, or in case of cloudy corneas, curling of the graft edges can be visualised by anterior segment OCT examination. If the curled edge of the graft is directed towards the anterior chamber, the graft orientation is wrong. In such cases surgical turning of the graft is a reasonable measure before considering graft replacement by re-DMEK.

When comparing with other techniques of corneal transplantation, the overall healing process is fastest after DMEK leading to a rapid and unsurpassed improvement in visual acuity. However, immunological considerations are even more decisive when considering to learn DMEK. *Graft rejection* which is the leading cause for graft failure after PK has lost its fright since the introduction of DMEK. It barely occurs after DMEK and can only be seen in about 1 % within the first two postoperative years. In contrast, the rate of graft rejection after DSEK and PK is 15-fold and 20-fold higher, respectively. The signs for graft rejection are usually weaker than those seen in PK patients. Some patients just show diffuse keratic precipitates without accompanying corneal edema. These patients might still have very good vision despite increasing amounts of precipitates over weeks or months. Commonly the precipitates can be observed on the graft itself, but since donor endothelial cells also migrate from the graft onto the neighbouring denuded corneal stroma, keratic precipitates can also be seen outside the graft in the context of DMEK graft rejection [25]. But also corneal edema and the formation of a Khodadoust line can occur in graft rejections after DMEK [26]. Similar to graft rejections after PK, the mainstay of treatment consists in high-frequency topical steroid application tapering over weeks or even months. In relapsing rejections systemic immunosuppressive treatment should be considered.

In case of (primary) graft failure, repeat DMEK (re-DMEK) should be considered. Primary graft failure is frequently associated with strong corneal edema. In such patients re-DMEK should be performed as soon as possible to avoid corneal ulcerations, infections or scaring. Overall, patients achieve very good vision after re-DMEK, but the results tend to be a little worse compared to corneas without previous DMEK [27]. Moreover, patients after re-DMEK are on higher risk for additional complications like primary or secondary graft failure, graft detachment, glaucoma or corneal ulceration meaning that these patients are in need of an intense postoperative follow-up. Technically the surgery is comparable to primary DMEK. Frequently, the corneas are very cloudy making a corneal abrasion or the intraoperative application of deswelling eye drops (e.g. glycerin eye drops) necessary.

In summary, cautious preoperative planning, standardised yet individualised surgery and careful postoperative monitoring can significantly reduce intra- and postoperative complications after DMEK [28, 29].

References

1. Kruse FE, Laaser K, Cursiefen C, Heindl LM, Schlotzer-Schrehardt U, Riss S, Bachmann BO. A stepwise approach to donor preparation and insertion increases safety and outcome of Descemet membrane endothelial keratoplasty. Cornea. 2011;30(5):580–7.
2. Siggel R, Heindl LM, Cursiefen C. Descemet membrane endothelial keratoplasty (DMEK) in phakic eyes with shallow anterior chamber. Graefes Arch Clin Exp Ophthalmol. 2015;253(5): 817–9.
3. Kobayashi A, Murata N, Yokogawa H, Yamazaki N, Masaki T, Sugiyama K. Evaluation of internationally shipped prestripped donor tissue for descemet membrane endothelial keratoplasty by vital dye staining. Cornea. 2015;34(2):225–7.
4. Park CY, Lee JK, Gore PK, Lim CY, Chuck RS. Keratoplasty in the United States: a 10-year review from 2005 through 2014. Ophthalmology. 2015;122(12):2432–42.
5. Lie JT, Lam FC, Groeneveld-van Beek EA, van der Wees J, Melles GR. Graft preparation for hemi-Descemet membrane endothelial keratoplasty (hemi-DMEK). Br J Ophthalmol. 2016; 100(3):420–4.

6. Dapena I, Moutsouris K, Droutsas K, Ham L, van Dijk K, Melles GR. Standardized "no-touch" technique for descemet membrane endothelial keratoplasty. Arch Ophthalmol. 2011; 129(1):88–94.
7. Dua HS, Faraj LA, Said DG, Gray T, Lowe J. Human corneal anatomy redefined: a novel pre-Descemet's layer (Dua's layer). Ophthalmology. 2013;120(9):1778–85.
8. Gamaleldin SA, Salama MM, Elshazly MI. Seven-day storage of pneumatically dissected Descemet's endothelial grafts with and without Dua's layer. Acta Ophthalmol. 2016;94(2): e130–4.
9. Schlotzer-Schrehardt U, Bachmann BO, Tourtas T, Cursiefen C, Zenkel M, Rossler K, Kruse FE. Reproducibility of graft preparations in Descemet's membrane endothelial keratoplasty. Ophthalmology. 2013;120(9):1769–77.
10. Tourtas T, Heindl LM, Kopsachilis N, Bachmann BO, Kruse FE, Cursiefen C. Use of accidentally torn descemet membrane to successfully complete descemet membrane endothelial keratoplasty. Cornea. 2013;32(11):1418–22.
11. Anshu A, Price MO, Price Jr FW. Risk of corneal transplant rejection significantly reduced with Descemet's membrane endothelial keratoplasty. Ophthalmology. 2012;119(3):536–40.
12. Tourtas T, Laaser K, Bachmann BO, Cursiefen C, Kruse FE. Descemet membrane endothelial keratoplasty versus descemet stripping automated endothelial keratoplasty. Am J Ophthalmol. 2012;153(6):1082–90.e2.
13. Heindl LM, Koch KR, Bucher F, Hos D, Steven P, Koch HR, Cursiefen C. Descemet membrane endothelial keratoplasty in eyes with glaucoma implants. Optom Vis Sci. 2013;90(9): e241–4; discussion 1029.
14. Bachmann BO, Laaser K, Cursiefen C, Kruse FE. A method to confirm correct orientation of descemet membrane during descemet membrane endothelial keratoplasty. Am J Ophthalmol. 2010;149(6):922–5.e2.
15. Isabel Dapena MD; Kyros Moutsouris ,... Arch Ophthalmol. 2011;129(1):88–94
16. Burkhart ZN, Feng MT, Price MO, Price FW. Handheld slit beam techniques to facilitate DMEK and DALK. Cornea. 2013;32(5):722–4.
17. Steven P, Le Blanc C, Velten K, Lankenau E, Krug M, Oelckers S, Heindl LM, Gehlsen U, Huttmann G, Cursiefen C. Optimizing descemet membrane endothelial keratoplasty using intraoperative optical coherence tomography. JAMA Ophthalmol. 2013;131(9):1135–42.
18. Stanzel TP, Ersoy L, Sansanayudh W, Felsch M, Dietlein T, Bachmann B, Cursiefen C. Immediate postoperative intraocular pressure changes after anterior chamber air fill in Descemet membrane endothelial keratoplasty. Cornea. 2016;35(1):14–9.
19. Price MO, Price Jr FW, Kruse FE, Bachmann BO, Tourtas T. Randomized comparison of topical prednisolone acetate 1% versus fluorometholone 0.1% in the first year after descemet membrane endothelial keratoplasty. Cornea. 2014;33(9):880–6.
20. Bucher F, Hos D, Muller-Schwefe S, Steven P, Cursiefen C, Heindl LM. Spontaneous long-term course of persistent peripheral graft detachments after Descemet's membrane endothelial keratoplasty. Br J Ophthalmol. 2015;99(6):768–72.
21. Heindl LM, Schlotzer-Schrehardt U, Cursiefen C, Bachmann BO, Hofmann-Rummelt C, Kruse FE. Myofibroblast metaplasia after descemet membrane endothelial keratoplasty. Am J Ophthalmol. 2011;151(6):1019–23.e2.
22. Tourtas T, Schlomberg J, Wessel JM, Bachmann BO, Schlotzer-Schrehardt U, Kruse FE. Graft adhesion in descemet membrane endothelial keratoplasty dependent on size of removal of host's descemet membrane. JAMA Ophthalmol. 2014;132(2):155–61.
23. Heinzelmann S, Maier P, Bohringer D, Huther S, Eberwein P, Reinhard T. Cystoid macular oedema following Descemet membrane endothelial keratoplasty. Br J Ophthalmol. 2015;99(1):98–102.
24. Hoerster R, Stanzel TP, Bachmann BO, Siebelmann S, Felsch M, Cursiefen C. Intensified topical steroids as prophylaxis for macular edema after posterior lamellar keratoplasty combined with cataract surgery. Am J Ophthalmol. 2016;163:174–9.e2.
25. Hos D, Heindl LM, Bucher F, Cursiefen C. Evidence of donor corneal endothelial cell migration from immune reactions occurring after descemet membrane endothelial keratoplasty. Cornea. 2014;33(4):331–4.

26. Dapena I, Ham L, Netukova M, van der Wees J, Melles GR. Incidence of early allograft rejection after Descemet membrane endothelial keratoplasty. Cornea. 2011;30(12):1341–5.
27. Baydoun L1, van Dijk K2, Dapena I2, Musa FU3, Liarakos VS2, Ham L1, Melles GR4. Repeat Descemet membrane endothelial keratoplasty after complicated primary Descemet membrane endothelial keratoplasty. Ophthalmology. 2015 Jan;122(1):8-16. doi: 10.1016/j.ophtha.2014.07.024. Epub 2014 Sep 5.
28. Maier P, Reinhard T, Cursiefen C. Descemet stripping endothelial keratoplasty–rapid recovery of visual acuity. Dtsch Arztebl Int. 2013;110(21):365–71.
29. Cursiefen C, Steven P, Roters S, Heindl LM. Prevention and management of complications in Descemet membrane endothelial keratoplasty (DMEK) and Descemet stripping automated endothelial keratoplasty (DSAEK). Ophthalmologe. 2013;110(7):614–21.

Chapter 11
DMEK: Step-by-Step Surgical Approach

Bindiya Hapani, M.O. Price, and F.W. Price Jr

Abbreviations

ABMD	Anterior basement membrane dystrophy
AC	Anterior chamber
BSS	Balanced salt solution
DALK	Deep anterior lamellar keratoplasty
DM	Descemet membrane
DMEK	Descemet membrane endothelial keratoplasty
DSEK	Descemet stripping endothelial keratoplasty
EK	Endothelial keratoplasty
FECD	Fuchs endothelial corneal dystrophy
I & A	Irrigation and Aspiration
IOL	Intraocular lens
IOP	Intraocular pressure
MMC	Mitomycin C
OCT	Optical coherence tomography
PI	Peripheral iridotomy
PK	Penetrating keratoplasty
PPV	Pars plana vitrectomy

B. Hapani, MS, FICO (✉)
Dr. Agarwal's Eye Hospital, Bangalore, India
e-mail: bindiyahapani@gmail.com

M.O. Price, PhD, MBA
Cornea Research Foundation of America,
9002 N. Meridian St., Suite 212, Indianapolis, IN 46260, USA
e-mail: mprice@cornea.org

F.W. Price Jr , MD
Price Vision Group, 9002 N. Meridian St., Suite 100, Indianapolis, IN 46260, USA
e-mail: fprice@pricevisiongroup.net

C. Cursiefen, A.S. Jun (eds.), *Current Treatment Options for Fuchs Endothelial Dystrophy*, DOI 10.1007/978-3-319-43021-8_11

11.1 Introduction

Endothelial keratoplasty (EK) has displaced penetrating keratoplasty as the treatment of choice for Fuchs endothelial corneal dystrophy (FECD) and other causes of endothelial cell dysfunction because EK provides rapid visual recovery, a stable corneal surface, and less risk of severe intra- and postoperative complications [5, 6, 17, 24, 26, 27, 41, 45–49, 53, 59].

Innovations in EK have transformed it from a procedure performed by only a few select surgeons because of its complex technique requirements into a surgery that can be performed in any regular ophthalmic surgical setup. While Descemet stripping endothelial keratoplasty (DSEK) is currently the most widely used method, Descemet membrane endothelial keratoplasty (DMEK) is gaining rapidly in popularity because it offers better visual recovery with reduced risk of rejection and lesser need of long-term topical corticosteroids [5, 6, 50–52] (Fig. 11.1).

In DMEK, healthy donor endothelium and Descemet membrane are implanted without the additional posterior donor stroma that is included with DSEK [41].

11.1.1 Advantages of DMEK Compared with DSEK or PK

- Nearly exact anatomic replacement of dysfunctional host endothelium.
- Better and faster visual recovery and more predictable refractive outcomes [5, 6, 13, 14, 18, 24–27, 34, 41, 43, 45, 46, 49, 53].

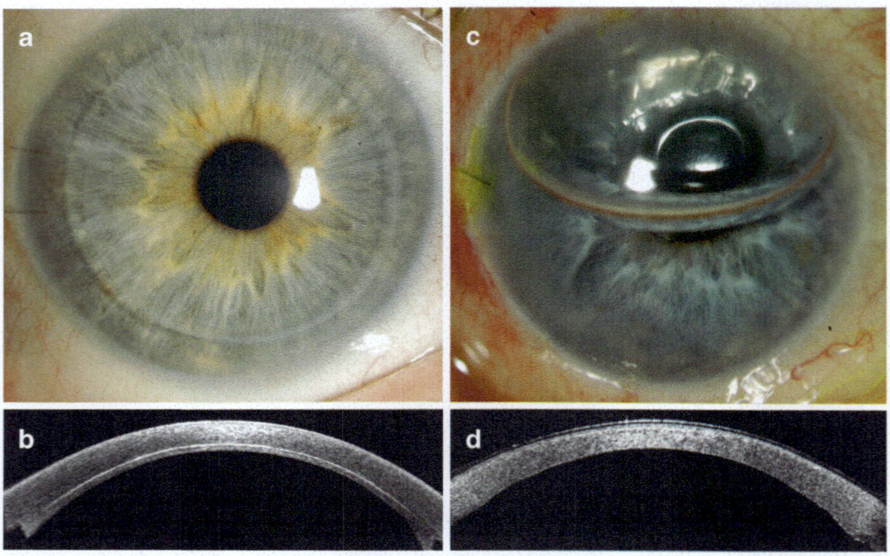

Fig. 11.1 (**a, b**) Slit-lamp image and anterior segment optical coherence tomography image 1 week after Descemet stripping endothelial keratoplasty (DSEK). (**c, d**) Slit-lamp image and anterior segment optical coherence tomography image 1 day after Descemet membrane endothelial keratoplasty (DMEK)

- Reduced risk of immunologic rejection, allowing less use of prophylactic topical corticosteroids and reduced risk of steroid-associated side effects [5, 6, 18, 26, 51, 52].
- No need for expensive instrumentation, such as the microkeratome typically used in DSEK tissue preparation, so it is readily accessible to corneal surgeons in any surgical setting.

11.2 Step-by-Step Approach for Success with DMEK

DMEK is generally considered more challenging than DSEK or PK. A structured approach with careful attention to the key elements discussed below will help ensure success.

11.2.1 Preparing DMEK Donor Tissue

The donor tissue can be prepared by the surgeon or by the eye bank [19]. Preparing the tissue ahead of time and preserving it in corneal storage medium saves time and reduces stress on the day of surgery [19, 21, 37].

The DMEK graft is quite thin and delicate, because it consists of DM and the endothelial layer without any stroma and the endothelium is on the outer or exposed surface, so proper handling is important to minimize endothelial cell loss and avoid inadvertent tears.

11.2.2 DMEK Donor Criteria

The tissue from older donors (over 40 or 50 years old) is easier to handle with DMEK. The thickness of DM is about 3 microns at birth increasing to about 20 microns in adulthood [29, 31]. In children, DM is more fragile and more tightly bound to the stroma. Also, the tissue harvested from young donors curls up tightly and can be difficult to unfold inside the eye [29].

The tissue from diabetic donors can be more prone to develop tears during preparation [23, 60]. However, since the prevalence of diabetes is so high among tissue donors (30% or higher), diabetic tissue cannot be completely excluded for DMEK. More careful characterization of donor diabetes is needed to determine whether certain thresholds of diabetes duration or degree of glycemic control should be exclusionary. Diabetic tissue may present more challenges because of glycation products from chronic hyperglycemia, which deposit between the posterior stroma and DM creating stronger adhesion, and the wide-spaced collagen present in the DM of diabetic corneas, which may have a deleterious effect on the tensile strength [23, 60].

11.2.3 Sizing the Graft

Measure the white-to-white diameter of the host cornea before choosing your donor punch. A small size graft in bigger host cornea may not be able to replace the required amount of endothelial cells especially in non-Fuchs endothelial decompensation when the entire cornea has decompensated.

A large donor graft might get stuck in the angle in a very small eye, and it might be hard to see the edges behind a very dense arcus. It is also important to consider that the paracentesis wound does not get covered up with the graft so that the irrigating cannula used to manipulate the graft with fluid has room to get into the anterior chamber without encountering the graft itself. A graft diameter of 8.0–9.0 mm is suitable in most cases.

11.3 Harvesting the Graft

Two general approaches have been used to isolate donor DM and endothelium: direct peeling and pneumatic separation. Direct peeling (https://itunes.apple.com/us/book/digital-manual-ophthalmic/id803683426?mt=13) is used more widely because many have achieved a higher success rate with less endothelial cell loss with this approach. Many variations have been developed within each general approach, and the exact techniques used by the Melles group [40–42], the Kruse group [32], the Ignatio group [30], and our group [57, 58] have been detailed in the literature.

We prefer the modified SCUBA (submerged cornea using backgrounds away) technique. This technique suspends the tissue with fluid above and below making it easy to visualize and handle during preparation [22, 57, 58].

Here we will discuss every step of DMEK graft harvesting, which starts with scoring of DM and ends with trephination and final peeling.

11.3.1 Scoring DM

Scoring is the process of bluntly marking the periphery of the posterior cornea. It can be done with a blunt tying forceps or a Y-hook with the donor corneoscleral rim placed on a cutting block or submerged in a donor tissue-viewing chamber (Krolman viewing chamber, K55-57007-23, Bausch & Lomb, Rochester, NY) [22, 58] (Fig. 11.2). The donor is fixated with a toothed forceps, while a peripheral break or "score" in the DM is created. A blunt Y-hook (9217E, Ambler Surgical, Exton, PA, 17157 Moria, Antony, France) can be used instead of tying forceps to create the initial score in the DM, because it produces a smoother break with fewer tears. The score line should be positioned just inside the trabecular meshwork.

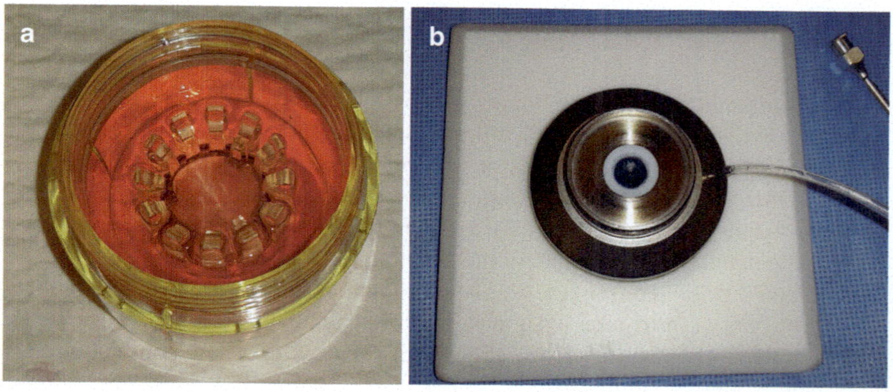

Fig. 11.2 (**a**) Krolman viewing chamber. (**b**) Cutting block

The Y-hook should be pressed firmly against the submerged corneoscleral rim to penetrate the DM without tearing the underlying stroma and can be lightly dragged along the periphery to propagate the score. Caution should be exercised not to press too hard or impale the delicate posterior stromal fibers. A blade should not be used to create this score to avoid cutting into the stroma, which would make it difficult to grasp or lift the DM without also grabbing the edge of the connected stroma. If counterpressure is needed to penetrate the DM, the centrally protruding viewing chamber pillar (Krolman viewing chamber) can be used with the tissue submerged, or the donor can be placed on a cutting block [57, 58].

11.3.2 Improving the View of the Scored Edge

To allow visualization of the scored edge, staining should be performed for 10 s using a 0.06 % trypan blue solution (VisionBlue; DORC, Zuidland, the Netherlands) after scoring is completed and before elevating the edge of DM. Trypan blue does not stain endothelial cells in their native healthy state when applied for a short time. During a 10-s exposure, only cells that are damaged by the scoring and exposed areas of DM itself will stain [32, 58].

VisionBlue improves the view of DM breaks and DM scarring (cataract wounds). "Snail tracks" in the endothelium from the donor harvest also stain, as do insufficient scoring strokes that only denuded endothelial cells. Such unscored zones can cause radial tears during the next step of lifting the edge of the DM.

Remove irregular DM tags outside the area of scoring. This improves the view of the DM edge to better see if radial tears are present, and it allows unsuccessful score zones to be discovered and rescored before radial tears develop [57, 58].

11.3.3 Lifting the Edge of DM

After scoring and staining, the donor corneoscleral rim is returned to the storage chamber for visualization under the microscope. The scored edge of the donor DM is lifted 360° with a small blunt instrument such as a microfinger (Moria, Antony, France) [58]. The tip of the microfinger is inserted 0.5 mm under the edge of DM and held against the stroma (Fig. 11.3a). The microfinger is glided circumferentially while maintaining the depth of the penetration to lift a consistent width of the DM. It should be glided from the area of minimum tension (loose DM attachment) toward the area of maximum tension (firm DM attachment). If a radial tear develops, it should first have the loose edges torn off leaving a new continuous torn edge. This converts the tear into a "crater" in the scored diameter. Then gently glide the microfinger back and forth along the free edges to lift the peripheral DM down to the circumference of the crater. The crater is lifted last. In lifting the crater, always carefully watch for further tearing. Each crater can limit the final diameter of the donor graft depending on its size and the diameter of the cornea with which you started.

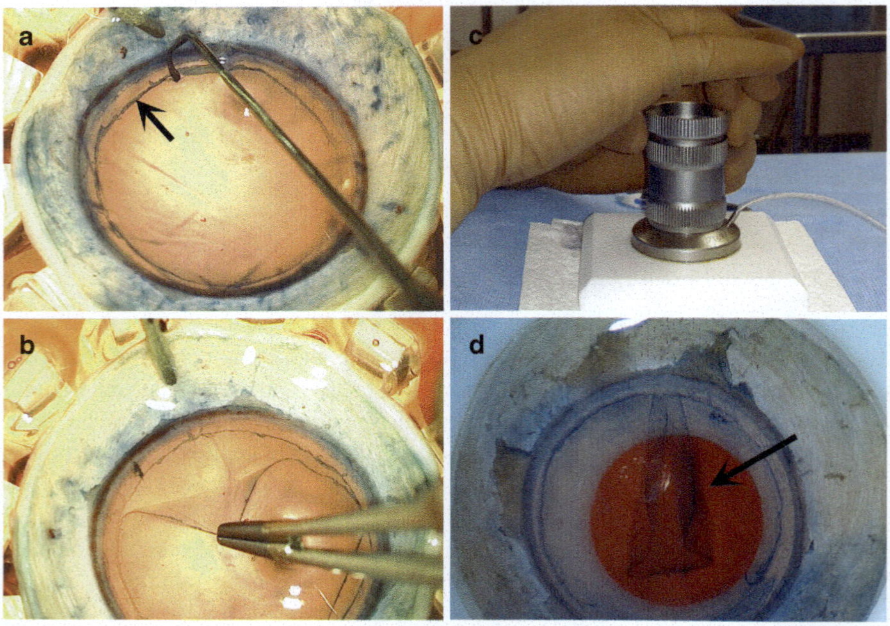

Fig. 11.3 (**a**) Using a microfinger to lift the scored edge of the graft. (**b**) Peeling off the donor Descemet membrane and endothelium while the tissue is submerged in storage medium. (**c**) Cutting block with trephine. (**d**) Donor Descemet membrane roll

11.3.4 Peeling DM

Before final trephination, 360° partial peeling of the DM is performed. This allows any zones of strong adhesions (which can develop tears) to be discovered. Such areas can be excluded from the final trephination depending on where they are located. The limbus is fixated with a toothed forceps, and the DM edge is grabbed with a Tubingen forceps (2457E, Ambler Surgical) or other large, smooth tiers, exactly central to fixation [58]. To avoid tears, the Tubingen forceps should not be twisted or elevated away from the cornea, because twisting can break DM just as forceps can do with suture. Each pull should be straight across [58]. A prominent stress line will appear if the pull deviates to the side.

The DM is peeled by quadrants ("corridor method", Fig. 11.3b). This technique minimizes tension by minimizing the width of the peel zone [57, 58]. The more centrally a peel is taken, the wider it gets, with increasing tension on the DM. The peel edge of the first quadrant is taken about halfway to the center of the cornea. Peel 2 should be started 180° away and also is taken halfway to the center. Peel 3 is started 90° to the left or the right of peel 2. A narrow corridor of unpeeled DM remains at this point. Because the peel zone now can get no wider than this corridor, the tension is low, making it safe to peel quadrant 3 close to the center of the cornea. Peel 4 (180° away from peel 3) is taken halfway to the center. Efforts should be made to grab a "peak," not a "crater" along the perimeter as the starting point of each pull. The meridian of peel 4 is marked as the intended start site for the final peel after trephination. Because peel 3 is taken close to the middle, the donor would fully separate from the stroma before the forceps advances over the opposing sclera (thus reducing the risk of endothelial touch).

Alternatively, one can peel DM by sequentially rotating the donor tissue 30–60° at a time and stripping partway across [22]. This technique is especially useful when encountering separation resistance. This can be felt as tension or seen as smile configuration or stress line as the tissue is being peeled. When the leading edge of the peel has minimal resistance, it forms a straight line. When the right and left edges of the peel lag behind the central portion (forming a "smile"), the resistance is high. In such circumstances, peel at 45° to both sides of this site, then the peel can be continued from the original site. This technique lessens tension by limiting the width of each peel.

11.3.5 Handling Horseshoe Tears

Continuing to pull after a horseshoe tear (HST) develops can tear the donor in half. Interestingly, "descemetoschisis," or "lamellar splitting" of the DM, can precede most HSTs as a tongue or triangular attachment of the anterior layers of the DM on the stroma. If an HST is suspected but hard to see as the tissue is being peeled, stop and apply focal VisionBlue staining. To complete the preparation in the presence of an HST, one strategy is to stop pulling at that site, partially peel all other quadrants, trephine, and then start the final donor peel 180° away from the HST [57, 58]. If two HSTs develop 180° apart, the tongue of one has to be lifted so that the peel can be continued through that HST. The centrally protruding Krolman viewing chamber pillar can be used for counterpressure to lift the tongue [57, 58]. The tissue with descemetoschisis or partial tears can still be used safely for DMEK [28].

11.3.6 Trephining DM

The trephine size should be selected based on the size of cornea and type of pathology. For FECD, an 8-mm graft diameter is sufficient, because FECD patients have healthy peripheral corneal endothelium. However, with pseudophakic bullous keratopathy or failed endothelial keratoplasty, a 9-mm graft will provide more healthy endothelial cells.

To trephine, the corneoscleral rim is placed on the cutting block and aligned with any imperfections outside the trephine zone. A cutting block with a marked central 8-mm area, such as the Hanna punch with a Price-cutting block (17169 & 630/660–7540, Moria), helps to get perfect alignment especially if the punch needs to be decentered [57, 58]. Suction is activated on the cutting block. The DM is checked to ensure that it is not curled. If it is curled, the storage solution is wicked from under the DM with a cellulose sponge so that the DM follows the fluid peripherally to lay flat. More fluid can be dripped on and soaked away as necessary. The guide cylinder is attached. The trephine punch cylinder is advanced into the guide until the blade makes contact with the cornea without rotating (Fig. 11.3c). The corneal thickness holds the punch cylinder up so that a small gap remains present between the guide and punch rims. The thumb and index finger of one hand is placed in this gap to hold the circumference of both rims to prevent rotation, while the other hand is used to lightly tap the punch in all four quadrants. When the gap is lessened, tapping is stopped so that the cornea is only penetrated but not perforated [57, 58].

11.3.7 Final Peel of the Donor

The donor is briefly restrained with VisionBlue, the sclera is grasped at the meridian of peel 4, submerged, and the peripheral rim of the DM beyond the trephine marks is removed with caution to separate sites with adhesions last. The final peel should be done at the same meridian where peel 4 is made, so the donor gets separated when the peel reaches the middle. When submerged, the donor forms a scroll with the endothelium on the outside [19, 40]. The scroll can be secured in the corneoscleral rim filled with the storage solution if it is to be used at that time (Fig. 11.3d).

It should be placed in a glass vial with smooth edges filled with the storage solution if it is intended to be used another day [57, 58].

[8] described making three semicircular orientation marks along the edge of the graft to help in later determining the anterior-posterior orientation of the donor graft while positioning it in the anterior chamber (AC). [61] described making an S-stamp on the donor tissue during preparation to confirm orientation after insertion into the eye.

11.4 Recipient Preparation

11.4.1 Preoperative Preparation

We prescribe topical ketorolac tromethamine 4 times a day for 2–3 days prior to surgery. This is especially useful if DMEK surgery is done under topical anesthesia, because it decreases the baseline level of prostaglandins in the eye and conjunctiva, which in turn reduces pain and discomfort during surgery [22].

11.4.2 Anesthesia

Anesthesia considerations include:

1. As in any ocular surgery, the patient's head and eye should remain still.
2. The eye should be soft with minimal back pressure.
3. Surgery may take longer for those new to the procedure.

We prefer to perform DMEK with topical anesthesia supplemented by intravenous sedation and intracameral lidocaine (non-preserved) to eliminate the risks associated with general anesthesia or a local block. We place scleral traction sutures with 4–0 silk at 6 and 12 o'clock to help prevent the patient from squeezing or moving the eye and facilitate eye positioning by the surgeon [22]. For those who prefer to use a peribulbar or retrobulbar block, it is necessary to achieve a soft eye by applying a Honan balloon or similar device for 30 min to avoid posterior (vitreous) pressure during the surgery.

11.4.3 DMEK Wound Construction

Create one self-sealing clear corneal incision (main incision) for donor insertion and two self-sealing paracentesis wounds for DM removal and donor manipulation. The corneal wound can be superior or temporal, and the paracentesis wounds should be 45° away from the main wound. The corneal incision can be created with 2.8 mm or smaller keratome knife and the paracentesis wounds with 75° super sharp paracentesis blades. It is helpful to mark the non-cutting edge of the blade with gentian violet prior to making incisions, because it allows easier identification of the incisions during the rest of the surgery. This is crucial in cases with cloudy corneas or loose epithelium. The paracentesis wounds should be self-sealing, but not so long as to be covered by the donor graft, to allow better manipulation of the graft in the eye with irrigating cannulas.

11.4.4 Removal of DM

Unlike DSEK, in DMEK the donor tissue does not stick easily with retained DM or endothelium [22], so thorough removal of host DM is essential. Before punching the donor, we use the trephine to indent the epithelium of the recipient to verify if the planned donor size is appropriate and to serve as a reference mark for DM removal. Next, we outline the area of DM to be removed (scoring) and strip DM from within that area using an inverted hook (Price Endothelial Keratoplasty Hook; Moria SA or reversed Sinskey hook, D.O.R.C. International, Zuidland, the Netherlands) introduced via paracentesis (Fig. 11.4a). Scoring and stripping can be done under viscoelastic, balanced salt solution (BSS) infusion, or air infusion. Air or viscoelastic provides better visualization than BSS and prevents increasing corneal edema during the stripping process. Viscoelastic provides a more rigid and stable chamber but is more expensive than BSS or air, and it needs to be completely removed before graft insertion, because residual viscoelastic in the interface prevents donor attachment and may lead to interface opacity [5, 6].

Air infusion is the most cost-effective method and provides the best contrast to ensure complete DM removal from within the planned graft area. The AC can be intermittently filled with air through a paracentesis or AC maintainer with an assistant injecting air as needed to keep the AC inflated.

After removing the host DM, it is advisable to spread it out on the surface of the cornea to make sure that it has actually all been retrieved. This is especially important for novice surgeons. Any retained DM can cause poor donor adhesion as well as visual aberration [33].

We recommend using VisionBlue after scoring and stripping of the DM to make sure there are no loose tags of DM or stroma or areas of attached DM (Fig. 11.4b). After removal of DM, fill the AC with BSS (first remove air or viscoelastic) and then inject VisionBlue. Let it stain for about a minute, and then irrigate the AC until it is clear. Areas of exposed DM will stain dense blue, those with exposed stroma will stain light blue, and those with attached DM will have minimal or no staining. Loose DM tags can be removed with irrigation and aspiration (I & A) or intraocular forceps after staining with trypan blue. Scissors can be used to cut off loose pieces of stroma. We create an inferior peripheral iridotomy (PI) with intraocular scissors or a vitrector in I & A/cutting mode and use bimanual I & A to aspirate the posterior pigment layer and ensure the PI is patent (Fig. 11.4c).

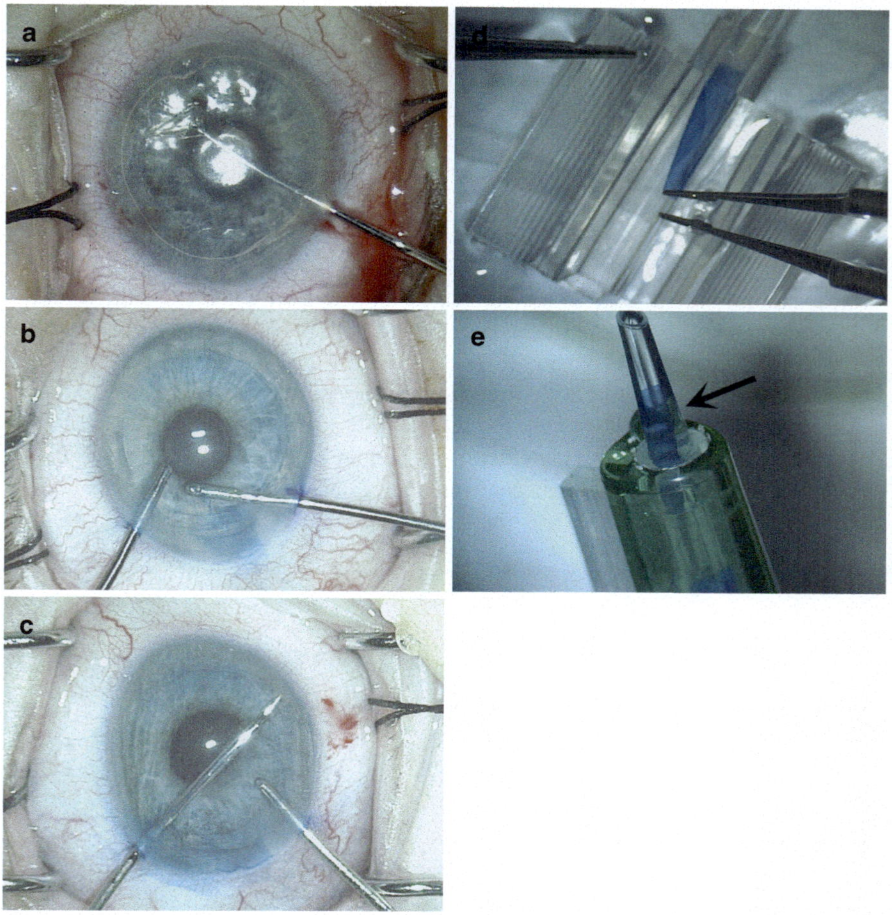

Fig. 11.4 (**a**) Air in the anterior chamber provides good contrast while removing the host Descemet membrane from the planned area where the graft will be placed. (**b**) After host Descemet membrane removal, the host cornea is stained with VisionBlue to help visualize any loose tags of host Descemet membrane or stroma. (**c**) A peripheral iridotomy is created with intraocular scissors; note that it is done inferiorly. (**d**) DMEK donor tissue being loaded into an intraocular lens cartridge. (**e**) Injector loaded with DMEK donor tissue

11.4.5 Inserting the Donor Tissue

1. Staining of donor tissue: After isolating the DM roll from the donor cornea, stain it with VisionBlue for about 60 s to make it more clearly visible during the process of insertion and orientation inside the AC.
2. Loading the tissue: The DMEK graft can be inserted into the eye with a glass pipette, intraocular lens (IOL) cartridge, or custom injector [19, 32, 45, 46]. An IOL cartridge provides a more controlled delivery than a glass pipette [49], but it

is important to use a cartridge that seals against the back pressure in the eye, because using viscoelastic to create a seal in the cartridge impairs graft attachment [45, 46]. Various IOL injectors can be used (VISCOJECT, Medicel AG, Switzerland; Carl Zeiss Meditec, Jena, Germany; Softec; Lenstec Inc., St. Petersburg, FL). The IOL injector needs to be modified by removing the plunger and spring and reattaching the plunger without spring. This prevents back suction and inadvertent damage to the donor graft. Fill the cartridge with BSS and keep it in a well or container filled with BSS. The cartridge will float in a container filled with BSS, so it needs to be stabilized or held with forceps. With the other hand, hold the edge of the stained donor tissue with a small tying forceps. Direct the donor tissue into the cartridge filled with BSS until it is halfway up the barrel tip (Fig. 11.4d). Assemble the cartridge to the injector. Make sure the donor tissue moves without getting stuck in the plunger, and move the plunger forward until it seals its tip with the sides of the cartridge (Fig. 11.4e).

3. Tissue insertion: Place the cartridge into the main wound with the bevel facing downward; insert the tube all the way into the AC and insert the donor (Fig. 11.5a).

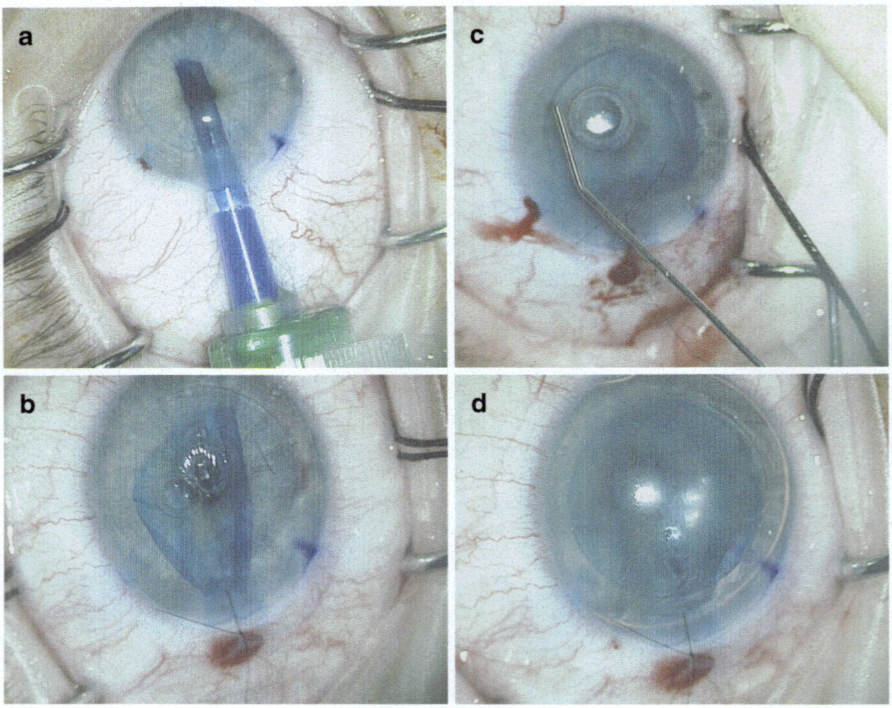

Fig. 11.5 (**a**) DMEK graft being inserted into the anterior chamber; note that the tip of the cartridge is well inside the anterior chamber. (**b**) Partially unwrapped graft with small air bubbles underneath; note that the anterior chamber is partially filled, and the wound has been sutured with 10–0 nylon. (**c**) Gentle strokes on the surface of the cornea with a hydrodissection cannula help center the DMEK graft. (**d**) The anterior chamber is filled with air, the DMEK graft is well centered, and the wound was sutured with 10–0 nylon

Wound-assisted insertion of the donor DM roll should be avoided because it can damage the donor endothelial cells. Before removing the cartridge, decompress the AC by venting a paracentesis wound with an instrument and push on the cornea just central to the wound to prevent donor ejection from the AC.

4. Suture wound: After insertion of donor tissue, the main wound may immediately be sutured with 10–0 nylon to prevent the graft from being expulsed from the AC.

11.4.6 Graft Orientation and Positioning

After the graft has been inserted, it may be loosely or tightly curled. Small intermittent bursts of BSS from a 10-ml syringe help in moving and rotating the donor tissue. With careful indirect manipulation of tissue with air and fluid, the graft can be oriented endothelial side down [19, 36, 41, 42]. The fluid can be directed to uncurl the donor. Before positioning the graft against the host cornea, it is important to confirm the orientation of the donor endothelium. The tissue can be pre-marked with an S-stamp or with asymmetrical orientation marks along the edge [32, 61]. Orientation can also be assessed by positioning the tip of a 30-gauge cannula on top of the membrane and underneath one of the peripheral curls [19]. We prefer to use a hand-held slit beam or intraoperative OCT to confirm which way the graft is curled inside the eye before fully unfolding it, knowing that the endothelium always faces outward [10, 54].

In the operating room, the portable slit lamp (510 L, Eidolon Optical LLC, Natick, MA) can be placed into the finger of a sterile glove for use during the case. With the overhead lights and operating microscope light turned off, the base of the slit lamp is twisted to turn on the beam. The beam width is adjusted using the twistable tip of the instrument, and the light is directed into the AC and onto the graft (Fig. 11.6). If the graft is properly positioned with the endothelium facing downward, it appears in the slit beam as two adjacent arcs representing the two scrolls, with the "connector" between them as a short beam segment posterior to the arcs. The central connecting part of DM can be difficult to see but is best seen over the pupil. If the graft is upside down, the slit beam shines on the "connector," which appears to the surgeon as a single broad arc in the AC just below the recipient cornea. If the correct configuration is seen, the surgeon knows that it is safe to proceed with further unfolding of the donor. If the upside-down configuration is seen, the surgeon must use the BSS cannula again to turn the graft over [10].

Once the orientation of the scrolled DM is clearly seen, it can be opened and positioned on the posterior stroma. [36] described four basic unfolding techniques as well as methods to center the graft and to release any peripheral inward folds. The technique we use was described by Giebel and modified by Price [22]. Once the graft is partially open and it has been confirmed that the endothelial side is facing downward, place a small air bubble under the donor (Fig. 11.5b). The air bubble secures the orientation and controls further unwrapping. Air should be placed slowly and in a controlled amount. Take a 1-mL tuberculin syringe on a 30-g cannula and place 0.02 mL of air underneath the partially unwrapped graft. Make sure that the bubble size is

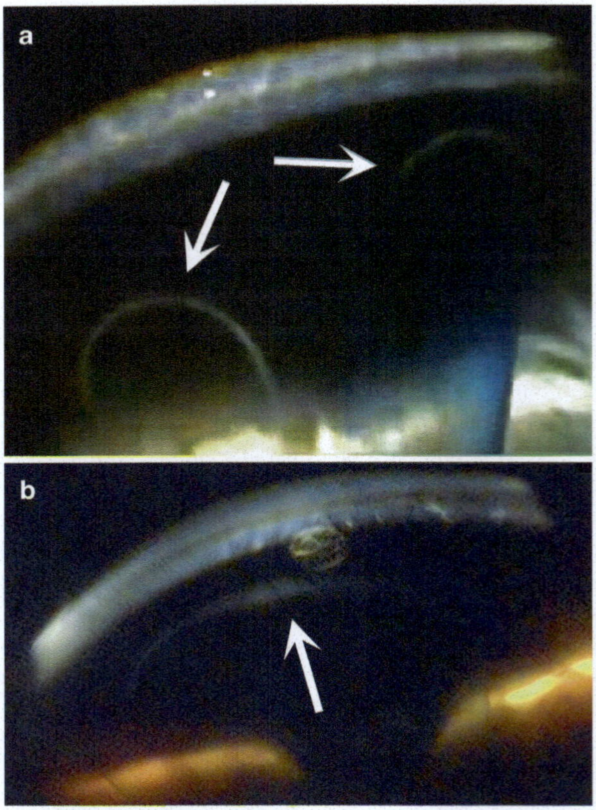

Fig. 11.6 (**a**) When the Descemet membrane double roll is correctly oriented, the slit beam shines on both scrolls of the graft, producing two anterior adjacent arcs of light. (**b**) In the case of an upside-down donor, the slit beam shines on the connector between the scrolls, seen by the surgeon as a single broad anterior arc

smaller than the edge of the unfolded part of the graft. While a small air bubble is maintaining the orientation of at least a partially unwrapped donor, tap on the cornea to allow the bubble to unroll the scrolled side. If the donor tends to curl back after each unwrapping maneuver, a small amount of air can be added under the donor to hold each successive amount of uncurling. This back and forth process between an unwrapping maneuver and an air injection continues until the membrane stays unwrapped.

The AC depth can affect the unwrapping and positioning of the graft. Leaky wounds can cause the chamber to shallow, resulting in a flatter bubble forcing a larger contact area between the host cornea and the donor membrane. The resulting interface friction can prevent further unwrapping or shifting of the graft position. Refilling the chamber with BSS will shrink the bubble and allow easier manipulation.

Once the graft is completely unwrapped, reposition it under the scored and stripped central cornea. A quick stroke of the cannula sweeping over the front of the cornea induces fluid waves in the interface that shifts the donor in the direction of the sweep (Fig. 11.5c). The strokes are very much like golf swings. Repeating these strokes as needed gets the donor in the correct position. If the donor is significantly off center and in the periphery, sometimes it is helpful to tilt the eye to get the initial bubble centered roughly under the donor. Positioning maneuvers are then able to move the donor out of the periphery. However, remember it is easier to move a donor with a small bubble under it than with a large bubble.

After the donor is well centered and totally unwrapped, the AC is filled up to 95 % with air (Fig. 11.5d). The air pressure should be enough to keep the graft in position, and at the same time it should not compress the optic nerve head and compromise its blood supply. That can be confirmed by checking if patient is able to perceive light or not. This is possible only if the surgery is done under topical anesthesia.

We apply one drop each of ketorolac tromethamine 0.4 %, homatropine 5 %, corticosteroid and antibiotic, give intravenous methyl prednisolone 125 mg, and apply a shield.

11.4.7 Postoperative Care

Patients should be advised to remain in a supine position for 60 min to allow the graft to adhere and should be instructed to avoid rubbing the eye because this can have an adverse effect on graft adherence. All patients should undergo a slit-lamp examination and IOP should be measured 1 h after supine positioning. If an air meniscus is occluding the iridotomy or the IOP is elevated, some air should be released. This can be done in a minor procedure room with the patient in a supine position. Partial, controlled AC decompression should be performed using a 30-gauge needle on a 1-ml syringe inserted through the cornea, taking care to avoid the graft edge. Usually the AC reforms spontaneously, but in some cases, BSS needs to be injected to provide a normal pressure to touch. The IOP should be measured, and the peripheral iridotomy should be rechecked at the slit lamp to ensure it is functioning properly before the patient leaves. Instruct the patient to lay face up as much as possible until examination the next day. Instruct the patient to call immediately if they experience marked pressure pain, because closure or blockage of the PI can occur from blood or inflammation a few hours after surgery. Serial examinations should be performed at days 1 and 2 and week 1 after surgery to assess graft adherence.

Postoperative antibiotic eye drops are used 4 times daily for 1 week, and topical corticosteroids are used on a tapering dose to prevent graft rejection. However, in eyes prone to inflammation, such as African Americans, increased steroid drops should be used for the first week or two to insure a quiet anterior chamber. Our steroid regimen for Caucasian patients is prednisolone acetate 1 % four times daily for 2 months, followed by use of a weaker steroid (fluorometholone 0.1 % or loteprednol 0.5 %) tapered from four times daily to once daily by 5 months, with continued once daily use. This regimen utilizes a stronger steroid initially to reduce postoperative inflammation and the risk of cystoid macular edema and then changes to a weaker steroid to reduce the risk of steroid-associated IOP elevation. We have found the risk of immunologic rejection to be extremely low with this regimen [5, 6, 50–52]. For non-Caucasian patients, we start with 6–8-times daily dosing of prednisolone acetate 1 % and taper more slowly, because increased pigment seems to be associated with increased anterior chamber reaction. In a DSEK study, we found that African Americans had 5 times higher risk than Caucasians of experiencing a rejection episode within the first 2 years after surgery [45, 46].

If a patient develops steroid-associated IOP elevation, antiglaucoma medication should be started. Treatment of early IOP rise usually involves use of topical beta-blockers (e.g., Timolol Maleate 0.5 %) followed by brimonidine and then prostamides. Carbonic anhydrase inhibitors should be the last resort, because they can decrease endothelial cell functioning. Before starting nonspecific topical beta-blockers, a history of asthma or cardiac arrhythmias should be ruled out, and their application should be followed by immediate punctal occlusion or lid closure for a period of 3 min to reduce systemic absorption. Prostaglandin analogs should be used only if needed, since their use has been associated with increased risk of cystoid macular edema. If the IOP cannot be managed adequately with glaucoma medication, the steroid strength or dosing frequency can also be reduced. Patients with a previous diagnosis of glaucoma are significantly more likely to experience IOP elevation than those without a previous glaucoma diagnosis.

If partial graft detachment is suspected on slit-lamp examination, anterior segment OCT can be used to facilitate visualization if the cornea is very cloudy. If detached areas seemed to be affecting vision or increasing in size, air should be reinjected to attain a faster and reliable visual recovery. Air reinjection should be done on the same day of the examination. Using a 30-gauge needle on a 1-ml syringe, the needle is inserted parallel to the iris with the bevel facing up, reaching up to the area of the residual air bubble (if it has not absorbed completely) to help minimize the chance of injecting between the graft and recipient cornea. Air is injected to enlarge the bubble to almost completely fill the AC. As the VisionBlue has leached out of the graft by this point, it can be hard to see the donor and make sure you have the needle under the graft for the air injection. Once air is injected, make sure you can see the circular outline of the donor edge against the recipient cornea. If you do not see it, you may have dislocated the donor with the air injection.

Subsequent follow-up examinations can be scheduled at 1, 3, 6, and 12 months after the surgery. Keep in mind that as long as patients are on topical steroids, they can have sudden and asymptomatic pressure increases. The higher the steroid dose, the greater the chance of increased pressure, so they may need to be checked every 3–4 months if still on topical steroids.

11.5 Epithelial Debridement with DMEK

FECD affected eyes can have corneal abnormalities such as anterior basement membrane changes, subepithelial haze, and scarring, either secondary to chronic corneal edema or because of coexisting anterior basement membrane dystrophy (ABMD). EK can effectively restore endothelial function and corneal clarity, but anterior cornea abnormalities may persist or limit complete visual recovery and require a separate surgical procedure to treat residual haze. DMEK can be combined with epithelial debridement with or without application of mitomycin C (MMC) in FECD affected eyes with preoperative subepithelial fibrosis or ABMD evident on slit-lamp examination [13, 14]

Immediately following a standard DMEK procedure and with the anterior chamber filled with air, the corneal epithelium is debrided using a cellulose sponge (Medtronic, Jacksonville, FL), and a Tooke knife is used to dissect off underlying scars in the central 8- to 9-mm area, leaving the Bowman layer intact. A cellulose sponge soaked with MMC (Accord, Intas Pharmaceuticals Ltd, Ahmedabad, India) at a concentration of 0.05 % is applied for 10–15 s and then irrigated off with BSS. A bandage soft contact lens is applied, and a drop of topical antibiotic and corticosteroid is instilled. The rest of the postoperative care remains the same. The bandage soft contact lens should be removed after the corneal surface has reepithelized, usually postoperative days 4–7.

11.6 Cataract Extraction with DMEK

Management of endothelial dysfunction with coexisting cataract requires concurrent or staged transplant and cataract extraction procedures. Like other intraocular procedures, DMEK accelerates cataract progression, especially in patients over 50 years of age [11].

Triple DMEK (DMEK combined with phacoemulsification and IOL implantation) is effective for rapid visual rehabilitation and offers the advantage of a single surgical procedure, with reduced risks and costs compared with staged procedures. Triple DMEK is not associated with any higher risk of complications or endothelial cell loss than DMEK alone [13, 14, 34, 39].

Advantages of DMEK triple procedure include:

1. Faster visual recovery
2. Avoids risk and costs of second surgical procedure
3. Avoids risk of further endothelial damage during cataract surgery

Concerns in triple DMEK include:

1. The viscoelastic used during cataract surgery can interfere with graft attachment, so complete removal of viscoelastic after descemetorhexis is imperative. [5, 6].
2. AC dynamics can fluctuate because of the instability of the newly implanted IOL. After IOL implantation and before insertion of the graft, intracameral injection of pilocarpine 0.5 % or carbachol helps maintain IOL stability and prevent inadvertent touch of the IOL and graft endothelium.

DMEK is not typically associated with significant refractive changes or prolonged visual rehabilitation and should be performed in all patients with concomitant endothelial dysfunction and cataract.

11.6.1 Contraindications for DMEK

Aphakia or large iridectomy are contraindications for DMEK, because of the high chance of the graft dislocating posteriorly during intraoperative manipulation unless the iris defect can be sutured during the same surgical session [18, 24].

11.6.2 Relative Contraindications for DMEK

1. After pars plana vitrectomy (PPV), because the AC will be very deep, it is often difficult to shallow the anterior chamber and keep the graft unrolled. It is even more difficult in cases with both a PPV and glued or scleral-fixated IOL [18, 24].
2. Heavy anticoagulation is a relative contraindication because of the risk of intraocular hemorrhage with tissue manipulation and reinjection of air. Reinjection of air postoperatively can stretch the anterior chamber angle leading to bleeding, just as with external trauma to the eye [18, 24].

11.7 Repeat DMEK

Indications

1. Upside-down graft
2. Endothelial cell failure
   A. Primary endothelial cell failure: graft attached but cornea does not clear up in 1 month
   B. Secondary endothelial cell failure: graft attached and cornea cleared initially but decompensated later in the postoperative period, with or without associated graft rejection or glaucoma filtering surgery.
3. Failure to adequately attach even after air reinjection

Technique

The technique is similar to primary DMEK. As we recommend for other EK surgeries, trypan blue may be applied to stain the primary DMEK graft or identify remnants left in situ. When a DMEK regraft is performed in an eye that developed a detachment of the initial DMEK graft, it may be especially important to meticulously scrape the recipient posterior stroma in the area of the detachment, to remove any endothelial cells that migrated over to cover the stromal defect, to enable better graft adherence.

The outcomes of secondary DMEK are comparable with those of primary DMEK when graft failure is treated promptly, i.e., within 1–2 months, to minimize the duration of corneal edema [51, 52, 62]. However, when secondary DMEK has been used to treat a primary graft that is decompensated for a prolonged period, the visual outcomes have not matched those achieved with primary DMEK [9, 15].

To summarize, a DMEK regraft can be done successfully with good long-term outcomes. The types of complications and incidences are comparable with the first surgery when intervention is done timely and wisely.

11.7.1 DMEK to Treat Failed PK

DSEK has been successfully performed for post-PK endothelial decompensation [16, 35, 44, 56] with good success and survival rates [4]. Likewise, DMEK can be performed for failed PK with endothelial decompensation if an acceptable refractive result was achieved with the PK prior to failure [7]. However, DMEK under failed PK is more challenging than DSEK under failed PK because of poor inherent adhesion of the donor DM to the PK stroma and the uneven posterior surface of the PK graft wound. Therefore, we recommend that surgeons should only undertake DMEK under failed PK after they are experienced with performing DMEK in virgin eyes.

In a post-PK cornea, DM stripping can be challenging because of DM adhesions at the PK wound and the need to avoid rupturing the PK wound. As mentioned previously, we recommend after the stripping is complete to check with trypan blue stain in the anterior chamber to identify remnants of retained DM or strands of loose stroma that should be removed or trimmed to allow better apposition of the graft to the recipient cornea.

Since it is harder to get a DMEK graft to stick over an irregular posterior cornea where the PK wound is, either make the diameter of the DMEK slight smaller than the PK diameter or 1.5–2 mm larger so the donor can extend out past the wound. It is also wise to advise the patient they may need one or more reinjections of air or gas to get the donor to stick properly on the eye with a failed PK.

11.8 Conclusion

DMEK is the ideal selective transplant procedure for endothelial disorders because it provides near normal anatomical replacement of the host endothelium. With faster and better visual rehabilitation, relatively predictable refractive outcomes and reduced risk of graft rejection, DMEK has many advantages over other keratoplasty procedures. In current ophthalmic surgery scenarios, faster rehabilitation and excellent refractive outcomes are the key requirements, and DMEK fulfills these demands. It is a surgery which is readily accessible to any cornea surgeon in any ophthalmic surgery setup. With the help of a standardized approach and when careful attention is given to surgical details, DMEK results are very promising. Taking a DMEK course and honing skills in a wet lab is highly recommended to reduce the learning curve.

11.9 Pre-Descemet's Endothelial Keratoplasty

In 2014 Agarwal et al. [1] described an alternative method of tissue preparation called pre-Descemet's endothelial keratoplasty (PDEK), based on evidence of a layer of collagenous tissue adjacent to and distinct from DM [20] and the suggestion that inclusion of this layer as a splint to DM and endothelium could facilitate tissue handling and unfolding. The donor graft is prepared by generating a type 1 big bubble, analogous to deep anterior lamellar keratoplasty (DALK) [3]. A corneoscleral donor tissue with a 2-mm scleral rim is placed with endothelial side facing up. Using a 5-mL air-filled syringe, a 30-G needle is inserted with the bevel up into the mid-periphery of the corneal stroma, and air is injected. Usually, a pre-Descemet's (type 1) bubble is created and can be expanded to about 7.5-mm diameter. Controlled injection is required for the bubble to form and expand, because sudden forceful injection can cause the bubble to form and pop. Placing the needle tip closer to DM improves the chance of achieving a type I bubble. In some cases a type II bubble (that extends to the limbus) forms. In that case the cleavage plane is the same as achieved with a DMEK direct peeling technique. Agarwal also suggests staining of donor tissue by injecting 0.06 % trypan blue solution into the periphery of the bubble. The donor tissue—that is, the cleaved posterior wall of the bubble—is then trephined with an appropriate size trephine. The PDEK tissue, like DMEK tissue, rolls with the endothelial cells on the outside of the roll, but the scroll tends to be looser and easier to uncurl. Therefore, young donor corneas can be used for PDEK [1, 2]. Further studies are needed to determine the relative tissue preparation success rate and endothelial cell loss with PDEK vs. DMEK. PDEK donor preparation techniques are similar to earlier hybrid endothelial techniques all of which had a portion of peripheral stroma attached to the central area of DM and endothelium. The hybrid techniques have essentially been abandoned because the tissue loss rates with big bubble separation techniques were significantly higher than with peeling methods [12, 38, 55].

References

1. Agarwal A, Dua HS, Narang P, Kumar DA, Agarwal A, Jacob S, Agarwal A, Gupta A. Pre-Descemet's endothelial keratoplasty (PDEK). Br J Ophthalmol. 2014;98:1181–5.
2. Agarwal A, Agarwal A, Narang P, Kumar DA, Jacob S. Pre-Descemet endothelial keratoplasty with infant donor corneas: a prospective analysis. Cornea. 2015;34:859–65.
3. Anwar M, Teichmann KD. Big-bubble technique to bare Descemet's membrane in anterior lamellar keratoplasty. J Cataract Refract Surg. 2002;28:398–403.
4. Anshu A, Price MO, Price FW. Descemet's stripping endothelial keratoplasty under failed penetrating keratoplasty: visual rehabilitation and graft survival rate. Ophthalmology. 2011; 118:2155–60.
5. Anshu A, Planchard B, Price MO, Pereira CR, Price Jr FW. A cause of reticular interface haze and its management after Descemet stripping endothelial keratoplasty. Cornea. 2012;31: 1365–8.

6. Anshu A, Price MO, Price Jr FW. Risk of corneal transplant rejection significantly reduced with Descemet's membrane endothelial keratoplasty. Ophthalmology. 2012;119:536–40.
7. Anshu A, Price MO, Price FW. Descemet membrane endothelial keratoplasty and hybrid techniques for managing failed penetrating grafts. Cornea. 2013;32:1–4.
8. Bachmann BO, Laaser K, Cursiefen C, Kruse FE. A method to confirm correct orientation of descemet membrane during descemet membrane endothelial keratoplasty. Am J Ophthalmol. 2010;149:922–5.
9. Baydoun L, Van Dijk K, Dapena I, Musa FU, Liarakos VS, Ham L, Melles GRJ. Repeat Descemet membrane endothelial keratoplasty after complicated primary Descemet membrane endothelial keratoplasty. Ophthalmology. 2015;122:8–16.
10. Burkhart ZN, Feng MT, Price MO, Price FW. Hand-held slit beam techniques to facilitate DMEK and DALK. Cornea. 2013;32:722–4.
11. Burkhart ZN, Feng MT, Price Jr FW, Price MO. One-year outcomes in eyes remaining phakic after Descemet membrane endothelial keratoplasty. J Cataract Refract Surg. 2014;40:430–4.
12. Busin M, Patel AK, Scorcia V, Galan A, Ponzin D. Stromal support for Descemet's membrane endothelial keratoplasty. Ophthalmology. 2010;117:2273–7.
13. Chaurasia S, Price Jr FW, Gunderson L, Price MO. Descemet's membrane endothelial keratoplasty, clinical results of single versus triple procedures (combined with cataract surgery). Ophthalmology. 2014;121:454–8.
14. Chaurasia S, Price MO, McKee Y, Price Jr FW. Descemet membrane endothelial keratoplasty combined with epithelial debridement and mitomycin-C application for Fuchs dystrophy with preoperative subepithelial fibrosis or anterior basement membrane dystrophy. Cornea. 2014;33:335–9.
15. Cirkovic A, Schlötzer-Schrehardt U, Weller JM, Kruse FK, Tourtas T. Clinical and ultrastructural characteristics of graft failure in DMEK: 1-year results after repeat DMEK. Cornea. 2015;34:11–7.
16. Covert DJ, Koenig SB. Descemet stripping and automated endothelial keratoplasty (DSAEK) in eyes with failed penetrating keratoplasty. Cornea. 2007;26:692–6.
17. Dapena I, Ham L, Netuková M, Van der Wees J, Melles GR. Incidence of early allograft rejection after Descemet membrane endothelial keratoplasty. Cornea. 2011;30:1341–5.
18. Dapena I, Ham L, Droutsas K, Dijk KV, Moutsouris K, Melles GR. Learning curve in Descemet's membrane endothelial keratoplasty, first series of 135 consecutive cases. Ophthalmology. 2011;118:2147–54.
19. Dapena I, Moutsouris K, Droutsas K, Ham L, Dijk KV, Melles GR. Standardized "no-touch" technique for Descemet membrane endothelial keratoplasty. Arch Ophthalmol. 2011;129:88–94.
20. Dua HS, Faraj LA, Said DG, Gray T, Lowe J. Human corneal anatomy redefined a novel pre-Descemet's layer (Dua's Layer). Ophthalmology. 2013;120:1778–85.
21. Feng MT, Burkhart ZN, Price Jr FW, Price MO. Effect of donor preparation-to-use times on Descemet membrane endothelial keratoplasty outcomes. Cornea. 2013;32:1080–2.
22. Giebel AW, Price Jr FW. Descemet's membrane endothelial keratoplasty (DMEK): the bare minimum. In: Price FW, Price MO, editors. DSEK: all you need to know about endothelial keratoplasty. Thorofare: Slack, Inc; 2008. p. 119–46.
23. Greiner MA, Rixen JJ, Wagoner MD, Schmidt GA, Stoeger CG, Straiko MD, Zimmerman MB, Kitzmann AS, Goins KM. Diabetes mellitus increases risk of unsuccessful graft preparation in Descemet membrane endothelial keratoplasty: a multicenter study. Cornea. 2014;33:1129–33.
24. Guerra FP, Anshu A, Price MO, Price FW. Endothelial keratoplasty: fellow eyes comparison of Descemet stripping automated endothelial keratoplasty and Descemet membrane endothelial keratoplasty. Cornea. 2011;30:1382–6.
25. Ham L, Van der Wees J, Melles GR. Causes of primary donor failure in Descemet membrane endothelial keratoplasty. Am J Ophthalmol. 2008;145:639–44.
26. Ham L, Balachandran C, Verschoor CA, Van der Wees J, Melles GRJ. Visual rehabilitation rate after isolated Descemet membrane transplantation: Descemet membrane endothelial keratoplasty. Arch Ophthalmol. 2009;127:252–5.

27. Ham L, Dapena I, van Luijk C, van der Wees J, Melles GRJ. Descemet membrane endothelial keratoplasty (DMEK) for Fuchs endothelial dystrophy: review of the first 50 consecutive cases. Eye (Lond). 2009;23:1990–8.
28. Heindl LM, Bucher F, Caramoy A, Hos D, Matthaei M, Cursiefen C. Safety of donor tissue preparation and use of descemetoschisis and torn tissue in descemet membrane endothelial keratoplasty. Cornea. 2014;33:e7–9.
29. Heinzelmann S, Huther S, Bohringer D, Eberwein P, Reinhard T, Maier P. Influence of donor characteristics on Descemet membrane endothelial keratoplasty. Cornea. 2014;33:644–8.
30. Ignacio TS, Nguyen TTB, Sarayba MA, Sweet PM, Piovanetti O, Chuck RS, Behrens A. A technique to harvest Descemet's membrane with viable endothelial cells for selective transplantation. Am J Ophthalmol. 2005;139:325–30.
31. Johnson DH, Bourne WM, Campbell RJ. The ultrastructure of Descemet's membrane. I. Changes with age in normal cornea. Arch Ophthalmol. 1982;100:1942–7.
32. Kruse FE, Laaser K, Cursiefen C, Heindl LM, Schlotzer-Schrehardt U, Riss S, Bachmann B. A stepwise approach to donor preparation and insertion increases safety and outcome of Descement membrane endothelial keratoplasty. Cornea. 2011;30:580–7.
33. Kymionis GD, Suh LH, Dubovy SR, Yoo SH. Diagnosis of residual Descemet's membrane after Descemet's stripping endothelial keratoplasty with anterior segment optical coherence tomography. J Cataract Refract Surg. 2007;33:1322–4.
34. Laaser K, Bachmann BO, Horn FK, Cursiefen C, Kruse FE. Descemet membrane endothelial keratoplasty combined with phacoemulsification and intraocular lens implantation: advanced triple procedure. Am J Ophthalmol. 2012;154:47–55.
35. Lee BS, Stark WJ, Jun AS. Descemet-stripping automated endothelial keratoplasty: a successful alternative to repeat penetrating keratoplasty. Clin Experiment Ophthalmol. 2011;39:195–200.
36. Liarakos VS, Dapena I, Ham L, Dijk KV, Melles GRJ. Intraocular graft unfolding techniques in Descemet membrane endothelial keratoplasty. Arch Ophthalmol. 2013;131:29–35.
37. Lie JT, Birbal R, Ham L, Wees JVD, Melles GRJ. Donor tissue preparation for Descemet membrane endothelial keratoplasty. J Cataract Refract Surg. 2008;34:1578–83.
38. McCauley MB, Price FW, Price MO. Descemet membrane automated endothelial keratoplasty: hybrid technique combining DSAEK stability with DMEK visual results. J Cataract Refract Surg. 2009;35:1659–64.
39. McKee Y, Price MO, Gunderson L, Price Jr FW. Rapid sequential endothelial keratoplasty with and without combined cataract extraction. J Cataract Refract Surg. 2013;39:1372–6.
40. Melles GR, Lander F, Rietveld FJ. Transplantation of Descemet's membrane carrying viable endothelium through a small scleral incision. Cornea. 2002;21:415–8.
41. Melles GR, Ong TS, Ververs B, Van der Wees J. Descemet membrane endothelial keratoplasty (DMEK). Cornea. 2006;25:987–90.
42. Melles GR, Ong TS, Ververs B, Van Der Wees J. Preliminary clinical results of Descemet membrane endothelial keratoplasty. Am J Ophthalmol. 2008;145:222–7.
43. Parker J, Dirisamer M, Naveiras M, Ham L, Melles GRJ. Endothelial cell density after Descemet membrane endothelial keratoplasty: 1- to 4-year follow-up. Am J Ophthalmol. 2011;151:1107.
44. Price FW, Price MO. Endothelial keratoplasty to restore clarity to a failed penetrating graft. Cornea. 2006;25:895–9.
45. Price MO, Giebel AW, Fairchild KM, Price Jr FW. Descemet's membrane endothelial keratoplasty: prospective multicenter study of visual and refractive outcomes and endothelial survival. Ophthalmology. 2009;116:2361–8.
46. Price MO, Jordan CS, Moore G, Price Jr FW. Graft rejection episodes after Descemet stripping with endothelial keratoplasty: part two: the statistical analysis of probability and risk factors. Br J Ophthalmol. 2009;93:391–5.
47. Price Jr FW, Price MO, editors. DSEK: what you need to know about endothelial keratoplasty. Thorofare: Slack Incorporated; 2009.

48. Price MO, Gorovoy M, Benetz BA, Price Jr FW, Menegay HJ, Debanne SM, Lass JH. Descemet's stripping automated endothelial keratoplasty outcomes compared with penetrating keratoplasty from the Cornea Donor Study. Ophthalmology. 2010;117:438–44.
49. Price MO, Price Jr FW. Descemet's membrane endothelial keratoplasty surgery: update on the evidence and hurdles to acceptance. Curr Opin Ophthalmol. 2013;24:329–35.
50. Price MO, Price Jr FW, Kruse FE, Bachmann BO, Tourtas T. Randomized comparison of topical prednisolone acetate 1% versus fluorometholone 0.1% in the first year after Descemet membrane endothelial keratoplasy. Cornea. 2014;33:880–6.
51. Price MO, Feng MT, Mckee Y, Price Jr FW. Repeat Descemet membrane endothelial keratoplasty: secondary grafts with early intervention are comparable with fellow-eye primary grafts. Ophthalmology. 2015;122:1639–44.
52. Price MO, Feng MT, Scanameo A, Price Jr FW. Loteprednol etabonate 0.5% gel vs. prednisolone acetate 1% solution after Descemet membrane endothelial keratoplasty: prospective randomized trial. Cornea. 2015;34:853–8.
53. Rudolph M, Laaser K, Bachmann BO, Cursiefen C, Epstein D, Kruse FE. Corneal higher-order aberrations after Descemet's membrane endothelial keratoplasty. Ophthalmology. 2012;119:528–35.
54. Steven P, Le Blanc C, Velten K, Lankenau E, Krug M, Oelckers S, Heindl LM, Gehlsen U, Hüttmann G, Cursiefen C. Optimizing descemet membrane endothelial keratoplasty using intraoperative optical coherence tomography. JAMA Ophthalmol. 2013;131:1135–42.
55. Studeny P, Farkas A, Vokrojova M, Liskova P, Jirsova K. Descemet membrane endothelial keratoplasty with a stromal rim (DMEK-S). Br J Ophthalmol. 2010;94:909–14.
56. Straiko MD, Terry MA, Shamie N. Descemet stripping automated endothelial keratoplasty under failed penetrating keratoplasty: a surgical strategy to minimize complications. Am J Ophthalmol. 2011;151:233–7.
57. Tenkman LR, Price FW. F169: SCUBA DMEK donor preparation: improving efficiency and managing difficult situations. Am Soc Cataract Refractive Surgeons Film Festival. 2012. http://ascrs2012.conferencefilms.com/
58. Tenkman LR, Price FW, Price MO. Descemet membrane endothelial keratoplasty donor preparation: navigating challenges and improving efficiency. Cornea. 2014;33:319–25.
59. Tourtas T, Laaser K, Bachmann BO, Cursiefen C, Kruse FE. Descemet membrane endothelial keratoplasty versus Descemet stripping automated endothelial keratoplasty. Am J Ophthalmol. 2012;153:1082–90.
60. Vianna LM, Stoeger CG, Galloway JD, Terry M, Cope L, Belfort Jr R, Jun AS. Risk factors for eye bank preparation failure of Descemet membrane endothelial keratoplasty tissue. Am J Ophthalmol. 2015;159:829–34.
61. Veldman PB, Dye PK, Holiman JD, Mayko ZM, Sáles CS, Straiko MD, Stoeger CG, Terry MA. Stamping an S on DMEK donor tissue to prevent upside-down grafts: laboratory validation and detailed preparation technique description. Cornea. 2015;34:1175–8.
62. Yoeruek E, Bartz-Schmidt KU. Secondary Descemet membrane endothelial keratoplasty after failed primary Descemet membrane endothelial keratoplasty: clinical results. Cornea. 2013;32:1414–7.

Chapter 12
Complications of Descemet Stripping Automated Endothelial Keratoplasty (DSAEK) Surgery

P. James Sanchez, Michael D. Straiko, and Mark A. Terry

12.1 Introduction

According to the [1], 13,817 endothelial keratoplasty surgeries were performed for Fuchs endothelial dystrophy as reported by associated eye banks, far surpassing penetrating keratoplasty as the most popular treatment for Fuchs dystrophy. DSAEK has been the standard of care for Fuchs for nearly 10 years, and because of its prevalence, the most common complications have been well documented and can be addressed by virtually any endothelial keratoplasty surgeon.

In this chapter we will outline the common complications associated with the DSAEK procedure and why they occur. If possible we describe ways to minimize complications, and when they do occur, what may be the appropriate response or treatment.

12.2 Intraoperative Complications of DSAEK

Intraoperative DSAEK complications begin with tissue preparation. For a variety of reasons including time of tissue preparation, tissue screening and testing, decrease tissue wastage, and quality control, the vast majority (82.8 %) of DSAEK surgeons in the United States utilize eye bank-prepared tissue (EBAA statistical report 2014). For surgeons who do perform their own preparations, microkeratome errors causing eccentric cuts are the leading cause of intraoperative complications.

P.J. Sanchez, MD (✉) • M.D. Straiko, MD • M.A. Terry, MD
Devers Eye Institute, 1040 N.W. 22nd Ave., Portland, OR 97210, USA
e-mail: pjamessanchez@gmail.com

C. Cursiefen, A.S. Jun (eds.), *Current Treatment Options for Fuchs Endothelial Dystrophy*, DOI 10.1007/978-3-319-43021-8_12

12.2.1 Failed Tissue Preparation and Eccentric Trephination

DSAEK lenticule trephination may rarely be complicated by an eccentric trephination resulting in a portion of the graft that is full thickness (Fig. 12.1). Full-thickness trephination has been demonstrated in multiple reports of graft failure with pathological evidence of epithelial ingrowth occupying the graft–host interface, preventing graft adherence [25, 34, 36]. This complication may be more easily avoided with the routine use of the operating microscope during donor lenticule preparation.

12.2.2 Retained Descemet Membrane

Incomplete descemetorhexis may result in retention of some or all of the host Descemet membrane. Occasionally, the retained host Descemet membrane may be associated with a fibrous membrane. The clinical significance of retained Descemet membrane is unknown; however, retained Descemet membrane has been demonstrated in pathologic specimens of failed DSAEK grafts [25, 34, 36]. Our group advocates careful inspection of the descemetorhexis edge utilizing either retroillumination with the red reflex or an air bubble in the anterior chamber to aid in visualization.

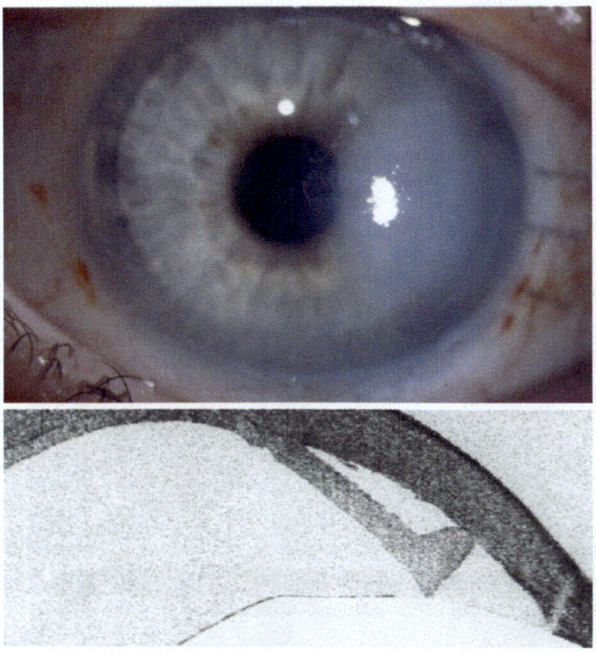

Fig. 12.1 Eccentric trephination of DSAEK graft. During preparation of the DSAEK lenticule, an eccentric trephination can lead to a full-thickness graft edge that will prevent full graft attachment and may lead to graft failure and the need for a repeat transplant. The authors advocate using the microscope and ink centration marks on the donor corneoscleral cap to prevent eccentric trephination

12.2.3 Intraoperative Posterior Graft Dislocation

One of the most feared intraoperative complications of DSAEK surgery is posterior dislocation of the donor lenticule in unicameral eyes. This complication has been reported in patients with a history of aphakia and scleral-sutured or iris-sutured intraocular lenses with a violated posterior capsule [37, 39, 40]. These reports showed that posterior dislocation of the DSAEK lenticule may result in proliferative vitreoretinopathy and subsequent tractional retinal detachment requiring surgical intervention. Surgeons have reported successful management of this complication with prompt pars plana vitrectomy with lenticule removal, but total retinal detachments with loss of light perception have also been reported [11, 39, 40].

12.2.4 Iatrogenic Primary Graft Failure: Graft Trauma

Iatrogenic primary graft failures (IPGFs) are graft failures caused by excessive trauma to the graft endothelium during DSAEK surgery. Endothelial damage can occur during tissue preparation, graft insertion, and graft centration and attachment maneuvers. There has been evidence to support increased graft trauma and endothelial cell loss when a smaller incision size is used. Independent laboratory and clinical studies have shown that a 5-mm incision is associated with less endothelial cell loss than a 3-mm incision using a variety of insertion techniques [27, 41].

12.2.5 Suprachoroidal Hemorrhage

One of the primary advantages of endothelial keratoplasty over penetrating keratoplasty is the much smaller incision size and the lack of a period of "open sky" during the procedure. Despite this advantage, suprachoroidal hemorrhage has been reported during DSAEK [34]. Treatment of suprachoroidal hemorrhage during DSAEK is the same as in other types of ocular surgery – rapid closure of all incisions and recovery of a physiologic intraocular pressure to tamponade the expanding hematoma.

12.2.6 Anterior Chamber Hemorrhage

An anterior chamber hemorrhage may arise either from iris trauma during phacoemulsification, fashioning of a peripheral iridectomy, or conjunctival hemorrhage tracking through one of the surgical incisions. If the hemorrhage is not removed from the anterior chamber prior to graft insertion and unfolding, the red blood cells and any associated fibrin may collect in the graft–host interface and result in postoperative interface haze, although this haze has been reported to clear 8 months after surgery [33]. Techniques to avoid hemorrhage include not performing an iridectomy at the time of DSAEK and pressurizing the eye when possible to prevent blood flow from the conjunctiva into the anterior chamber. Once the hemorrhage has started, pressurizing the eye with BSS or viscoelastic can tamponade the bleeding and allow coagulation while other steps of the procedure are performed. It is essential to remove all viscoelastic prior to inserting the graft to prevent graft detachment and interface haze.

12.2.7 Interface Fluid

Persistent interface fluid after insertion of the graft can make centration of the donor difficult and may result in early dislocation. A number of strategies to reduce interface fluid after filling the anterior chamber with air have been developed. Sweeping the corneal surface from the center of the donor disk to the edge under a full air fill pushes interface fluid to the edge of the graft, where it is released into the anterior chamber [42]. Venting incisions in the donor cornea overlying pockets of interface fluid allows for direct drainage of interface fluid through the incision [30]. Filling the anterior chamber completely with air under normal, elevated intraocular pressure may also decrease the magnitude of interface fluid, although the effect on postoperative dislocations rates is not known [46].

12.2.8 Upside-Down Graft

Although rare, the DSAEK lenticule may be unfolded and positioned on the host stroma upside down, with the donor endothelium against the host stroma (Fig. 12.2). A number of techniques are currently used to avoid this complication, including the

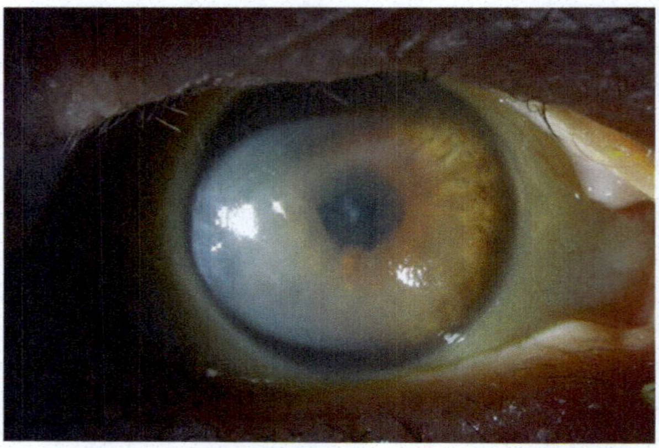

Fig. 12.2 Upside-down graft. If the orientation of the graft is lost after insertion of the lenticule, the graft may be inadvertently floated against the stroma upside down resulting in graft failure. This complication may be prevented with the use of an asymmetric fold technique and careful anterior chamber manipulation with slow opening of the graft

use of an under- or overfold technique and marking the donor lenticule with trypan or gentian violet on the stromal surface. Although trypan blue has been shown to be safe on the endothelium at commercially available concentrations and durations of exposure, gentian violet has been shown to cause localized endothelial damage following a stromal mark [14]. While marking the tissue for correct orientation is possible and may benefit surgeons new to the procedure, most forgo the additional tissue damage with increased experience. Once the upside-down orientation of the tissue is diagnosed, the graft may be replaced with a new tissue.

12.3 Early Postoperative Complications of DSAEK

Early postoperative complications usually occur within 1 day to 1 month after surgery depending on the complication. Our practice has set follow-up periods at 1 day, 1 week, and 1 month to try and identify any complications as early as possible. Regular use of anterior segment OCT, careful clinical examination, and a standardized medication regimen may lead to early identification and/or prevention of many complications.

12.3.1 Graft Dislocation

The most common reported complication following DSAEK surgery is graft dislocation (Fig. 12.3), which has been reported in 1.5–35 % of cases [17, 20, 35, 39, 40, 42, 43]. The causes for graft detachments and complete dislocations vary widely, and surgeons have published mixed results regarding the association between previous glaucoma surgery and DSAEK graft dislocation. Some surgeons report no significant difference in dislocation (15 % in eyes with a history of glaucoma surgery vs 13 % without – Wiaux et al. 2011), while others report a significant association (9 % dislocation with a history of glaucoma surgery vs 2 % with no history of glaucoma surgery – Goshe et al. [10]). It is likely that both patient demographics and surgical technique play a role. However, within the group of patients with a history of glaucoma surgery, there appears to be a strong correlation between postoperative hypotony and graft detachment [10]. The surgical learning curve and associated trouble

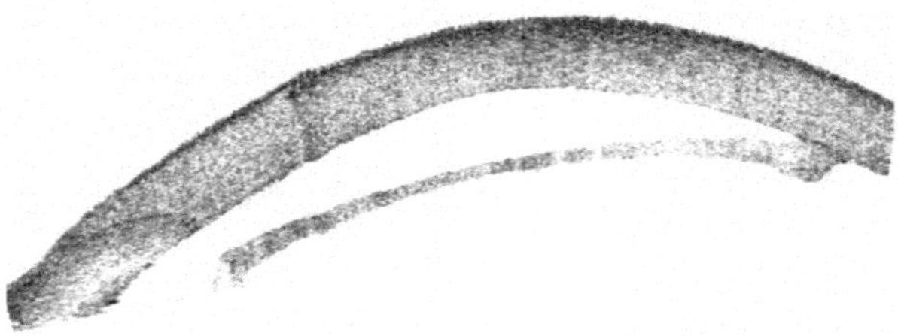

Fig. 12.3 Graft dislocation. Postoperative graft dislocation is the most common complication of DSAEK surgery. The majority of cases can be managed with a single rebubble procedure

with graft manipulation and air bubble management have been shown to lead to higher detachment rates in early cases which may decrease over time [30]. Other risk factors to which graft detachment is often attributed include eye rubbing, interface fluid remaining at the end of surgery, retained interface viscoelastic, and folds of retained Descemet membrane. DSAEK surgery for penetrating keratoplasty failure presents the unique challenge of matching the DSAEK lenticule to the posterior graft–host junction of the full-thickness corneal graft (Fig. 12.4). Sizing the graft so that the diameter is smaller than the penetrating graft and careful centration during surgery has been associated with a low rate of postoperative graft dislocation [38] However, Price et al. have also shown that making the graft larger than the diameter of the overlying PK has also yielded a low detachment rate [28]. The key to success appears to be to not make the DSAEK graft the same diameter as the overlying failed PK in order to avoid the edge protuberances of the PK edges from pushing the graft edges down and creating edge separations.

The management of partial or complete graft detachment is the placement of a new air bubble in the anterior chamber with subsequent face-up patient positioning to support the graft tissue. This is performed either in a minor procedure room or in the operating room. The operating room may be preferred in the case of the need for more significant surgical manipulation. Graft reattachment occurs in the majority of grafts which undergo rebubble [30, 39, 42, 43]. In the minority of eyes which do not achieve successful attachment after several rebubble attempts, iatrogenic primary graft failure is often declared, and either a repeat DSAEK or PKP can be performed.

12.3.2 Iatrogenic Primary Graft Failure

Failure of initial corneal clearance after any form of endothelial keratoplasty is usually attributable to excessive manipulation of the donor tissue during surgery, and this has been termed *iatrogenic* primary graft failure. If donor characteristics or tissue preparation techniques are suspected of being responsible for graft failure, then true *primary* graft failure can be declared in the absence of excessive surgical

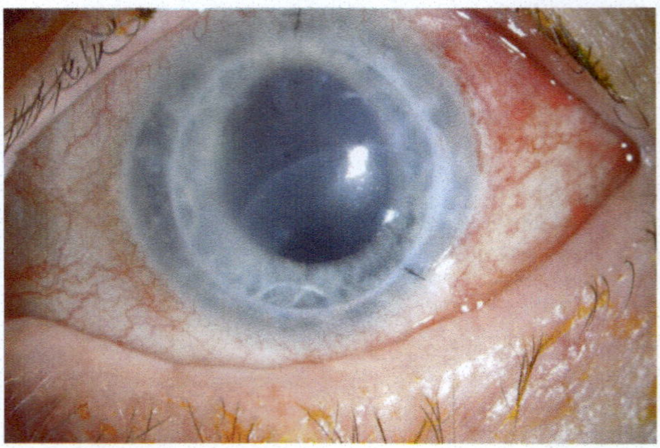

Fig. 12.4 DSAEK dislocation under PKP. DSAEK grafts placed under a PKP must be carefully sized and centered to avoid abutting the posterior graft–host junction of the PKP, which could lead to graft detachment and failure

manipulation. The rates of iatrogenic primary graft failure vary widely in the published DSAEK reports from as low as 0% [42, 43] to as high as 17% [39, 40]. In most cases graft replacement with a new DSAEK lenticule is the treatment of choice. However, in situations where patient comorbidities may be responsible for increased risk of dislocation such as the inability to maintain anterior chamber air due to glaucoma surgery or a history of vitrectomy in a unicameral eye, the procedure of choice for DSAEK graft failure may be penetrating keratoplasty.

12.3.3 Pupil Block/Urrets-Zavalia Syndrome

The placement of a large air bubble in the anterior chamber at the end of the DSAEK surgery may lead to pupil block and occasionally permanent vision loss due to optic neuropathy or a fixed dilated pupil due to Urrets-Zavalia syndrome [5]. Although most large series have not reported pupil block after DSAEK, there have been some reports of this complication in the literature [39, 40]. The routine use of mydriatic drops at the end of the surgery and titration of an air bubble that can clear the edge of the dilated pupil has been associated with elimination of this complication in a large series [42, 43]. The placement of an inferior peripheral iridectomy prior to placement of the air bubble may also prevent pupil block. Cases of pupil block may be treated with the release of air from the anterior chamber. However, it is important to identify the complication early in its course to prevent prolonged elevated intraocular pressure and its sequelae.

12.3.4 Endophthalmitis

Endophthalmitis following DSAEK surgery is exceedingly rare, but has been reported (Fig. 12.5). Responsible organisms include *Mycobacterium abscessus* [7], *Candida* spp. [8], and *Streptococcus pneumoniae* [35]. A unique characteristic of postoperative infections following DSAEK is the possibility of keratitis involving

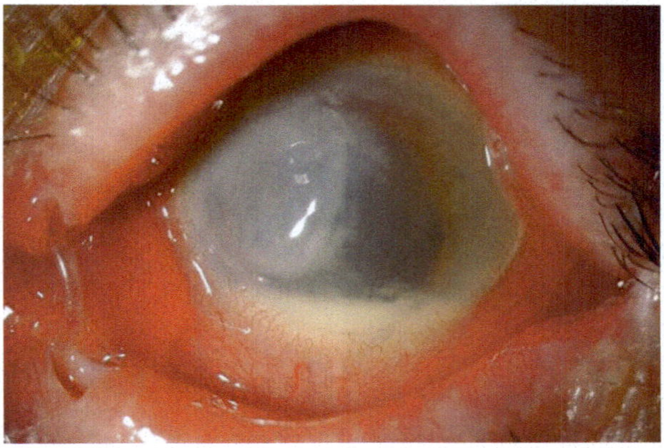

Fig. 12.5 Endophthalmitis following DSAEK surgery. Endophthalmitis is a rare postoperative complication of DSAEK, but has the unique possibility of involving infection of the stromal graft–host interface, making the choice of primary treatment especially difficult

the graft–host interface. Possible treatments include topical antimicrobials, injection of antimicrobials into the interface, or removal of the DSAEK lenticule with placement of a new DSAEK graft or penetrating keratoplasty. Theoretically, donor rim cultures could be used to guide therapy of post-DSAEK infections; however, this topic remains controversial.

12.3.5 Fungal Infections

Fungal infections following a DSAEK transplant are exceedingly rare, but have been reported [19]. These infections tend to involve the graft–host stromal interface [24]. The most commonly reported causative organism is *Candida albicans*. Depending on local climate, the risk may increase with increased exposure by donors. Many surgeons will test donor tissue for the presence of potential pathogenic microbes by culturing the donor corneal-scleral rim tissue left over after trephination, but often the culture reports will only be available a week or more after transplantation. Even in cases where a positive fungal growth from the donor rim tissue is identified, an infection usually will not develop. However, in the face of a positive donor rim culture and a clinical picture of increasing inflammation of the eye, early identification of the causative organism allows faster and more appropriately targeted therapy. If a fungal infection is identified by culture and clinically manifests in the interface or graft itself, eradication may require a combination of topical, oral, and intracameral antifungal therapy and often ultimately results in removal of the infected graft.

12.4 Late Postoperative Complications of DSAEK

There will always be a risk of postoperative complications post EK surgery. However, with close patient follow-up and strict return precautions, the risks can be minimized. Our practice observes patients at a minimum on an annual basis for the longevity of the graft.

12.4.1 Late Graft Failure

Endothelial cell density decreases over time following DSAEK surgery, with the greatest decline occurring in the first year after surgery. Continued decline at a slower rate has been demonstrated up to 5 years following transplantation. Late graft failure has been reported in 6–8 % of patients 5 years after undergoing DSAEK [28, 32]. At 5 years after surgery, patients with a history of pseudophakic or aphakic bullous keratopathy have a greater risk of late graft failure (24 %) compared to patients with Fuchs dystrophy (5 %). In addition, long-term graft survival in eyes with prior glaucoma surgery is worse than with Fuchs dystrophy eyes [28]. Contrary to surgeon biases, the characteristics of donor tissue that passes EBAA standards have no relationship to graft survival or postoperative cell counts. Tissue that is "young, fresh, and with a high cell count" does not improve the postoperative outcomes or health of the DSAEK graft. In large studies, preoperative donor endothelial cell density, death-to-preservation time, donor age, and recipient age have not been associated with decreased postoperative endothelial cell density or late graft failure [42, 43]. The most important preventable causes of late graft failure are endothelial cell loss from traumatic surgical implantation and immunologic rejection. Late graft failures may be reduced by adhering to careful surgical technique with a 5-mm incision, gentle treatment of the endothelial layer, and close postoperative care to monitor for and treat immunologic rejection episodes as expediently as possible.

12.4.2 Rejection

Endothelial immunologic rejection is an important treatable cause of endothelial cell loss and late graft failure. Cumulative rates of rejection have been reported at 1 year between 6.0 and 7.6%, at 2 years between 12 and 14%, and at 3 years 22% [15, 29, 48]. The peak time for immunologic rejection occurs between 12 and 18 months following DSAEK surgery [21]. Patients generally present with corneal edema, keratic precipitates, and decreased visual acuity (Fig. 12.6). Approximately one third of patients are asymptomatic at the time of presentation. Risk factors for immunologic rejection include stopping topical corticosteroids and being of African-American descent [29]. Endothelial rejection is treated with frequent topical corticosteroids and can be followed with pachymetry and clinical exam. Most patients are treated successfully with medication alone, but 7–26% eventually require graft replacement. Some studies have suggested that DSAEK grafts are less likely to fail as a result of immunologic rejection than PKP grafts [4]. In order to minimize the occurrence of immunologic rejection following DSAEK surgery, we recommend continuing corticosteroid therapy until at least 2 years following

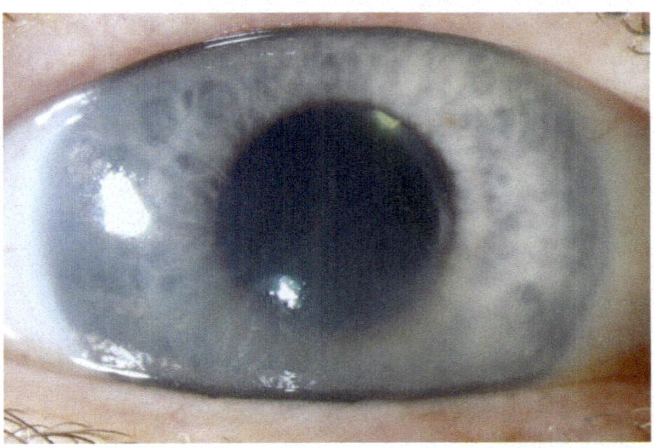

Fig. 12.6 DSAEK rejection. Although less common than after PKP, endothelial rejection following DSAEK surgery may result in graft failure

transplant, strict return precautions for telltale symptoms of rejection, and monitoring patients frequently during the first 2 years after surgery to ensure that they do not suffer significant cell loss from subclinical rejection episodes.

12.4.3 Glaucoma

In addition to the risk of acute pupil block glaucoma from the anterior chamber air bubble in the early postoperative period, there is also the risk of iatrogenic glaucoma following DSAEK due to prolonged corticosteroid use. Elevation of intraocular pressure following DSAEK is twice as common at 41 % in patients with a history medically managed glaucoma, than in patients with a history of glaucoma surgery (24 %) or in patients with no history of glaucoma (20 %) [2]. Among all DSAEK patients, the need for addition of a medication to control postoperative pressure elevation has been reported to be as high as 11 % [35]. Among patients with a history of glaucoma, the percent requiring the addition of medication to control the intraocular pressure is as high as 62 %, with 28 % requiring surgical intervention for their glaucoma [31] (Fig. 12.7).

12.4.4 Cataract

Phakic patients undergoing DSAEK surgery for indications such as CHED or early-onset Fuchs dystrophy often do not have visually significant cataract at the time of transplant. Small series of these cases have suggested a rate of cataract formation following phakic DSAEK surgery of 17–40 % [13, 45].

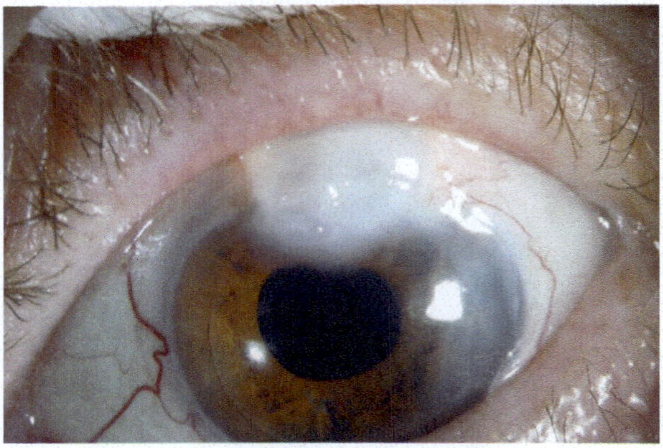

Fig. 12.7 DSAEK in a post-trabeculectomy eye. Performing DSAEK surgery in an eye with a history of trabeculectomy presents a unique set of challenges including difficulty maintaining an anterior chamber air bubble, blockage of the trabeculectomy site with air resulting in elevated IOP, and an increased risk of postoperative hypotony which could lead to graft failure

12.4.5 Intraocular Lens Opacification

Opacification of a newly implanted or preexisting intraocular lens (IOL) has been described following DSAEK surgery [3]. The rate of IOL opacification is greater in patients who undergo rebubble for a dislocated graft, implying that prolonged exposure of the IOL to air or gas may be responsible. These opacifications can become visually significant (Fig. 12.8), and laboratory analysis of explanted IOLs has shown that the opaque deposits consist of calcium [47]. The development of opaque IOL deposits following DSAEK is most commonly associated with hydrophilic IOLs [23]. We would suggest that the preoperative history includes identification of the type of IOL material if the patient is pseudophakic in order to prepare the patient for the possibility of IOL opacification. If a triple procedure is planned, hydrophilic IOL material should be avoided.

12.4.6 Refractive Shift

DSAEK surgery has been shown to induce a hyperopic refractive shift of 0.9–1.5 diopters [26, 49]. A number of theories to explain this hyperopic shift have been proposed, including the nonuniform shape of microkeratome-prepared grafts, which tend to be thinner in the center [9, 16] and then a thickening of the graft noted at the perimeter [12]. Astigmatic shift following DSAEK surgery has also been shown to be minimal, with no statistically significant shift in magnitude of astigmatism with either a scleral tunnel [41, 44] or clear corneal approach

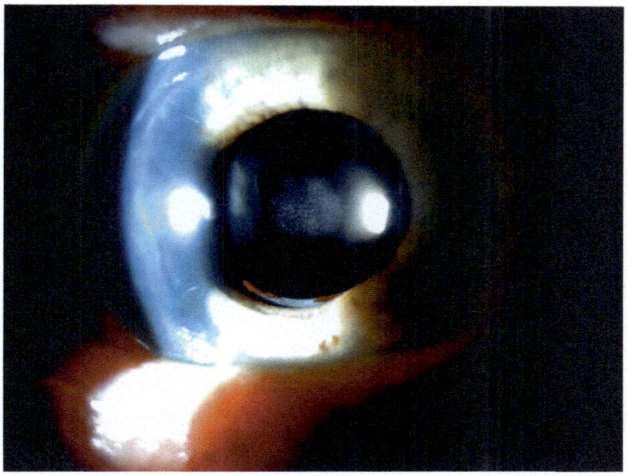

Fig. 12.8 Opacification of a hydrophilic IOL following DSAEK. Opacification of intraocular lenses has been reported following DSAEK surgery. Hydrophilic acrylic lens material and repeated exposure to air or gas have been associated with increased risk of this complication. Opacification may become visually significant and require intraocular lens exchange (Photo courtesy of Albert Jun, M.D., Ph.D.)

[18]. It is important to account for the predicted hyperopic shift when combining DSAEK with cataract surgery in order to avoid a refractive surprise.

12.4.7 *Retinal Detachment*

Retinal detachment has been reported following DSAEK surgery in up to 4 % of patients [39, 40]. Postoperative retinal detachment has been associated with a history of retinal detachment, previous ocular surgery, and intraoperative posterior dislocation of intraocular lens or DSAEK lenticule [37].

12.4.8 *Epithelial Ingrowth*

Epithelial ingrowth can occur either due to the migration of epithelial cells with the graft at the time of surgery or migration of cells through a non-apposing incision after surgery such as a gaping venting incision [39, 40, 35]. Epithelial ingrowth can range from a small nest in the interface to a prodigious sheet associated with graft nonadherence and failure (Fig. 12.9). Treatment may range from observation of small, noncentral epithelial nests to graft removal and replacement for more advanced cases. Presence of implanted epithelium can be readily identified on histopathological analysis of the explanted graft [50]. There are also recent reports of successfully using YAG laser to destroy epithelial ingrowth under a laser-assisted in situ keratomileusis (LASIK) flap, which might also be applicable for post-DSAEK interface epithelial ingrowth [6]. Avoiding the use of venting incisions and careful closure of all surgical incisions may help prevent this complication.

12.4.9 *Cystoid Macular Edema*

Cystoid macular edema (CME) has been reported in as many as 5 % of patients receiving DSAEK surgery [39, 40]. Macular edema has been shown to resolve with topical nonsteroidal anti-inflammatory or intravitreal corticosteroid therapy. In one prospective case series, a significant increase in macular thickness was observed at 1 and 3 months following surgery in patients undergoing DSAEK combined with cataract surgery, but not in patients undergoing DSAEK alone [22]. Many surgeons routinely prescribe nonsteroidal anti-inflammatory drops along with topical corticosteroids in order to minimize the risk of postoperative macular edema.

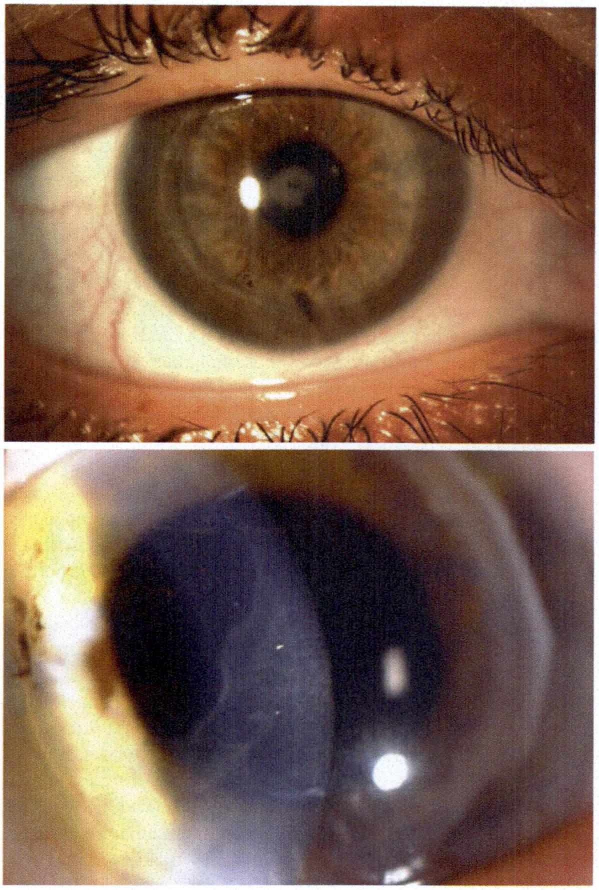

Fig. 12.9 DSAEK epithelial ingrowth. Epithelial ingrowth through an incision or epithelium inadvertently introduced to the stromal surface of the graft during insertion may lead to epithelial growth in the interface

12.5 Conclusion

DSAEK surgery is an exceedingly safe and successful treatment for endothelial dysfunction due to a variety of causes. DSAEK results in faster visual rehabilitation, better visual acuity, and lower risk of rejection than penetrating keratoplasty. Nevertheless, there are a number of complications associated with DSAEK that may result in temporary or permanent vision loss for the patient. With careful attention to patient selection, operative technique, and postoperative care, many of these complications can be minimized or prevented completely. Although DMEK is emerging as the treatment of choice for endothelial dysfunction for many indications, DSAEK will surely continue to be an important skill for corneal surgeons around the world.

Financial Interests MAT receives small royalties from Bausch and Lomb Surgical (St Louis, MO) on the DSAEK instruments that he designed. MAT also receives unrestricted educational funding from Bausch and Lomb Surgical (St. Louis, MO) and Moria (Antoin, FR) for the annual Endothelial Keratoplasty Group breakfast.

References

1. EBAA Statistical Report 2014. Eye Bank Association of America. Online. Accessed: http://www.restoresight.org/wpcontent/uploads/2015/03/2014_Statistical_Report-FINAL.pdf.
2. Aldave AJ, Chen JL, Zaman AS, Deng SX, Yu F. Outcomes after DSEK in 101 eyes with previous trabeculectomy and tube shunt implantation. Cornea. 2014;33(3):223–9.
3. Ahad MA, Darcy K, Cook SD, Tole DM. Intraocular lens opacification after Descemet stripping automated endothelial keratoplasty. Cornea. 2014;33(12):1307–11.
4. Allan BD, Terry MA, Price Jr FW, Price MO, Griffin NB, Claesson M. Corneal transplant rejection rate and severity after endothelial keratoplasty. Cornea. 2007;26(9):1039–42.
5. Anwar DS, Chu CY, Prasher P, Bowman RW, Mootha VV. Features of Urrets-Zavalia syndrome after Descemet stripping automated endothelial keratoplasty. Cornea. 2012;31(11):1330–4.
6. Ayala MJ, Alió JL, Mulet ME, De La Hoz F. Treatment of laser in situ keratomileusis interface epithelial ingrowth with neodymium: yttrium–aluminum–garnet laser. Am J Ophthalmol. 2008;145(4):630–4.
7. Chang V, Karp CL, Yoo SH, Ide T, Budenz DL, Kovach JL, Suh LH. Mycobacterium abscessus endophthalmitis after Descemet's stripping with automated endothelial keratoplasty. Cornea. 2010;29(5):586–9.
8. Chew AC, Mehta JS, Li L, Busmanis I, Tan DT. Fungal endophthalmitis after Descemet stripping automated endothelial keratoplasty-a case report. Cornea. 2010;29(3):346–9.
9. Dupps WJ, Qian Y, Meisler DM. Multivariate model of refractive shift in Descemet-stripping automated endothelial keratoplasty. J Cataract Refract Surg. 2008;34(4):578–84.
10. Goshe JM, Terry MA, Li JY, Straiko MD, Davis-Boozer D. Graft dislocation and hypotony after Descemet's stripping automated endothelial keratoplasty in patients with previous glaucoma surgery. Ophthalmology. 2012;119(6):1130–33.
11. Grueterich M, Messmer E, Kampik A. Posterior lamellar disc dislocation into the vitreous cavity during Descemet stripping automated endothelial keratoplasty. Cornea. 2009;28(1):93–6.
12. Holz HA, Meyer JJ, Espandar L, Tabin GC, Mifflin MD, Moshirfar M. Corneal profile analysis after Descemet stripping endothelial keratoplasty and its relationship to postoperative hyperopic shift. J Cataract Refract Surg. 2008;34(2):211–4.
13. Huang T, Luo Y, Wang Y, Hu A, Gao N. Descemet's stripping with endothelial keratoplasty for special Fuchs' endothelial dystrophy in phakic eyes. Ophthalmic Res. 2011;46(1):44–9.
14. Ide T, Yoo SH, Kymionis GD, Perez VL, Goldman JM, O'Brien TP. Descemet-stripping automated endothelial keratoplasty (DSAEK): effect of nontoxic gentian violet marking pen on DSAEK donor tissue viability by using vital dye assay. Cornea. 2008;27(5):562–4.
15. Jordan CS, Price MO, Trespalacios R, Price FW. Graft rejection episodes after Descemet stripping with endothelial keratoplasty: part one: clinical signs and symptoms. Br J Ophthalmol. 2009;93(3):387–90.
16. Jun B, Kuo AN, Afshari NA, Carlson AN, Kim T. Refractive change after descemet stripping automated endothelial keratoplasty surgery and its correlation with graft thickness and diameter. Cornea. 2009;28(1):19–23.
17. Koenig SB, Covert DJ. Early results of small-incision Descemet's stripping and automated endothelial keratoplasty. Ophthalmology. 2007;114(2):221–6.
18. Koenig SB, Covert DJ, Dupps Jr WJ, Meisler DM. Visual acuity, refractive error, and endothelial cell density six months after Descemet stripping and automated endothelial keratoplasty (DSAEK). Cornea. 2007;26(6):670–4.

19. Lee WB, Foster JB, Kozarsky AM, Zhang Q, Grossniklaus HE. Interface fungal keratitis after endothelial keratoplasty: a clinicopathological report. Ophthalmic Surg Lasers Imaging Off J Int Soc Imaging Eye. 2010;42:e44–8.
20. Lee WB, Jacobs DS, Musch DC, Kaufman SC, Reinhart WJ, Shtein RM. Descemet's stripping endothelial keratoplasty: safety and outcomes: a report by the American Academy of Ophthalmology. Ophthalmology. 2009;116(9):1818–30.
21. Li JY, Terry MA, Goshe J, Shamie N, Davis-Boozer D. Graft rejection after Descemet's stripping automated endothelial keratoplasty: graft survival and endothelial cell loss. Ophthalmology. 2012;119(1):90–4.
22. Mashor RS, Nasser O, Sansanayudh W, Rootman DS, Slomovic AR. Changes in macular thickness after descemet stripping automated endothelial keratoplasty. Am J Ophthalmol. 2015;159(3):415–8.
23. Morgan-Warren PJ, Andreatta W, Patel AK. Opacification of hydrophilic intraocular lenses after Descemet stripping automated endothelial keratoplasty. Clin Ophthalmol (Auckland, NZ). 2015;9:277.
24. Ortiz-Gomariz A, Higueras-Esteban A, Gutiérrez ÁR, González-Méijome JM, Arance-Gil A, Villa-Collar C. Late-onset Candida keratitis after Descemet stripping automated endothelial keratoplasty: clinical and confocal microscopic report. Eur J Ophthalmol. 2011;21(4): 498–502.
25. Oster SF, Ebrahimi KB, Eberhart CG, Schein OD, Stark WJ, Jun AS. A clinicopathologic series of primary graft failure after Descemet's stripping and automated endothelial keratoplasty. Ophthalmology. 2009;116(4):609–14.
26. Price MO, Baig KM, Brubaker JW, Price FW. Randomized, prospective comparison of precut vs surgeon-dissected grafts for descemet stripping automated endothelial keratoplasty. Am J Ophthalmol. 2008;146(1):36–41.
27. Price MO, Bidros M, Gorovoy M, Price Jr FW, Benetz BA, Menegay HJ, Lass JH. Effect of incision width on graft survival and endothelial cell loss after DSAEK. Cornea. 2010;29(5): 523.
28. Price MO, Fairchild KM, Price DA, Price FW. Descemet's stripping endothelial keratoplasty: five-year graft survival and endothelial cell loss. Ophthalmology. 2011;118(4):725–9.
29. Price MO, Jordan CS, Moore G, Price FW. Graft rejection episodes after Descemet stripping with endothelial keratoplasty: part two: the statistical analysis of probability and risk factors. Br J Ophthalmol. 2009;93(3):391–5.
30. Price FW, Price MO. Descemet's stripping with endothelial keratoplasty in 200 eyes: early challenges and techniques to enhance donor adherence. J Cataract Refract Surg. 2006;32(3): 411–8.
31. Quek DT, Wong T, Tan D, Mehta JS. Corneal graft survival and intraocular pressure control after Descemet stripping automated endothelial keratoplasty in eyes with pre-existing glaucoma. Am J Ophthalmol. 2011;152(1):48–54.e2.
32. Ratanasit A, Gorovoy MS. Long-term results of Descemet stripping automated endothelial keratoplasty. Cornea. 2011;30(12):1414–8.
33. Schmitt AJ, Feilmeier MR, Piccoli FV, Ide T, Yoo SH. Interface blood after Descemet stripping automated endothelial keratoplasty. Cornea. 2011;30(7):815–7.
34. Suh LH, Dawson DG, Mutapcic L, Rosenfeld SI, Culbertson WW, Yoo SH, Dubovy SR. Histopathologic examination of failed grafts in Descemet's stripping with automated endothelial keratoplasty. Ophthalmology. 2009;116(4):603–8.
35. Shih CY, Ritterband DC, Rubino S, Palmiero PM, Jangi A, Liebmann J, Ritch R, Seedor JA. Visually significant and nonsignificant complications arising from Descemet stripping automated endothelial keratoplasty. American journal of ophthalmology. 2009;148(6):837–43.
36. Shulman J, Kropinak M, Ritterband DC, Perry HD, Seedor JA, McCormick SA, Milman T. Failed descemet-stripping automated endothelial keratoplasty grafts: a clinicopathologic analysis. Am J Ophthalmol. 2009;148(5):752–9.
37. Singh A, Gupta A, Stewart JM. Posterior dislocation of descemet stripping automated endothelial keratoplasty graft can lead to retinal detachment. Cornea. 2010;29(11):1284–6.

38. Straiko MD, Terry MA, Shamie N. Descemet stripping automated endothelial keratoplasty under failed penetrating keratoplasty: a surgical strategy to minimize complications. Am J Ophthalmol. 2011;151(2):233–7.
39. Suh LH, Yoo SH, Deobhakta A, Donaldson KE, Alfonso EC, Culbertson WW, O'Brien TP. Complications of Descemet's stripping with automated endothelial keratoplasty: survey of 118 eyes at one institute. Ophthalmology. 2008;115(9):1517–24.
40. Suh LH, Kymionis GD, Culbertson WW, O'Brien TP, Yoo SH. Descemet stripping with endothelial keratoplasty in aphakic eyes. Arch Ophthalmol. 2008;126(2):268–70.
41. Terry MA, Saad HA, Shamie N, Chen ES, Phillips PM, Friend DJ, Stoeger C. Endothelial keratoplasty: the influence of insertion techniques and incision size on donor endothelial survival. Cornea. 2009;28(1):24–31.
42. Terry MA, Shamie N, Chen ES, Hoar KL, Friend DJ. Endothelial keratoplasty: a simplified technique to minimize graft dislocation, iatrogenic graft failure, and pupillary block. Ophthalmology. 2008;115(7):1179–86.
43. Terry MA, Shamie N, Chen ES, Hoar KL, Phillips PM, Friend DJ. Endothelial keratoplasty: the influence of preoperative donor endothelial cell densities on dislocation, primary graft failure, and 1-year cell counts. Cornea. 2008;27(10):1131–7.
44. Terry MA, Shamie N, Chen ES, Phillips PM, Hoar KL, Friend DJ. Precut tissue for Descemet's stripping automated endothelial keratoplasty: vision, astigmatism, and endothelial survival. Ophthalmology. 2009;116(2):248–56.
45. Tsui JY, Goins KM, Sutphin JE, Wagoner MD. Phakic descemet stripping automated endothelial keratoplasty: prevalence and prognostic impact of postoperative cataracts. Cornea. 2011;30(3):291–5.
46. Vaddavalli PK, Diakonis VF, Canto AP, Kankariya VP, Pappuru RR, Ruggeri M, Yoo SH. Factors affecting DSAEK graft lenticle adhesion: an in vitro experimental study. Cornea. 2014;33(6):551–4.
47. Werner L, Wilbanks G, Nieuwendaal CP, Dhital A, Waite A, Schmidinger G, Mamalis N. Localized opacification of hydrophilic acrylic intraocular lenses after procedures using intracameral injection of air or gas. J Cataract Refract Surg. 2015;41(1):199–207.
48. Wu EI, Ritterband DC, Yu G, Shields RA, Seedor JA. Graft rejection following descemet stripping automated endothelial keratoplasty: features, risk factors, and outcomes. Am J Ophthalmol. 2012;153(5):949–57.
49. Yoo SH, Kymionis GD, Deobhakta AA, Ide T, Manns F, Culbertson WW, Alfonso EC. One-year results and anterior segment optical coherence tomography findings of descemet stripping automated endothelial keratoplasty combined with phacoemulsification. Arch Ophthalmol. 2008;126(8):1052–5.
50. Zhang Q, Randleman JB, Stulting RD, Lee WB, Stone DU, Kozarsky AM, Grossniklaus HE. Clinicopathologic findings in failed Descemet stripping automated endothelial keratoplasty. Arch Ophthalmol. 2010;128(8):973–80.

Chapter 13
Revision Surgical Options for Failed PK in FED

Danny Mitry and Bruce Allan

13.1 Introduction

Since 2000, endothelial keratoplasty (EK) in its various forms has largely eclipsed penetrating keratoplasty (PK) as the procedure of choice in the primary treatment for corneal endothelial failure secondary to Fuchs dystrophy [1]. Advantages include safer surgery under local anaesthetic and early functional visual rehabilitation – both of particular benefit in the older age group comprising the majority of patients with endothelial failure. Additional advantages include preservation of eye wall strength, refractive shape, and freedom from suture-related complications. Although primary transplantation for Fuchs dystrophy is now predominantly by EK, a sizeable cohort of Fuchs dystrophy cases treated initially with PK remains. The advantages of primary EK mostly hold true for EK surgery after failed PK, but a number of additional considerations apply in surgical planning [1–5]. Here we will explore results for EK after PK, surgical variations, and an algorithm for procedure choice.

D. Mitry, PhD, FRCOphth
Moorfields Eye Hospital NHS Foundation Trust, London, UK

B. Allan, MD, FRCOphth (✉)
Moorfields Eye Hospital NHS Foundation Trust, London, UK

Moorfields and University College London NIHR Biomedical Research Centre in Ophthalmology, London, UK
e-mail: bruce.allan@ucl.ac.uk

C. Cursiefen, A.S. Jun (eds.), *Current Treatment Options for Fuchs Endothelial Dystrophy*, DOI 10.1007/978-3-319-43021-8_13

13.2 EK After PK Versus PK After PK

If the initial refractive shape of a failed PK was good and opacification within the stroma is potentially reversible (oedema rather than scarring), EK has clear advantages as a revision transplantation modality. But does EK graft survival after PK match or improve on PK survival after reoperation for failed PK?

Graft registry studies, led by the Australian Corneal Graft Registry [6], have transformed our understanding of corneal transplantation outcomes. The paradigm is simple: surgeons return structured feedback on outcomes for individual cases to a central registry at key time points, survival analysis (Kaplan–Meier) is used to describe the likelihood of transplant failure at key time points, and a variant of multivariate regression modelling applicable to survival data (Cox proportional hazards) is used to identify clinical risk factors for graft failure at a given time point. Cox proportional hazard modelling, as the name suggests, will generate 'hazard ratios', quantifying the reduction in survival probability associated with a particular risk factor versus that for eyes undergoing transplantation without this risk. Hazard ratios are normally tabulated against risk factors included in the model together with confidence intervals and p values and help to allow both surgeons and patients to make informed choices prior to surgical intervention. Examples of Kaplan–Meier survival data and hazard ratios detailing risk factors for graft failure from a multicentre study of EK after PK for all indications [5] are given in Fig. 13.1 and Table 13.1. Key conclusions from this study were:

- 5-year survival for EK after PK is approximately 50 % (similar to PK after PK).
- Visual outcomes in EK after PK are similar to those for PK after PK.
- Preoperative predictors of graft failure in EK after PK were young age, previous glaucoma tube surgery, and endothelial rejection prior to PK failure.
- Rejection prior to PK failure increases the risk of rejection in EK after PK, and rejection in the EK increases the risk of graft failure.
- Surgery in high-volume, single surgeon centres had a protective effect.

Transplant registries are yet to report on the outcomes of EK after PK. Even when these data do emerge, as illustrated by the centre effect above, it may initially be difficult to tease out the learning curve from the true clinical potential for new EK techniques. At this stage, it is probably safe to conclude that the advantages of early visual rehabilitation and closed eye surgery (relative safety under local anaesthetic) are a rational basis for choosing EK after PK in suitable cases of failed primary PK for Fuchs dystrophy, but final visual results and graft survival have not yet been shown to be superior.

Outcome data reported to date are results for Descemet stripping automated EK (DSAEK) rather than Descemet membrane endothelial keratoplasty (DMEK). Since techniques for graft preparation and implantation in DMEK have become better understood in the last 5 years, many EK surgeons have switched to DMEK [7]. Potential advantages for DMEK in the context of EK after PK are reduced rejection risk [8, 9] and reduced graft detachment in association with an irregular posterior corneal contour.

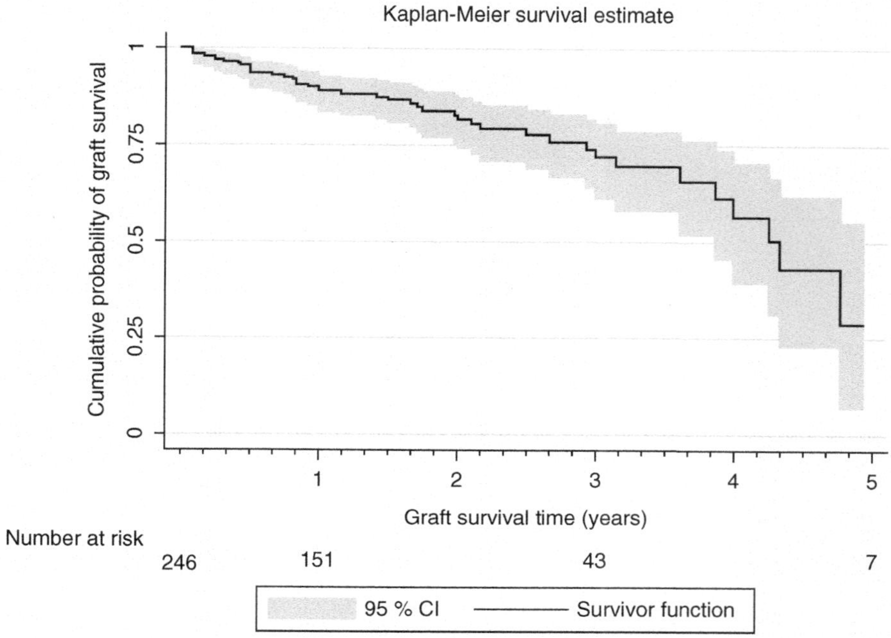

Fig. 13.1 Endothelial keratoplasty after failed penetrating keratoplasty – graft survival. Median survival time was 57 months (interquartile range, 36–70.8 months). The region in *grey* represents the 95 % confidence interval for the probability estimate with vertical inflexions indicating censored data (Reproduced with permission from Mitry et al. [5])

13.3 Rejection Prophylaxis

In primary transplantation for Fuchs dystrophy, 2-year rejection probabilities for PK and DSAEK appear to be similar at approximately 10–20 %. Rates are an order of magnitude lower (1–2 %) for DMEK [8, 9]. It is not yet clear whether this reduced rejection risk translates to DMEK after failed PK, but it would be surprising if a tenfold reduction in rejection risk only applied to primary transplantation. Inflammation at the time of transplantation is an important risk factor for rejection and subsequent graft failure. Pretreatment with topical steroids to minimize any residual inflammation in cases of transplant failure secondary to endothelial rejection is therefore a logical step.

The role of tissue matching in keratoplasty remains poorly defined, and any benefits for matching strategies in high-risk PK may not apply to DMEK [10]. Similarly, although systemic immunosuppression is widely used with the aim of reducing the risk of transplant rejection in high-risk PK cases, particularly those with multiple failed grafts, the evidence base supporting this additional intervention remains weak [11]. As with the protective effect observed for DMEK in primary transplantation, it is not clear whether benefits observed in some high-risk PK series will translate to DMEK after PK, and all systemic immunosuppressive drugs have a significant side-effect profile. Another factor to consider in DMEK after PK before exposing

Table 13.1 Hazard ratios and associated confidence intervals for pre- and postoperative risk factors for DSAEK failure after PK

Pre- and postoperative risk factors for DSAEK failure		
		p-value
Age		
≥80 years	1	
60–79 years	2.38(0.89–6.30)	0.082
40–59 years	3.98(1.40–11.37)	0.010
<39 years	8.42(2.23–31.69)	0.002
Centre		
1	1	
2	0.15(0.06–0.39)	<0.001
3	0.57(0.14–2.26)	0.43
4	0.11(0.03–0.37)	<0.001
5	0.16(0.06–0.40)	<0.001
6	0.54(0.16–1.85)	0.32
Previous glaucoma surgery		
None	1	
Trabeculectomy	2.12(0.78–5.75)	0.14
Shunt drainage	4.12(1.63–10.41)	0.003
Rejection episodes prior to PK failure		
No episodes	1	
Rejection episodes	2.41(1.02–5.70)	0.04
Post-DSAEK rejection		
No	1	
Yes	2.49(1.18–5.26)	0.01

patients to potentially hazardous drug treatment is the relative ease of repeat surgery. DMEK can be performed through a 2.4-mm self-sealing incision under local anaesthetic, and the risks to the eye from repeat surgery are relatively well contained.

Clear, evidence-based thresholds for additional interventions to prevent rejection in high-risk repeat transplantation using EK are unlikely to emerge in the near future. Surgeons must therefore take an educated guess at the best approach for avoiding rejection in individual cases. A switch to DMEK and pretreatment with topical steroids to minimize inflammation prior to surgery are both low-risk alternatives which may be beneficial, whereas systemic immunosuppression [11] or keratoprosthesis surgery [12] can be considered after multiple graft failures.

13.4 Glaucoma

Secondary glaucoma is second only to repeated rejection as a risk factor for corneal transplant failure [6]. Poor intraocular pressure control on medication prior to transplantation is likely to be exacerbated by steroid use after surgery, and glaucoma

drainage surgery after transplantation may be damaging to the endothelium. It is therefore logical to offer glaucoma drainage surgery prior to transplantation in cases with preexisting problems with intraocular pressure control. Once filtration surgery has been performed, topical steroids can be used with relative impunity and may even help to reduce the risk of filtration failure.

Trabeculectomy results are relatively poor after corneal transplantation. For this reason, primary tube drainage surgery is often preferred [13]. The 'catch 22' here is that whilst tube drainage surgery should help to control intraocular pressure, thereby reducing the risk of graft failure, tube surgery itself is a risk factor for graft failure in EK after PK. Tube drainage devices may damage the endothelium directly. This risk can be mitigated by aiming for a relatively posterior placement of the tube entry site in a deep anterior chamber or vitrectomy and placement in the posterior chamber. Air may also escape into the tube at surgery or soon after, reducing the efficacy of graft tamponade in EK.

13.5 Posterior Corneal Contour

There is commonly a step in the sectional profile through the posterior cornea after PK at the donor/host wound edge. This can be problematic for EK adhesion in revision transplantation surgery. The common practice for DSAEK after PK has been to undersize or oversize the donor diameter relative to the diameter of the original PK to help avoid edge lift in association with a posterior wound edge step. Preoperative optical coherence tomography can be useful to help anticipate this problem. Ultrathin DSAEK or DMEK may drape more effectively in cases of shape mismatch, and undersized grafts (0.5 mm smaller than the original PK) can be used in cases with a large posterior step [14].

In DMEK in particular, edge lift can also be caused by tags at the margins of the Descemet rhexis. Wound healing at the posterior donor/host junction can make a clean Descemet rhexis extending to the posterior margin of the PK difficult to achieve. In EK after PK, a Descemet rhexis may not be necessary. No effect was observed in a recent multicentre study in which regression modelling was used to examine whether leaving the failed endothelium in place had any influence on revision EK graft survival [5].

13.6 Anterior Corneal Contour

Knowledge of the corrected distance visual acuity – the most important functional measure of irregular astigmatism after transplantation in cases without significant visual comorbidity – and manifest refraction prior to transplant failure is an important guide to when repeat PK may be a better option than EK after PK. If the astigmatic outcome from the original transplant was poor, the fastest route to effective visual rehabilitation is likely to be a repeat PK.

PK after PK is also generally a better option if there is significant stromal opacity, although variations including femtosecond laser-assisted DLEK [15] can be useful if the anterior corneal contour is good and the opacity is confined to the posterior stroma.

13.7 Poor Visual Potential

If there is significant visual comorbidity and the visual potential is poor, the anterior contour becomes less relevant. If the aims are simply to restore good comfort and good cosmesis in bullous keratopathy after a failed PK, a Gundersen conjunctival flap can achieve both without repeat transplantation and the risk of subsequent further graft failure. However, a flap can be difficult to mobilize if there has been previous glaucoma filtration surgery, particularly a tube drainage device. So EK can still be a good alternative after failed PK even in cases with poor visual potential.

13.8 Unicameral Eyes

Techniques for unfolding DMEK donor scrolls in the presence of an anterior chamber lens are becoming better established, but in eyes with a large lens/iris diaphragm defect, DSAEK with a stay suture [16] may be preferable to avoid posterior dislocation.

13.9 Summary

Endothelial failure is the leading indication for repeat keratoplasty in Fuchs dystrophy. The advent of EK and DMEK in particular offers surgeons a minimally invasive and easily repeatable surgical revision option. Although not applicable to all cases (Fig. 13.2), DMEK is likely to emerge as the modality of choice in repeat keratoplasty, not least because the rejection risk may be lower where less corneal tissue is transplanted.

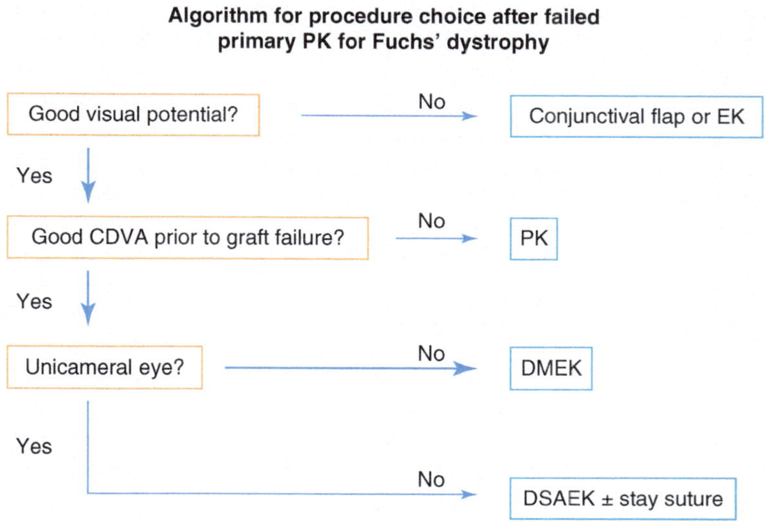

Fig. 13.2 Algorithm summarizing procedure choice after failed primary penetrating keratoplasty for Fuchs dystrophy

References

1. Ang M, Ho H, Wong C, Htoon HM, Mehta JS, Tan D. Endothelial keratoplasty after failed penetrating keratoplasty: an alternative to repeat penetrating keratoplasty. Am J Ophthalmol. 2014;158(6):1221–7.e1.
2. Clements JL, Bouchard CS, Lee WB, Dunn SP, Mannis MJ, Reidy JJ, et al. Retrospective review of graft dislocation rate associated with descemet stripping automated endothelial keratoplasty after primary failed penetrating keratoplasty. Cornea. 2011;30(4):414–8.
3. Heitor de Paula F, Kamyar R, Shtein RM, Sugar A, Mian SI. Endothelial keratoplasty without Descemet stripping after failed penetrating keratoplasty. Cornea. 2012;31(6):645–8.
4. Jangi AA, Ritterband DC, Wu EI, Mehta VV, Koplin RS, Seedor JA. Descemet stripping automated endothelial keratoplasty after failed penetrating keratoplasty. Cornea. 2012;31(10):1148–53.
5. Mitry D, Bhogal M, Patel AK, Lee BS, Chai SM, Price MO, et al. Descemet stripping automated endothelial keratoplasty after failed penetrating keratoplasty: survival, rejection risk, and visual outcome. JAMA Ophthalmol. 2014;132(6):742–9.
6. Williams KA, Lowe M, Bartlett C, Kelly TL, Coster DJ, All C. Risk factors for human corneal graft failure within the Australian corneal graft registry. Transplantation. 2008;86(12):1720–4.
7. Kruse FE, Schrehardt US, Tourtas T. Optimizing outcomes with Descemet's membrane endothelial keratoplasty. Curr Opin Ophthalmol. 2014;25(4):325–34.
8. Anshu A, Price MO, Price Jr FW. Risk of corneal transplant rejection significantly reduced with Descemet's membrane endothelial keratoplasty. Ophthalmology. 2012;119(3):536–40.
9. Dapena I, Ham L, Netukova M, van der Wees J, Melles GR. Incidence of early allograft rejection after Descemet membrane endothelial keratoplasty. Cornea. 2011;30(12):1341–5.
10. Bohringer D, Schwartzkopff J, Maier PC, Reinhard T. HLA matching in keratoplasty: lessons learned from lamellar techniques. Klin Monbl Augenheilkd. 2013;230(5):490–3.
11. Abudou M, Wu T, Evans JR, Chen X. Immunosuppressants for the prophylaxis of corneal graft rejection after penetrating keratoplasty. Cochrane Database Syst Rev. 2015;(8):CD007603.

12. Srikumaran D, Munoz B, Aldave AJ, Aquavella JV, Hannush SB, Schultze R, et al. Long-term outcomes of boston type 1 keratoprosthesis implantation: a retrospective multicenter cohort. Ophthalmology. 2014;121(11):2159–64.
13. Tandon A, Espandar L, Cupp D, Ho S, Johnson V, Ayyala RS. Surgical management for post-keratoplasty glaucoma: a meta-analysis. J Glaucoma. 2014;23(7):424–9.
14. Straiko MD, Terry MA, Shamie N. Descemet stripping automated endothelial keratoplasty under failed penetrating keratoplasty: a surgical strategy to minimize complications. Am J Ophthalmol. 2011;151(2):233–7.e2.
15. Alio Del Barrio JL, Ziaei M, Bhogal M, Allan BD. Femtosecond laser-assisted deep lamellar endothelial keratoplasty: a new approach to a forgotten technique. Cornea. 2015;34:1369–74.
16. Eguchi H, Miyamoto T, Hotta F, Tomida M, Inoue M, Mitamura Y. Descemet-stripping automated endothelial keratoplasty for vitrectomized cases with traumatic aniridia and aphakic bullous keratopathy. Clin Ophthalmol. 2012;6:1513–8.

Chapter 14
Long-Term Clear Graft Survival and Chronic Endothelial Cell Loss Following Posterior Lamellar Keratoplasty

Philip Maier and Thomas Reinhard

14.1 Introduction

Diseases of the corneal endothelium (Fuchs endothelial dystrophy, bullous keratopathy, and endothelial failure following penetrating keratoplasty) count for the most frequent indications for corneal transplantation. Instead of replacing all five layers of the cornea (epithelium, Bowman layer, stroma, Descemet membrane, endothelium) by penetrating keratoplasty (PK), which has first been performed by Eduard Zirm [1–3] in 1905, nowadays techniques for the selective replacement of the diseased corneal endothelium are preferred. This has first been suggested by Tillet in 1956 [4] to avoid characteristical complications following PK (e.g. high irregular astigmatism and wound healing problems). The technical principle of this kind of posterior lamellar keratoplasty or endothelial keratoplasty (EK) was to excise the host's posterior stroma including Descemet membrane and endothelium and to replace it by identical lamellar graft prepared from the donor lamella. However, due to interface irregularities between host and donor stroma the visual results were not satisfying for the patients. One important technical step in improving posterior lamellar keratoplasty was the introduction of descemetorhexis by Melles et al. [5], where the stroma of the recipients cornea is not manipulated and only the Descemet membrane including the diseased endothelial cells is removed completely [6]. By avoiding manipulations of the recipient's posterior stroma the clinical results could be improved as the lamellar graft could be attached to a smooth surface of the posterior stroma. In case of Descemet stripping endothelial keratoplasty (DSEK) the lamellar graft is manually prepared and consists of posterior stroma, Descemet membrane, and endothelium of the donor. It is transferred into the anterior chamber via a corneoscleral or clear cornea incision using special surgical instruments, unfolded and sutureless attached to

P. Maier • T. Reinhard (✉)
Eye Center, Faculty of Medicine, University Hospital Freiburg, Killianstr. 5, 79106 Freiburg, Germany
e-mail: philip.maier@uniklinik-freiburg.de

C. Cursiefen, A.S. Jun (eds.), *Current Treatment Options for Fuchs Endothelial Dystrophy*, DOI 10.1007/978-3-319-43021-8_14

the posterior stroma of the recipient's cornea by an air bubble. Regarding DSEK one problem is the manual preparation process of the lamellar graft leading to graft preparation failures in some cases [7]. To overcome these problems of complete manual graft preparation the separation of the stromal lamellae can be performed using a microkeratome, by which a 400–500 μm thick layer of the anterior part of the donor cornea can be cut leaving a 80–150 μm thick lamella consisting of posterior stroma, Descemet membrane, and endothelium (Descemet stripping automated endothelial keratoplasty, DSAEK). The characteristic advantages of DSEK/DSAEK compared to PK are a suture-free graft adaptation and a faster improvement of visual acuity without a change of the refractive status. On the other hand, due to more intensive graft manipulations during graft preparation, implantation, and adaptation, the early endothelial cell loss following DSEK/DSAEK seems to be higher than that after PK. Furthermore, patients following DSEK/DSAEK often do not reach the maximum possible visual acuity which may be explained by optical phenomena caused by graft-host-interface reactions [8]. To reach the respective advantages of DSEK/DSAEK but to avoid graft-host-interface problems, Descemet membrane endothelial keratoplasty (DMEK) has been developed where the corneal graft consists only of Descemet membrane and endothelial cells without corneal stroma [9]. For DMEK graft preparation Descemet membrane including the endothelium is manually peeled off the donor's posterior stroma using fine forceps. Following complete peeling off Descemet membrane forms a roll with the endothelial cells on the exterior. This graft roll can then be implanted into the anterior chamber through a small clear cornea incision and attached to the posterior recipient's stroma by using an air bubble after the graft has been carefully unfolded. As no stromal tissue of the donor is grafted the primary anatomical situation is restored by DMEK leading to the maximum reachable visual acuity. However, one disadvantage of DMEK is that macroscopically invisible collagen fibres of the donor stroma can insert into Descemet membrane causing tears in the thin graft leading to graft preparation failures [10]. Furthermore, the unfolding of the graft may also be much more difficult than in DSAEK potentially leading to more intraoperative endothelial cell damage and more primary graft failures [3, 11].

The following chapter will focus on the long-term follow-up after DSEK/DSAEK/DMEK compared to each other and to PK with respect to clear graft survival and chronic endothelial cell loss.

14.2 Graft Failure

14.2.1 Primary Graft Failure

Primary graft failures (failure within 6 months following surgery) are not associated with endothelial graft rejections but are caused by endothelial insufficiency from insufficient tissue quality, complicated recipient factors (inflammation, interface problems, infection, flat anterior chamber, previous surgeries, etc.) or problems with

Table 14.1 Factors associated and not associated with an increased endothelial cell loss following DSAEK

Factors associated with increased cell loss	Factors not associated with increased cell loss
Smaller incisions [51]	Donor tissue storage time [25, 52]
Longer incisions [53]	Graft diameter [25, 54]
Larger area of tissue compression by forceps [53]	Preoperative ECD [55]
Donor tissue dislocation [53]	Manual versus microkeratome preparation of the donor tissue [53]
	Use of pre-cut versus surgeon-cut tissue [56]
	Use of graft delivery devices [57, 58]

the surgical technique. Primary graft failure following posterior lamellar keratoplasty can also be due to primary malfunction of the donor endothelium, but it more often is explained by a high endothelial cell loss due to intensive manipulation of the graft during surgery. Therefore, in some reports this kind of failure is named as iatrogenic primary graft failure. Various comparative cohort studies show that the risk for early/primary graft failure is lower after PKP (0–3 %) than after DSAEK (0–29 %) as well as after DMEK (0–9 %, see Table 14.2). Besides these results of various cohort and case control studies, Monnereau et al. [12] give an overview on real-life data when they published the results from 18 surgeons performing DMEK with different techniques. They included in total 431 cases of DMEK and found 1.2 % intraoperative failures and 10 % surgery associated primary graft failures.

14.2.2 Midterm and Long-Term Clear Graft Survival

In the Cornea Donor Study clear graft survival following PK for endothelial insufficiency was 86 % after 5 years [13], and the clear graft survival rate was better for patients with Fuchs dystrophy (93 %) than for patients with pseudophakic or aphakic corneal oedema [14]. For PK the 10-year failure rate for Fuchs dystrophy ranges between 10 and 20 % [15–17]. From the Irish keratoplasty registry a clear graft survival rate of 93 % after 1 year was reported [18], and in the Swedish Corneal Transplant Register a graft survival rate of 90 % after 2 years was found [19]. Thompson et al. [17] reported on 90 % clear graft survival 5 years after PK. Regarding late endothelial graft failure the recipient bed endothelial reservoir seems to play an important role on the long-term prognosis following PK as, for example patients with keratoconus (92 %) have a much better prognosis regarding 15-year long-term clear graft survival than patients with bullous keratopathy (67 %) [20].

For posterior lamellar keratoplasty such long-term survival data are not available. However, large register data from the United Kingdom [21] and from Australia [22] show that early and midterm to long-term graft survival following posterior lamellar keratoplasty is worse compared to PK. These register data seem to mirror the real-life situation including a lot of learning curves from different surgeons. In the analysis of the Australian registry [22] the authors included the clinical course after 13920 penetrating keratoplasties (2965 were performed in Fuchs endothelial dystrophy or bullous keratopathy) and 2287 endothelial keratoplasties performed between 1996 and 2013. Primary (within 1 month after surgery) as well as overall graft survival was worse following posterior lamellar keratoplasty compared to PK. If primary graft failures were excluded from the analysis, as they may be correlated to surgical effects, grafts following endothelial keratoplasty in patients with Fuchs endothelial dystrophy still had worse survival rates than grafts following PK. The analysis included data from 74 surgeons performing endothelial keratoplasty and found that graft survival was better for more experienced surgeons that had performed 100 or more endothelial keratoplasties. A similar surgeon's experience effect regarding endothelial keratoplasty was found in the analysis of the registry data from the United Kingdom [21] where 2074 cases of endothelial keratoplasty performed between 2006 and 2011 were compared to 2622 cases of penetrating keratoplasty performed between 2000 and 2005 for Fuchs endothelial dystrophy or bullous keratopathy. The authors also found an overall worse survival rate after 2 years for endothelial keratoplasty compared to PK. Besides donor's endothelial cell count, donor age, and glaucoma at the time of surgery the surgical experience was also a statistically significant factor influencing clear graft survival following endothelial keratoplasty. Akanda et al. [23] performed a systematic review on the available literature regarding graft rejection and graft failure following PK compared to EK. For posterior lamellar procedures they included seven studies and found that the pooled odds ratio for graft failure of PK versus posterior lamellar procedures was 2.09 (95 % CI: 0.57–7.59) demonstrating a statistically non-significant difference. From various cohort studies, it was reported that clear graft survival following DSAEK with follow-ups from 12 to 24 months ranges from 55 to 100 % (for literature see Table 14.1). Up to now the study with the longest follow-up after DSAEK comprises 5 years. Ratanasit and Gorovoy found that 92 % of the 51 included DSAEK grafts were clear and Price et al. reported on 93 % cumulative 5-year clear graft survival [24, 25]. As for PK Price et al. found a better clear graft survival for patients with Fuchs dystrophy (95 % cumulative 5-year clear graft survival) compared to pseudophakic bullous keratopathy (76 % cumulative 5-year clear graft survival) and also as for PK [26, 27] they found pre-existing glaucoma as a significant risk factor for graft failure. In their study 3.6 % of graft failed due to endothelial decompensation and 3 % of patients were regrafted for unsatisfactory corrected distance visual acuity [25].

Following DMEK only data on midterm clear graft survival with 12 months follow-up are available where graft survival rates were between 99.3 and 100 % [28, 29]. Regarding the data from the Australian register it is important to notice that the number of included DMEK cases is very small (129 out of 1214 cases of endothelial keratoplasty). As it could be shown the success rates of DMEK increase with more experience [30], these follow-up data on DMEK have to be interpreted with caution as the learning curves of different surgeons are included in this small number of cases. Our own experience shows that during the first 2 years following surgery the graft failure rate was higher following EK than following PK, where PK (2 %) had the lowest graft failure rate followed by DMEK (7 %) and DSAEK (20 %) [31]. However, graft failure was also defined as repeat keratoplasty due to unsatisfying visual results following EK, which was higher following DSAEK compared to DMEK.

14.3 Endothelial Cell Loss

14.3.1 Physiologic Endothelial Cell Loss

Human corneal endothelial cells may be able to proliferate in vitro but they rarely show mitotic activity in vivo [32, 33]. Therefore, during lifetime a yearly chronic endothelial cells loss of about 0.6 % can be observed [34]. This cell loss does not lead to malfunction of a healthy endothelium if there is no additional condition causing a decrease in endothelial cell density like Fuchs dystrophy, trauma, inflammation or iatrogenic cell damage [35–37].

14.3.2 Endothelial Cell Loss Following Penetrating Keratoplasty

The yearly decrease of endothelial cells in the first year following PK is in the mean 4–16 % [15, 20, 38], but this chronic endothelial cell loss slows down during long-term follow-up. However, the individual endothelial cell loss varies widely [39, 40]. One reason for this may be the migration capability of the recipient's peripheral endothelium as Reinhard et al. found a higher yearly endothelial cell loss for patients with bullous keratopathy (29.4 ± 17.6 %) compared to patients with Fuchs dystrophy (17.0 ± 19.1 %) or keratoconus (14.0 ± 19.0 %) [41]. The measurement of endothelial cell densities in the first years following PK can be more useful as a predictor for late endothelial graft failure as the preoperative endothelial cell counts [20, 40, 42]. The overall endothelial cell loss 5 years following PK lies in the range of 59–70 % [43, 44].

14.3.3 Endothelial Cell Loss Following Endothelial Keratoplasty

In the age of posterior lamellar keratoplasty it seems important to differentiate between the early endothelial cell loss that can be associated to the surgical trauma and the chronic endothelial cell loss in long-term follow-up.

14.3.4 Early Endothelial Cell Loss up to Six Months Following Posterior Lamellar Keratoplasty

In the early post-operative follow-up the endothelial cell decrease is higher following EK than after PK, which can be associated to more intensive surgical manipulations of the graft during EK. In a systematic review of the literature including 19 trials Lee et al. [45] reported on an early endothelial cell loss within 6 months between 25 and 54 % after DSAEK with a mean endothelial cell loss of 37 %. When comparing DSAEK and PK, Price et al. [46] found a statistically significant lower endothelial cell loss 6 months following PK compared to DSAEK (11 ± 20 % vs. 34 ± 22 %, respectively, $p < 0.001$). For their multi-centre case series Monnereau et al. [12] found an overall decrease in ECD of 47 % (SD 20 %) 6 months following DMEK. In a large single centre series on 500 DMEK cases Rodríguez-Calvo-de-Mora et al. [30] report on an average endothelial cell loss 6 months following DMEK of 37 ± 18 %. In a direct comparison of DSAEK and DMEK comparable rates of early endothelial cell loss within 6 months following surgery were found (41 % for DSAEK and 39 % for DMEK) [47]. Regarding the early, most probably surgery associated endothelial cell loss, it has to be considered that the extent of the early endothelial cell loss may depend on the learning curve and the experience of the surgeon [48]. One other important factor regarding the early endothelial cell loss following posterior lamellar keratoplasty is the dislocation of the lamellar graft which is the most frequent post-surgical complication following endothelial keratoplasty. Graft dislocations are treated by a repeat air fill of the anterior chamber (so called rebubbling), which may be required in 1–82 % of cases following DSAEK [49] and even more often after DMEK (33–81 %) [28, 47]. The risk of graft dislocation seems to be lower using grafts that have been stored in organ culture, which is the case in most European eye banks, than using grafts stored in short-term culture, which is the case in most American eye banks [50]. Finally, for all studies comparing pre- vs. post-operative endothelial cell loss the reported figures have to be interpreted with caution as in many cases the technique of measuring the endothelial cell density of the graft in the eye bank and of the recipient following surgery varies so that there might be a systematic error in these comparisons.

Several factors have been identified that are associated with an increased early endothelial cell loss following DSAEK. These factors are summarised in Table 14.1.

14.3.5 Chronic Endothelial Cell Loss Following Posterior Lamellar Keratoplasty

The high endothelial cell loss in the early post-operative period following EK seems to stabilise over time with longer follow-up what further supports the important influence of the surgical manipulations regarding the early endothelial cell loss. When looking at the systematic review of Lee at al. [45] they reported on an endothelial cell loss at 1 year after DSAEK from 24 to 61 %, with an average of 41 % which was only a slight increase compared to the endothelial cell loss after 6 months (mean 37 %). Similar data were found by Price et al. [46] with an endothelial cell loss of 38 ± 22 % 1 year after DSAEK compared to 20 ± 23 % after PK where the increase of cell loss within 6–12 months after surgery was higher in the PK group compared to the DSAEK group. This observation could also be found 3 years following keratoplasty, when the mean endothelial cell loss was 39–46 % after DSAEK and 47–51 % after PKP [59, 60]. Van Dooren et al. [61] presented their 3 years follow-up data of 39 DSAEK versus 33 PK patients and calculated a regression model for the decrease in endothelial cell density. They found in their statistical model that the early endothelial cell loss was higher following DSAEK compared to PK but is slower in the long run so that the endothelial cell densities seem to converge after a certain time of follow-up. It seems as if the chronic endothelial cell loss, which is a characteristical property of PK grafts, may be slower after DSAEK. This hypothesis can be strengthened by the longest available follow-up data for 51 patients 5 years following DSAEK where the mean endothelial cell density decreased from 2700 (2500–3000) cells mm^2 to 1312 (374–2927) cells/mm^2 which is a mean cell loss of about 49 % [24]. Price et al. also reported on 5-year follow-up after DSAEK and found a mean endothelial cell loss of 53 % [25]. Comparing these results to the data of the Cornea Donor Study shows that the endothelial cell loss 5 years after DSAEK (49–53 %) was lower than that 5 years after PK (70 %) [24, 25, 44].

For DMEK less information regarding the chronic endothelial cell loss is available as the technique is evolutionary younger. After 12 months the endothelial cell loss varies between 19 and 40 % [29, 62]. However, it seems that in the long run the chronic endothelial cell loss after DMEK is comparable to that after DSAEK and therefore slower than after PK, so that the endothelial cell densities may also converge about 2 years after surgery [63]. Up to date the longest follow-up period following DMEK is 5 years where the loss of endothelial cells was high early after DMEK with 38 % after 1 year but 55 % after 5 years meaning a mean decrease of endothelial cells of around 7 % per year after the first year [64].

Figure 14.1 shows a comparison of the chronic endothelial cell loss up to 5 years following PK (data extracted from the younger cohort (<66 years of age) of the Cornea Donor Study Investigator Group), DSAEK (data extracted from Price et al. [25]), and DMEK (data extracted from Baydoun et al. [64]) demonstrating the high endothelial cell loss early after endothelial keratoplasty whereas the chronic endothelial cell loss seems to slow down so that in the long run the endothelial cell density may be higher after endothelial keratoplasty compared to the endothelial cell density following PK. Furthermore, Quilendrino et al. [65] created a mathematical model for the estimation of the increase in posterior corneal surface area associated with post-operative corneal deturgescence and its effect on ECD measurements. From this theoretical model they found that the endothelial cell loss following DMEK may be overestimated by about 8 % due to the increased posterior corneal surface area associated with post-operative corneal deturgescence. However, the reason for the slower chronic endothelial cell loss following either DSAEK or DMEK compared to PK is

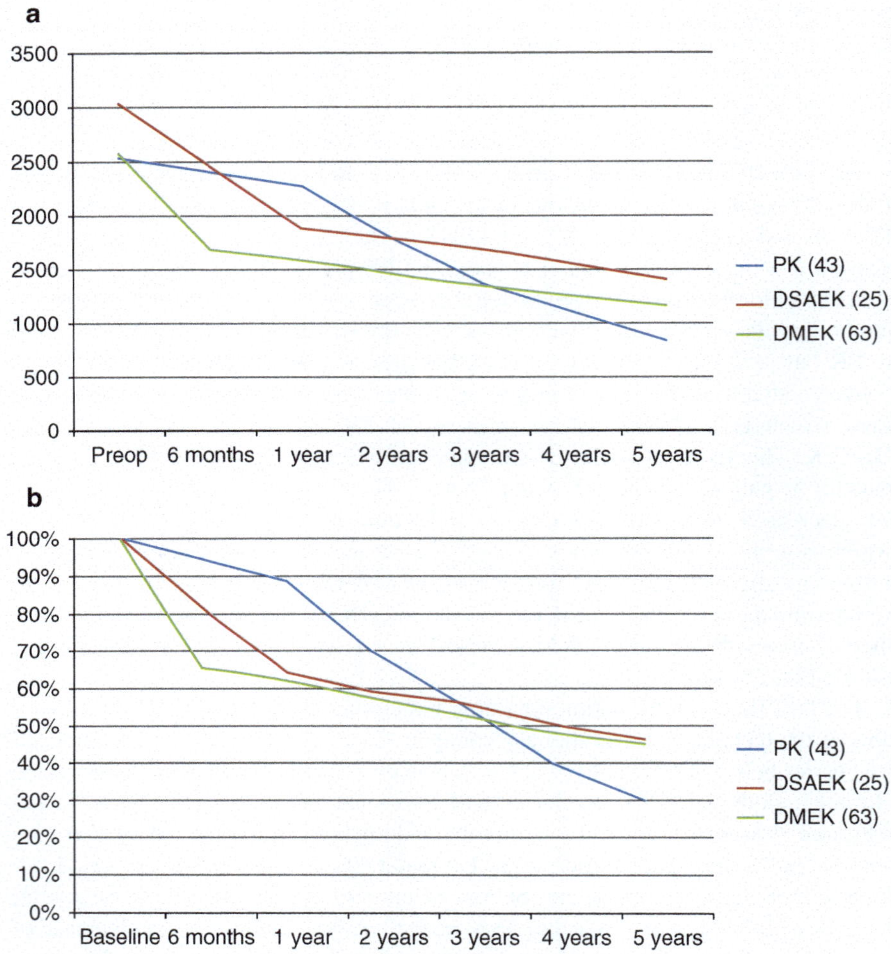

Fig. 14.1 Decrease of the median absolute endothelial cell density (**a**) respectively the ratio of endothelial cell survival (**b**) as a function of time following penetrating keratoplasty (PK) extracted from the younger donor cohort (<66 years of age) of the Cornea Donor Study Investigator Group [44] versus Descemet stripping endothelial keratoplasty (DSAEK) extracted from Price et al. [25] versus Descemet membrane endothelial keratoplasty (DMEK) extracted from Baydoun et al. [64]

not fully understood. One explanation could be the reduced risk of endothelial immune reactions following DMEK, which still is the most important cause of graft failure after PK [19]. In the available literature the following risks of endothelial graft rejection within 2 years after transplantation have been reported: 0–23 % for PK, 0–14 % for DSAEK, and 1–3 % for DMEK (Table 14.2). In their systematic review Akanda et al. [23] included seven publications on the risk of graft rejection comparing PK and EK and found that a pooled odds ratio for rejection of PK over EK was 1.52 (95 % CI: 1.00–2.32) demonstrating a statistically significantly reduced

Table 14.2 Data from the literature on primary graft failure, mid-to long-term clear graft survival, chronic endothelial cell loss, and the risk of endothelial immune reactions for PK, DSAEK, and DMEK, respectively

	PKP	DSAEK	DMEK
Primary graft failure	0–3 % [15, 30]	0–29 % [15, 19, 27, 30, 34, 38, 40, 71, 73–76]	0–9 % [11, 12, 72, 77, 78]
Overall mid- to long-term graft failure	86–90 % after 5 years [13–19]	55–100 % after 12–24 months [53, 55–57, 72, 79–85]	99.3–100 % after 12 months [29, 62]
Endothelial cell loss after 5 years	70 % [43, 44]	49–53 % [24, 25]	55 % [37]
Risk of graft rejection within 2 years	0.5–23.3 % [15–17, 30, 40, 41, 59, 86–88]	0–14 % [11, 15, 19, 30, 34, 40, 67, 68, 71, 86]	1–3 % [11, 68, 72, 89]

risk of graft rejection following posterior lamellar keratoplasty. However, data from the registry of the United Kingdom [21] could not demonstrate a difference in the risk of endothelial immune reactions comparing 1961 PK versus 1525 EK for either Fuchs endothelial dystrophy or bullous keratopathy. However, in this study there was no differentiation between DSAEK and DMEK for EK, and it seems obvious that most included cases were DSAEK and not DMEK. As the risk for endothelial rejections following DSAEK seems to be in the same range as for PK, it does not seem surprising that no difference in the risk of immune reaction could be found. The reason for the reduced risk of rejection following DMEK is not completely understood; however, it seems that the risk increases with the amount of grafted tissue. Further evidence for this observation can be found in the mouse experiments from Hori et al. where they found that alloimmunogenicity of the normal cornea resides within its epithelial and stromal layers, whereas immune privilege arises from the endothelium [66, 67]. Besides the corneal epithelium, which seems to play the major role in allograft sensitisation [68], it has also been found that corneal stroma cells are able to inhibit the production of anti-inflammatory cytokines [69]. This experimental data may help to explain the clinically observed reduced risk of endothelial immune reaction following DMEK compared to DSAEK and PK.

14.4 Perspective

During the last years PK for patients with endothelial insufficiency has been replaced by posterior lamellar keratoplasty techniques like DSAEK and nowadays more and more DMEK. Various case series could demonstrate that better visual results without or with only minor changes of the refractive status can be reached faster following endothelial keratoplasty than after PK. However, compared to PK DSAEK and DMEK have higher reoperation rates (i.e. rebubbling) and more primary graft failures. Up to now no long-term follow-up data on posterior lamellar keratoplasty are available (maximum follow-up of case series for DSAEK and DMEK is 5 years) to give sufficient information for comparison of chronic endothelial cell loss or long-term clear graft survival of endothelial grafts compared with PK. Therefore, in a recent Cochrane review Nanavaty and Shortt [70, 71] draw the conclusion that randomized controlled trials with long-term follow-up are needed to make a decision on which surgical technique gives the best clinical results for which individual patient not only in short term but especially in the long-term follow-up.

References

1. Zirm EK. Eine erfolgreiche totale Keratoplastik (A successful total keratoplasty). 1906. Refract Corneal Surg. 1989;5(4):258–61.
2. Cursiefen C, Seitz B, Kruse F. Hornhauttransplantation: Glänzende Bilanz und viele Perspektiven. Dtsch Arztebl. 2005;102(45):A–3078/B–2603/C–2445.
3. Maier P, Reinhard T, Cursiefen C. Descemet stripping endothelial keratoplasty – rapid recovery of visual acuity. Dtsch Arztebl Int. 2013;110(21):365–71.
4. Tillet C. Posterior lamellar keratoplasty. Am J Ophthalmol. 1956;41:530–3.
5. Melles GRJ, Wijdh RHJ, Nieuwendaal CP. A technique to excise the descemet membrane from a recipient cornea (descemetorhexis). Cornea. 2004;23(3):286–8.
6. Heindl LM, Hofmann-Rummelt C, Schlötzer-Schrehardt U, Kruse FE, Cursiefen C. Histologic analysis of descemet stripping in posterior lamellar keratoplasty. Arch Ophthalmol. 2008;126(4):461–4.
7. Price MO, Price Jr FW. Descemet's stripping with endothelial keratoplasty: comparative outcomes with microkeratome-dissected and manually dissected donor tissue. Ophthalmology. 2006;113(11):1936–42.
8. Heinzelmann S, Böhringer D, Maier PC, Reinhard T. Correlation between visual acuity and interface reflectivity measured by pentacam following DSAEK. Acta Ophthalmol. 2013; 92(1):e1–4.
9. Melles GRJ, Ong TS, Ververs B, van der Wees J. Descemet membrane endothelial keratoplasty (DMEK). Cornea. 2006;25(8):987–90.
10. Schlötzer-Schrehardt U, Bachmann BO, Laaser K, Cursiefen C, Kruse FE. Characterization of the cleavage plane in DESCemet's membrane endothelial keratoplasty. Ophthalmology. 2011;118(10):1950–7.
11. Heinzelmann S, Maier P, Reinhard T. Perspectives of posterior lamellar keratoplasty. In search of the perfect lamella. Ophthalmologe. 2011;108(9):825–32.
12. Monnereau C, Quilendrino R, Dapena I, Liarakos VS, Alfonso JF, Arnalich-Montiel F, et al. Multicenter study of descemet membrane endothelial keratoplasty: first case series of 18 surgeons. JAMA Ophthalmol. 2014;132(10):1192–8.
13. Cornea Donor Study Investigator Group, Gal RL, Dontchev M, Beck RW, Mannis MJ, Holland EJ, et al. The effect of donor age on corneal transplantation outcome results of the cornea donor study. Ophthalmology. 2008;115(4):620–6.e6.
14. Sugar A, Tanner JP, Dontchev M, Tennant B, Schultze RL, Dunn SP, et al. Recipient risk factors for graft failure in the cornea donor study. Ophthalmology. 2009;116(6):1023–8.
15. Ing JJ, Ing HH, Nelson LR, Hodge DO, Bourne WM. Ten-year postoperative results of penetrating keratoplasty. Ophthalmology. 1998;105(10):1855–65.
16. Pineros O, Cohen EJ, Rapuano CJ, Laibson PR. Long-term results after penetrating keratoplasty for Fuchs' endothelial dystrophy. Arch Ophthalmol. 1996;114(1):15–8.
17. Thompson RW, Price MO, Bowers PJ, Price FW. Long-term graft survival after penetrating keratoplasty. Ophthalmology. 2003;110(7):1396–402.

18. Guerin M, O' Connell E, Walsh C, Fulcher T. Visual outcomes and graft survival following corneal transplants: the need for an Irish National Corneal Transplant Registry. Ir J Med Sci. 2008;177(2):107–10.
19. Claesson M, Armitage WJ, Fagerholm P, Stenevi U. Visual outcome in corneal grafts: a preliminary analysis of the Swedish Corneal Transplant Register. Br J Ophthalmol. 2002; 86(2):174–80.
20. Böhringer D, Böhringer S, Poxleitner K, Birnbaum F, Schwartzkopff J, Maier P, et al. Long-term graft survival in penetrating keratoplasty: the biexponential model of chronic endothelial cell loss revisited. Cornea. 2010;29(10):1113–7.
21. Greenrod EB, Jones MNA, Kaye S, Larkin DFP, National Health Service Blood and Transplant Ocular Tissue Advisory Group and Contributing Ophthalmologists (Ocular Tissue Advisory Group Audit Study 16). Center and surgeon effect on outcomes of endothelial keratoplasty versus penetrating keratoplasty in the United Kingdom. Am J Ophthalmol. 2014;158(5): 957–66.
22. Coster DJ, Lowe MT, Keane MC, Williams KA, Australian Corneal Graft Registry Contributors. A comparison of lamellar and penetrating keratoplasty outcomes: a registry study. Ophthalmology. 2014;121(5):979–87.
23. Akanda ZZ, Naeem A, Russell E, Belrose J, Si FF, Hodge WG. Graft rejection rate and graft failure rate of penetrating keratoplasty (PKP) vs lamellar procedures: a systematic review. PLoS One. 2015;10(3):e0119934.
24. Ratanasit A, Gorovoy MS. Long-term results of Descemet stripping automated endothelial keratoplasty. Cornea. 2011;30(12):1414–8.
25. Price MO, Fairchild KM, Price DA, Price FW. Descemet's stripping endothelial keratoplasty five-year graft survival and endothelial cell loss. Ophthalmology. 2011;118(4):725–9.
26. Reinhard T, Böhringer D, Sundmacher R. Accelerated chronic endothelial cell loss after penetrating keratoplasty in glaucoma eyes. J Glaucoma. 2001;10(6):446–51.
27. Reinhard T, Kallmann C, Cepin A, Godehardt E, Sundmacher R. The influence of glaucoma history on graft survival after penetrating keratoplasty. Graefes Arch Clin Exp Ophthalmol. 1997;235(9):553–7.
28. Guerra FP, Anshu A, Price MO, Giebel AW, Price FW. Descemet's membrane endothelial keratoplasty: prospective study of 1-year visual outcomes, graft survival, and endothelial cell loss. Ophthalmology. 2011;118(12):2368–73.
29. Reid RA, Craig EA, Suleman H. Descemet's membrane endothelial keratoplasty (DMEK): first UK prospective study of 1-year visual outcomes, graft survival and endothelial cell count. Br J Ophthalmol. 2015;99(2):166–9.
30. Rodríguez-Calvo-de-Mora M, Quilendrino R, Ham L, Liarakos VS, van Dijk K, Baydoun L, et al. Clinical outcome of 500 consecutive cases undergoing Descemet's membrane endothelial keratoplasty. Ophthalmology. 2015;122(3):464–70.
31. Heinzelmann S, Böhringer D, Eberwein P, Reinhard T, Maier P. Outcomes of Descemet membrane endothelial keratoplasty, Descemet stripping automated endothelial keratoplasty and penetrating keratoplasty from a single centre study. Graefes Arch Clin Exp Ophthalmol. 2016;254(3):515–22. doi: 10.1007/s00417-015-3248-z. Epub 2016 Jan 7.
32. Engelmann K, Bednarz J, Böhnke M. Endothelial cell transplantation and growth behavior of the human corneal endothelium. Ophthalmologe. 1999;96(9):555–62.
33. Senoo T, Joyce NC. Cell cycle kinetics in corneal endothelium from old and young donors. Invest Ophthalmol Vis Sci. 2000;41(3):660–7.
34. Bourne WM, Nelson LR, Hodge DO. Central corneal endothelial cell changes over a ten-year period. Invest Ophthalmol Vis Sci. 1997;38(3):779–82.
35. Armitage WJ, Dick AD, Bourne WM. Predicting endothelial cell loss and long-term corneal graft survival. Invest Ophthalmol Vis Sci. 2003;44(8):3326–31.
36. Bourne WM, Nelson LR, Hodge DO. Continued endothelial cell loss ten years after lens implantation. Ophthalmology. 1994;101(6):1014–22; discussion 1022–1023.

37. Bourne WM, Nelson LR, Buller CR, Huang PT, Geroski DH, Edelhauser HF. Long-term observation of morphologic and functional features of cat corneal endothelium after wounding. Invest Ophthalmol Vis Sci. 1994;35(3):891–9.
38. Böhringer D, Reinhard T, Spelsberg H, Sundmacher R. Influencing factors on chronic endothelial cell loss characterised in a homogeneous group of patients. Br J Ophthalmol. 2002; 86(1):35–8.
39. Patel SV, Hodge DO, Bourne WM. Corneal endothelium and postoperative outcomes 15 years after penetrating keratoplasty. Am J Ophthalmol. 2005;139(2):311–9.
40. Patel SV, Diehl NN, Hodge DO, Bourne WM. Donor risk factors for graft failure in a 20-year study of penetrating keratoplasty. Arch Ophthalmol. 2010;128(4):418–25.
41. Reinhard T, Böhringer D, Hüschen D, Sundmacher R. Chronic endothelial cell loss of the graft after penetrating keratoplasty: influence of endothelial cell migration from graft to host. Klin Monbl Augenheilkd. 2002;219(6):410–6.
42. Lass JH, Sugar A, Benetz BA, Beck RW, Dontchev M, Gal RL, et al. Endothelial cell density to predict endothelial graft failure after penetrating keratoplasty. Arch Ophthalmol. 2010; 128(1):63–9.
43. Bourne WM, Hodge DO, Nelson LR. Corneal endothelium five years after transplantation. Am J Ophthalmol. 1994;118(2):185–96.
44. Cornea Donor Study Investigator Group, Lass JH, Gal RL, Dontchev M, Beck RW, Kollman C, et al. Donor age and corneal endothelial cell loss 5 years after successful corneal transplantation. Specular microscopy ancillary study results. Ophthalmology. 2008;115(4):627–32.e8.
45. Lee WB, Jacobs DS, Musch DC, Kaufman SC, Reinhart WJ, Shtein RM. Descemet's stripping endothelial keratoplasty: safety and outcomes: a report by the American Academy of Ophthalmology. Ophthalmology. 2009;116(9):1818–30.
46. Price MO, Gorovoy M, Benetz BA, Price Jr FW, Menegay HJ, Debanne SM, et al. Descemet's stripping automated endothelial keratoplasty outcomes compared with penetrating keratoplasty from the Cornea Donor Study. Ophthalmology. 2010;117(3):438–44.
47. Tourtas T, Laaser K, Bachmann BO, Cursiefen C, Kruse FE. Descemet membrane endothelial keratoplasty versus descemet stripping automated endothelial keratoplasty. Am J Ophthalmol. 2012;153(6):1082–90.e2.
48. Koenig SB, Covert DJ, Dupps Jr WJ, Meisler DM. Visual acuity, refractive error, and endothelial cell density six months after Descemet stripping and automated endothelial keratoplasty (DSAEK). Cornea. 2007;26(6):670–4.
49. Arenas E, Esquenazi S, Anwar M, Terry M. Lamellar corneal transplantation. Surv Ophthalmol. 2012;57(6):510–29.
50. Laaser K, Bachmann BO, Horn FK, Schlötzer-Schrehardt U, Cursiefen C, Kruse FE. Donor tissue culture conditions and outcome after descemet membrane endothelial keratoplasty. Am J Ophthalmol. 2011;151(6):1007–18.e2.
51. Price MO, Bidros M, Gorovoy M, Price Jr FW, Benetz BA, Menegay HJ, et al. Effect of incision width on graft survival and endothelial cell loss after Descemet stripping automated endothelial keratoplasty. Cornea. 2010;29(5):523–7.
52. Terry MA, Li J, Goshe J, Davis-Boozer D. Endothelial keratoplasty: the relationship between donor tissue size and donor endothelial survival. Ophthalmology. 2011;118(10):1944–9.
53. Price MO, Price Jr FW. Endothelial cell loss after descemet stripping with endothelial keratoplasty influencing factors and 2-year trend. Ophthalmology. 2008;115(5):857–65.
54. Terry MA. Endothelial keratoplasty: a comparison of complication rates and endothelial survival between precut tissue and surgeon-cut tissue by a single DSAEK surgeon. Trans Am Ophthalmol Soc. 2009;107:184–91.
55. Terry MA, Shamie N, Chen ES, Hoar KL, Phillips PM, Friend DJ. Endothelial keratoplasty: the influence of preoperative donor endothelial cell densities on dislocation, primary graft failure, and 1-year cell counts. Cornea. 2008;27(10):1131–7.
56. Price MO, Baig KM, Brubaker JW, Price Jr FW. Randomized, prospective comparison of precut vs surgeon-dissected grafts for descemet stripping automated endothelial keratoplasty. Am J Ophthalmol. 2008;146(1):36–41.

57. Busin M, Bhatt PR, Scorcia V. A modified technique for descemet membrane stripping automated endothelial keratoplasty to minimize endothelial cell loss. Arch Ophthalmol. 2008;126(8):1133–7.
58. Khor W-B, Mehta JS, Tan DT-H. Descemet stripping automated endothelial keratoplasty with a graft insertion device: surgical technique and early clinical results. Am J Ophthalmol. 2011;151(2):223–32.e2.
59. Ang M, Mehta JS, Anshu A, Wong HK, Htoon HM, Tan D. Endothelial cell counts after Descemet's stripping automated endothelial keratoplasty versus penetrating keratoplasty in Asian eyes. Clin Ophthalmol. 2012;6:537–44.
60. Price MO, Gorovoy M, Price FW, Benetz BA, Menegay HJ, Lass JH. Descemet's stripping automated endothelial keratoplasty: three-year graft and endothelial cell survival compared with penetrating keratoplasty. Ophthalmology. 2013;120(2):246–51.
61. Dooren BTHV, Saelens IEY, Bleyen I, Mulder PGH, Bartels MC, Rij GV. Endothelial cell decay after descemet's stripping automated endothelial keratoplasty and top hat penetrating keratoplasty. Invest Ophthalmol Vis Sci. 2011;52(12):9226–31.
62. Gorovoy IR, Gorovoy MS. Descemet membrane endothelial keratoplasty postoperative year 1 endothelial cell counts. Am J Ophthalmol. 2015;159(3):597–600.e2.
63. Cursiefen C, Kruse FE. DMEK: Descemet membrane endothelial keratoplasty. Ophthalmologe. 2010;107(4):370–6.
64. Baydoun L, Tong CM, Tse WW, Chi H, Parker J, Ham L, et al. Endothelial cell density after Descemet membrane endothelial keratoplasty: 1 to 5-year follow-up. Am J Ophthalmol. 2012;154(4):762–3.
65. Quilendrino R, Höhn H, Tse WHW, Chi H, Dapena I, Ham L, et al. Do we overestimate the endothelial cell "loss" after descemet membrane endothelial keratoplasty? Curr Eye Res. 2013;38(2):260–5.
66. Hori J, Joyce NC, Streilein JW. Immune privilege and immunogenicity reside among different layers of the mouse cornea. 2000. Ocul Immunol Inflamm. 2007;15(3):225–39.
67. Hori J, Joyce NC, Streilein JW. Immune privilege and immunogenicity reside among different layers of the mouse cornea. Invest Ophthalmol Vis Sci. 2000;41(10):3032–42.
68. Hori J, Streilein JW. Role of recipient epithelium in promoting survival of orthotopic corneal allografts in mice. Invest Ophthalmol Vis Sci. 2001;42(3):720–6.
69. Holán V. Corneal stromal cells selectively inhibit the production of certain anti-inflammatory cytokines. Expert Rev Clin Immunol. 2006;2(1):101–8.
70. Nanavaty MA, Wang X, Shortt AJ. Endothelial keratoplasty versus penetrating keratoplasty for Fuchs endothelial dystrophy. Cochrane Database Syst Rev. 2014;2:CD008420.
71. Nanavaty MA, Shortt AJ. Endothelial keratoplasty versus penetrating keratoplasty for Fuchs endothelial dystrophy. Cochrane Database Syst Rev. 2011;7:CD008420.
72. Bahar I, Kaiserman I, McAllum P, Slomovic A, Rootman D. Comparison of posterior lamellar keratoplasty techniques to penetrating keratoplasty. Ophthalmology. 2008;115(9):1525–33.
73. Foster JB, Vasan R, Walter KA. Three-millimeter incision descemet stripping endothelial keratoplasty using sodium hyaluronate (healon): a survey of 105 eyes. Cornea. 2011;30(2):150–3.
74. Chen ES, Terry MA, Shamie N, Hoar KL, Friend DJ. Descemet-stripping automated endothelial keratoplasty: six-month results in a prospective study of 100 eyes. Cornea. 2008;27(5):514–20.
75. Shih CY, Ritterband DC, Rubino S, Palmiero P-M, Jangi A, Liebmann J, et al. Visually significant and nonsignificant complications arising from Descemet stripping automated endothelial keratoplasty. Am J Ophthalmol. 2009;148(6):837–43.
76. Suh LH, Yoo SH, Deobhakta A, Donaldson KE, Alfonso EC, Culbertson WW, et al. Complications of Descemet's stripping with automated endothelial keratoplasty: survey of 118 eyes at One Institute. Ophthalmology. 2008;115(9):1517–24.
77. Heindl LM, Kruse FE, Cursiefen C. Complications after posterior lamellar keratoplasty (DSAEK): prevention, detection and treatment. Klin Monbl Augenheilkd. 2010;227(6):478–82.

78. Price MO, Giebel AW, Fairchild KM, Price Jr FW. Descemet's membrane endothelial keratoplasty: prospective multicenter study of visual and refractive outcomes and endothelial survival. Ophthalmology. 2009;116(12):2361–8.
79. Gorovoy MS. Descemet-stripping automated endothelial keratoplasty. Cornea. 2006;25(8):886–9.
80. Bahar I, Kaiserman I, Sansanayudh W, Levinger E, Rootman DS. Busin guide vs forceps for the insertion of the donor lenticule in descemet stripping automated endothelial keratoplasty. Am J Ophthalmol. 2009;147(2):220–6.e1.
81. Mearza AA, Qureshi MA, Rostron CK. Experience and 12-month results of descemet-stripping endothelial keratoplasty (DSEK) with a small-incision technique. Cornea. 2007;26(3): 279–83.
82. Sarnicola V, Toro P. Descemet-stripping automated endothelial keratoplasty by using suture for donor insertion. Cornea. 2008;27(7):825–9.
83. Terry MA, Chen ES, Shamie N, Hoar KL, Friend DJ. Endothelial cell loss after Descemet's stripping endothelial keratoplasty in a large prospective series. Ophthalmology. 2008;115(3): 488–96.e3.
84. Wylegała E, Tarnawska D. Management of pseudophakic bullous keratopathy by combined Descemet-stripping endothelial keratoplasty and intraocular lens exchange. J Cataract Refract Surg. 2008;34(10):1708–14.
85. Yoo SH, Kymionis GD, Deobhakta AA, Ide T, Manns F, Culbertson WW, et al. One-year results and anterior segment optical coherence tomography findings of descemet stripping automated endothelial keratoplasty combined with phacoemulsification. Arch Ophthalmol. 2008;126(8):1052–5.
86. Allan BDS, Terry MA, Price Jr FW, Price MO, Griffin NB, Claesson M. Corneal transplant rejection rate and severity after endothelial keratoplasty. Cornea. 2007;26(9):1039–42.
87. Seitz B, Langenbucher A, Diamantis A, Cursiefen C, Küchle M, Naumann GO. Immunological graft reactions after penetrating keratoplasty – a prospective randomized trial comparing corneal excimer laser and motor trephination. Klin Monbl Augenheilkd. 2001;218(11):710–9.
88. Hjortdal J, Pedersen IB, Bak-Nielsen S, Ivarsen A. Graft rejection and graft failure after penetrating keratoplasty or posterior lamellar keratoplasty for fuchs endothelial dystrophy. Cornea. 2012;32(5):e60–3.
89. Anshu A, Price MO, Price Jr FW. Risk of corneal transplant rejection significantly reduced with Descemet's membrane endothelial keratoplasty. Ophthalmology. 2012;119(3):536–40.

Chapter 15
Immune Reactions and Dry Eye After Posterior Lamellar Keratoplasty

Philipp Steven, Sebastian Siebelmann, Deniz Hos, Franziska Bucher, and Claus Cursiefen

15.1 Introduction

Posterior lamellar keratoplasty has been demonstrated to be a successful, increasingly applied surgical method to replace diseased endothelial cells of the human cornea. Potential immune reactions may occur following DMEK or DSAEK with different clinical phenotypes, reasons, and risk factors that accompany graft failure. In addition in this chapter the clinically relevant yet only rudimentarily investigated development of dry eye disease following posterior lamellar keratoplasty is outlined.

This chapter is meant to give an overview of potential immune reactions that may occur following any of the two techniques and to discuss clinical phenotypes, reasons, and risk factors that accompany graft failure. In addition, the clinically relevant yet only rudimentarily investigated development of dry eye disease is outlined.

P. Steven, MD (✉) • S. Siebelmann
Department of Ophthalmology, University of Cologne, Medical Faculty, Cologne, Germany

Cluster of Excellence: Cellular Stress Responses in Aging-associated Disease (CECAD), University of Cologne, Cologne, Germany

Ocular Surface Group, Ocular GvHD Competence Center, Department of Ophthalmology, University of Cologne, Kerpenerstr. 62, 50937 Cologne, Germany
e-mail: philipp.steven@uk-koeln.de

D. Hos • F. Bucher • C. Cursiefen
Department of Ophthalmology, University of Cologne, Medical Faculty, Cologne, Germany

C. Cursiefen, A.S. Jun (eds.), *Current Treatment Options for Fuchs Endothelial Dystrophy*, DOI 10.1007/978-3-319-43021-8_15

15.2 Corneal Graft Rejection

In addition to postoperative complications such as graft detachment, immediate graft failure, and misalignment that may all be treated by either air/gas reinjections or regrafting, immune reactions following posterior lamellar keratoplasty are often difficult to detect and to treat.

Immune reactions that lead to corneal graft rejection were extensively studied in mouse models of penetrating keratoplasty (PK). Based on the concept of the so-called ocular immune privilege, the high acceptance rates of corneal allografts could be elucidated by: (i) avascularity (both blood and lymphatic vessels) of the recipient cornea, (ii) absence of mature donor-derived antigen-presenting cells (APCs), (iii) expression of FAS ligand, and (iv) capacity of corneal allografts to induce immune deviation through regulatory T-cells, downregulation of delayed-type hypersensitivity, and production of non-complement-fixing antibodies (the latter process called anterior chamber-associated immune deviation ACAID) [4].

15.3 Rejection Rates in Penetrating Keratoplasty

Rejection of full corneal grafts may occur if one or more of the described mechanisms are compromised, by, for example, vascularization of the graft bed [5], which then leads to a "high-risk" situation and increased rejection rates. In fact, rejection rates in patients increase with the number of corneal quadrants being pathologically vascularized [6].

Regarding "normal-risk" keratoplasty, rejection rates of approximately 5–10 % are documented within the first 3–5 years after transplantation, with much higher rates up to 100 % depending on the individual recipient's corneal situation (e.g., vascularization) and the number of previous transplantations [7].

15.4 Rejection Rates in Posterior Lamellar Keratoplasty

The rate of endothelial rejection in Descemet stripping automated endothelial keratoplasty (DSAEK) is comparable to rates of perforating keratoplasties, with approximately 7 % after 1 year and 12 % after 2 years [2, 8]. However, clinical features of the rejection are much more subtle than in PK, whereas Descemet membrane endothelial keratoplasty (DMEK) demonstrates almost full acceptance rates [1, 9]. In our last 1000 DMEKs at the Department of Ophthalmology at the University of Cologne, only 1 % experienced an immune reaction (Hos, D. et al. 2016).

Several authors have presented explanations for reduced rejection rates, for example, that anteriorly located APCs would not get access to the transplanted tissue [10] or that the amount of antigen transplanted in DMEK would be too little to induce immune rejections [11]. However immune reactions leading to rejection still occur in both techniques that need to be explained. In fact the clinical observation of low if any immune reaction after DMEK compared to PK nicely fits to experimental data of Hori et al. of murine composite corneal transplants: immunogenicity resided within corneal epithelium and to lesser extent in the stroma [12]. In contrast corneal endothelium conferred immune protection [13]. Since clinical data on corneal endothelial cell changes after DMEK [14] do not rule out a slight but progressive endothelial cell loss over time, it may still be the case that after DMEK mild and subclinical forms of immune destruction occur.

15.5 Clinical Findings

Clinical findings of endothelial rejection also differ between DSAEK and DMEK. In DSAEK endothelial rejection appears milder than in PK. In a study by Price and coworkers from 2009, 35 % of patients with detected immune rejections were asymptomatic [15]. Also, isolated endothelial precipitates, diffuse edema, or both were not present in all cases. Classic Khodadoust line was only reported in each of a single case of DSAEK [16] and DMEK [11]. Interestingly precipitates may also be detected in denuded areas, onto which graft endothelial cells had migrated over time. This finding simultaneously showed proof of endothelial cell migration across the graft perimeter [17] (Fig. 15.1). These clinical findings correlate with experimental studies by Khodadoust and Silverstein from 1969, in which they demonstrated endothelial rejections of solely endothelial transplants in rabbit eyes [18].

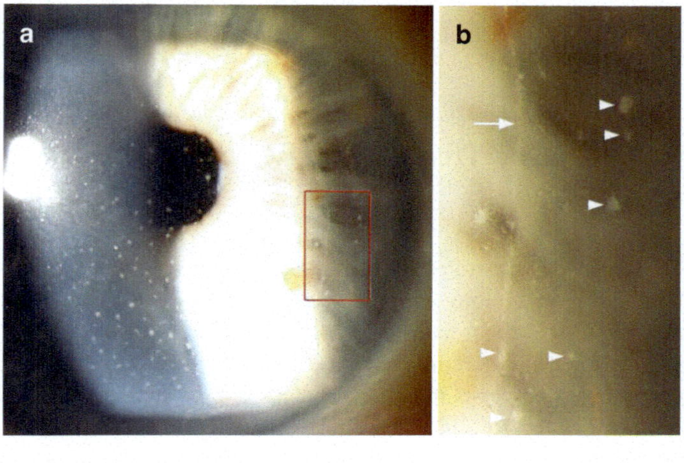

Fig. 15.1 (**a**) Endothelial precipitates following DMEK for treatment of Fuchs endothelial dystrophy in a 71-year-old individual. (**b**) Precipitates (*arrowheads*) also extend toward the initially denuded area demonstrating migration of donor-derived endothelial cells across the perimeter of the graft (*arrows*) (From Hos et al. [17]; reprint with kind permission)

15.6 Hypothesis for Less Rejection in DMEK Than in DSAEK

Besides the immunological reasons speculated on above, the (obvious) difference between DMEK and DSAEK is the disposition of stroma at Descemet membrane in DSAEK. It has been hypothesized that stromal and to a lesser extent endothelial antigen is responsible for initiating the immune response that then may lead to higher rejection rates in DSAEK than in DMEK (see above). However novel experimental findings might give reason for another hypothesis for increased rejection rates in DSAEK than in DMEK. Slnoniecka and coworkers recently published a study that demonstrated that the injury of the corneal stroma induces the secretion of substance P (SP) by corneal keratocytes [19]. Consecutively SP stimulation induces the secretion of interleukin 8, a pro-inflammatory chemokine. Together with the highly interesting finding of Paunicka et al. from 2015, in which the authors demonstrated that a substance P burst, deriving from nerve damage in the published experiments led to abolition of immune privilege, also on the contralateral eye, introducing the term "sympathetic loss of immune privilege" (SLIP) [20]. In the context of posterior lamellar keratoplasty, localized nerve damage occurs through the corneal incisions which would induce an initial SP burst. In DSAEK other than in DMEK, the remnant stroma and keratocytes are traumatized at time point of dissection and may therefore induce another (potentially chronic) SP secretion that would then abolish immune privilege and may lead to endothelial rejection, though weaker in characteristics than those in PK. In DMEK however, an additional SP burst is missing due to the lack of keratocytes which would be the reason for almost no endothelial rejections. To test this hypothesis on the one hand, animal models as described by Khodadoust and Silverstein in the 1960s could be used, but on the other hand, SP levels could be measured in DSAEK and DMEK specimens in vitro as first steps toward understanding the role of SP and SLIP in posterior lamellar keratoplasty.

15.7 Prevention and Treatment of Rejection in DMEK and DSAEK

Several studies have demonstrated that long-term low-dose therapy with topical steroids is successful in preventing endothelial rejection in PK. In a prospective study with more than 400 eyes that received a "normal-risk" PK, a once daily topical 1 % prednisolone acetate was demonstrated to significantly reduce the risk of graft rejection in comparison to eyes in which topical steroids were terminated 6 months after transplantation [7]. Another study further demonstrated a positive effect of long-term 0.1 % fluorometholone (up to 9 years after PK) regarding the risk of endothelial corneal rejection [21].

For posterior lamellar keratoplasty, no comparable prospective studies are available. In terms of DSAEK which demonstrates clinically less severe though similar rates of rejection compared to PK, long-term use of topical steroids, e.g., once daily or every other day, seems reasonable. In DMEK, with only occasional rejection rates, careful consideration of benefits and potential side effects should be performed. However from our experience, continuation or early restart of topical steroids (unpreserved prednisolone acetate or dexamethasone) is recommended once immune cells or presumed immune cells are visible at the endothelium in routine slit lamp examinations, even if other signs of rejection such as edema or Khodadoust line are lacking.

15.8 Graft Failure or Immune Reaction?

It is currently unclear whether late-onset graft failures, accompanied with ongoing loss of endothelial cells, is caused by either previously undetected diseases of the donor endothelium or by subclinical immune reactions, in other words subclinical graft rejection. In this context better and more accurate noninvasive methods are necessary that would enable functional analysis of the graft: (i) to reliably detect and characterize immune cells in close proximity to endothelial cells, (ii) to measure endothelial cell function, and (iii) to detect early morphological changes of the donor endothelium accompanied with immune reactions or degenerative diseases such as Fuchs dystrophy. To achieve this, imaging methods with higher resolution than specular microscopy, for example, confocal laser scanning microscopy (CLSM), optical coherence microscopy [22], and two-photon microscopy (2 PM) [23, 24], would be suitable. All three technologies, potentially in combination, would enable imaging the transplanted endothelium at resolutions of approximately 1 µm (Fig. 15.2a) together with the option to use autofluorescence detection of intrinsic fluorophores to characterize immune cells and to quantify their activation

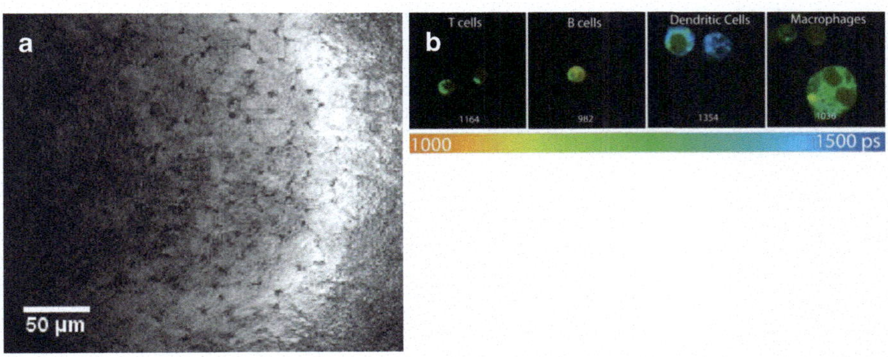

Fig. 15.2 (**a**) En-face optical coherence microscopy (OCM) of pig corneal endothelium allowing detection of hexagonal cellular borders and subcellular details. (**b**) Autofluorescence signal of different immune cells allows differentiation by means of two-photon microscopy (From Gehlsen et al. [23], Copyright Wiley-VCH Verlag GmbH & Co. KGaA. Reproduced with kind permission)

state in 2 PM (Fig. 15.2b). In this context the most obvious technique, since already available in the clinic, would be CLSM. CLSM could give information on the morphology of endothelial precipitates in DMEK and DSAEK and potentially allow for easier decision-making regarding onset, duration, and intensity of an immunosuppressive therapy. A recent study by Monnereau et al. in 2014 demonstrated early changes of endothelial cells as a prequel of graft rejection in DMEK; however no immune cells or precipitates were detected and analyzed [25].

15.9 Dry Eye Disease

Dry eye disease (DED) belongs among the most common ophthalmic conditions worldwide. It is generally accepted that the dysfunction of the lacrimal functional unit [26] leads to inflammation of the ocular surface as one of the core pathomechanisms of DED and consecutively to blurred vision, burning sensation, redness, tired eyes, and other symptoms. One reason for onset or exacerbation of DED is corneal refractive surgery such as LASIK or PTK [27, 28] and cataract surgery [29]. In particular following refractive surgery, the dissection of corneal nerves interrupts the corneal reflex arc, thereby reducing lacrimation and at the same time triggering an inflammatory response through the release of neuron-derived peptides such as substance P and CGRP [30]. The same may be hypothesized following perforating keratoplasty because all corneal nerves are dissected during trephination. Interestingly until now, only little information on DED following PK has been available, possibly because of consecutive anesthesia of the cornea and therefore lack of subjective symptoms. One study by Kuechle et al. demonstrated that dry eye disease is a risk factor for graft rejection in PK [31]. However, it is still unclear to what extent DED develops following PK.

Regarding DSAEK and DMEK, no information on DED either before or after surgery is available. Recently we demonstrated by means of CLSM that corneal incisions during DMEK surgery lead to a significant alteration of the density and function of the subbasal nerve plexus of the cornea [32] (Fig. 15.3). Although all parameters tested (including corneal sensitivity) recovered within 4–10 months, it is likely that during this recovery period or beyond, DED may be present and like in PK might have an influence on subclinical or clinical graft rejection.

Overall prospective clinical trials are needed to investigate the role of preexisting DED in the context of corneal transplantation and in particular its influence on graft survival.

15.10 Summary

Regarding immune reactions following corneal transplantation, DMEK surgery demonstrates advantages through very limited rejection episodes in comparison to DSAEK, which shows almost similar rejection rates as PK. Several explanations

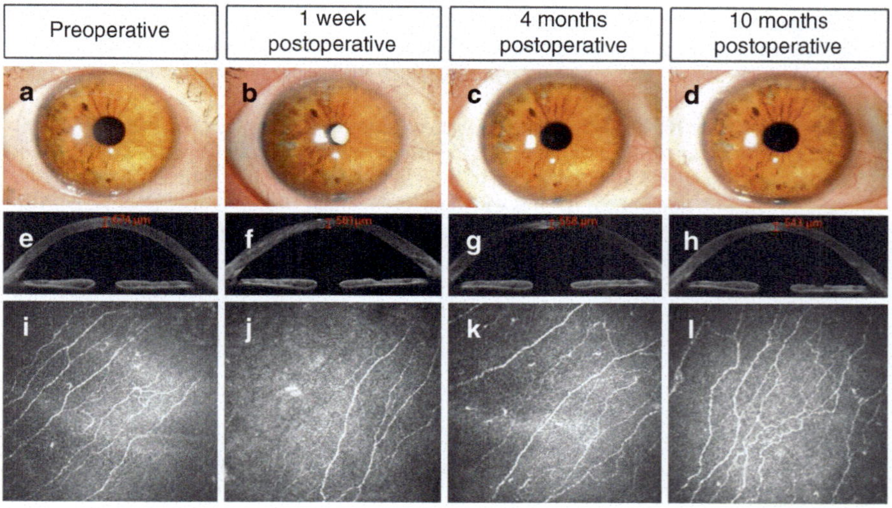

Fig. 15.3 Corneal nerve alterations following DMEK. (**a**–**d**) Anterior segment photographies. (**e**–**h**) Anterior segement optical coherence tomography and (**i**–**l**) CLSM imaging of subbasal nerve plexus demonstrates reduction of nerve length, number, and branches at 1 week after surgery which fully recover at 4 and 10 months post surgery (From Bucher et al. [32], reprint with kind permission)

and hypotheses exist that could explain reduced rejection rates in DMEK and less severe immune responses in DSAEK that imply potential benefit of prolonged topical steroids. In the future, additional basic immunological and clinical studies together with novel imaging technologies will enable earlier and more accurate diagnosis of graft rejection. These approaches will allow differentiation of nonimmunological graft failures and more appropriate application of immunosuppressive therapy. The role of DED in the context of posterior lamellar keratoplasty needs to be elucidated and might have an influence on graft survival as demonstrated for PK.

References

1. Melles GR, Ong TS, Ververs B, van der Wees J. Descemet membrane endothelial keratoplasty (DMEK). Cornea. 2006;25(8):987–90. doi:10.1097/01.ico.0000248385.16896.34 [published Online First: Epub Date].
2. Maier P, Reinhard T, Cursiefen C. Descemet stripping endothelial keratoplasty–rapid recovery of visual acuity. Dtsch Arztebl Int. 2013;110(21):365–71. doi:10.3238/arztebl.2013.0365 [published Online First: Epub Date].
3. Tourtas T, Laaser K, Bachmann BO, Cursiefen C, Kruse FE. Descemet membrane endothelial keratoplasty versus descemet stripping automated endothelial keratoplasty. Am J Ophthalmol. 2012;153(6):1082–90 e2. doi:10.1016/j.ajo.2011.12.012 [published Online First: Epub Date].
4. Niederkorn JY. Corneal transplantation and immune privilege. Int Rev Immunol. 2013;32(1):57–67. doi:10.3109/08830185.2012.737877 [published Online First: Epub Date].
5. Bock F, Maruyama K, Regenfuss B, et al. Novel anti(lymph)angiogenic treatment strategies for corneal and ocular surface diseases. Prog Retin Eye Res. 2013;34:89–124. doi:10.1016/j.preteyeres.2013.01.001 [published Online First: Epub Date].

6. Bachmann B, Taylor RS, Cursiefen C. Corneal neovascularization as a risk factor for graft failure and rejection after keratoplasty: an evidence-based meta-analysis. Ophthalmology. 2010;117(7):1300–5 e7. doi:10.1016/j.ophtha.2010.01.039 [published Online First: Epub Date].
7. Nguyen NX, Seitz B, Martus P, Langenbucher A, Cursiefen C. Long-term topical steroid treatment improves graft survival following normal-risk penetrating keratoplasty. Am J Ophthalmol. 2007;144(2):318–9. doi:10.1016/j.ajo.2007.03.028 [published Online First: Epub Date].
8. Steven P, Hos D, Heindl LM, Bock F, Cursiefen C. [Immune reactions after DMEK, DSAEK and DALK]. Klin Monbl Augenheilkd. 2013;230(5):494–9. doi:10.1055/s-0032-1328257 [published Online First: Epub Date].
9. Price MO, Jordan CS, Moore G, Price Jr FW. Graft rejection episodes after Descemet stripping with endothelial keratoplasty: part two: the statistical analysis of probability and risk factors. Br J Ophthalmol. 2009;93(3):391–5. doi:10.1136/bjo.2008.140038 [published Online First: Epub Date].
10. Yamagami S, Amano S. Role of resident corneal leukocytes and draining cervical lymph nodes in corneal allograft rejection. Cornea. 2003;22(7 Suppl):S61–5.
11. Dapena I, Ham L, Netukova M, van der Wees J, Melles GR. Incidence of early allograft rejection after Descemet membrane endothelial keratoplasty. Cornea. 2011;30(12):1341–5. doi:10.1097/ICO.0b013e31820d8540 [published Online First: Epub Date].
12. Hori J, Streilein JW. Survival in high-risk eyes of epithelium-deprived orthotopic corneal allografts reconstituted in vitro with syngeneic epithelium. Invest Ophthalmol Vis Sci. 2003;44(2):658–64.
13. Hori J, Joyce NC, Streilein JW. Immune privilege and immunogenicity reside among different layers of the mouse cornea. Invest Ophthalmol Vis Sci. 2000;41(10):3032–42.
14. Chaurasia S, Price Jr FW, Gunderson L, Price MO. Descemet's membrane endothelial keratoplasty: clinical results of single versus triple procedures (combined with cataract surgery). Ophthalmology. 2014;121(2):454–8. doi:10.1016/j.ophtha.2013.09.032 [published Online First: Epub Date].
15. Jordan CS, Price MO, Trespalacios R, Price Jr FW. Graft rejection episodes after Descemet stripping with endothelial keratoplasty: part one: clinical signs and symptoms. Br J Ophthalmol. 2009;93(3):387–90. doi:10.1136/bjo.2008.140020 [published Online First: Epub Date].
16. Saelens IE, Bleyen I, Bartels MC, Van Rij G. A posterior khodadoust line in a graft rejection episode after descemet stripping automated endothelial keratoplasty. Cornea. 2011;30(2):245–6. doi:10.1097/ICO.0b013e3181ec9080 [published Online First: Epub Date].
17. Hos D, Heindl LM, Bucher F, Cursiefen C. Evidence of donor corneal endothelial cell migration from immune reactions occurring after descemet membrane endothelial keratoplasty. Cornea. 2014;33(4):331–4. doi:10.1097/ICO.0000000000000054 [published Online First: Epub Date].
18. Khodadoust AA, Silverstein AM. Transplantation and rejection of individual cell layers of the cornea. Invest Ophthalmol. 1969;8(2):180–95.
19. Sloniecka M, Le Roux S, Zhou Q, Danielson P. Substance P enhances keratocyte migration and neutrophil recruitment through interleukin-8. Mol Pharmacol. 2016;89(2):215–25. doi:10.1124/mol.115.101014 [published Online First: Epub Date].
20. Paunicka KJ, Mellon J, Robertson D, Petroll M, Brown JR, Niederkorn JY. Severing corneal nerves in one eye induces sympathetic loss of immune privilege and promotes rejection of future corneal allografts placed in either eye. Am J Transplant Official J Am Soc Transplant Am Soc Transplant Surg. 2015;15(6):1490–501. doi:10.1111/ajt.13240 [published Online First: Epub Date].
21. Shimazaki J, Iseda A, Satake Y, Shimazaki-Den S. Efficacy and safety of long-term corticosteroid eye drops after penetrating keratoplasty: a prospective, randomized, clinical trial. Ophthalmology. 2012;119(4):668–73. doi:10.1016/j.ophtha.2011.10.016 [published Online First: Epub Date].
22. Ansari R, Myrtus C, Aherrahrou R, Erdmann J, Schweikard A, Huttmann G. Ultrahigh-resolution, high-speed spectral domain optical coherence phase microscopy. Opt Lett. 2014;39(1):45–7. doi:10.1364/OL.39.000045 [published Online First: Epub Date].

23. Gehlsen U, Szaszak M, Gebert A, Koop N, Huttmann G, Steven P. Non-invasive multi-dimensional two-photon microscopy enables optical fingerprinting (TPOF) of immune cells. J Biophotonics. 2015;8(6):466–79. doi:10.1002/jbio.201400036 [published Online First: Epub Date].
24. Steven P, Muller M, Koop N, Rose C, Huttmann G. Comparison of Cornea Module and DermaInspect for noninvasive imaging of ocular surface pathologies. J Biomed Opt. 2009;14(6):064040. doi:10.1117/1.3275475 [published Online First: Epub Date].
25. Monnereau C, Bruinsma M, Ham L, Baydoun L, Oellerich S, Melles GR. Endothelial cell changes as an indicator for upcoming allograft rejection following descemet membrane endothelial keratoplasty. Am J Ophthalmol. 2014;158(3):485–95. doi:10.1016/j.ajo.2014.05.030 [published Online First: Epub Date].
26. Stern ME, Gao J, Siemasko KF, Beuerman RW, Pflugfelder SC. The role of the lacrimal functional unit in the pathophysiology of dry eye. Exp Eye Res. 2004;78(3):409–16.
27. Wilson SE. Laser in situ keratomileusis-induced (presumed) neurotrophic epitheliopathy. Ophthalmology. 2001;108(6):1082–7.
28. Albietz JM, Lenton LM, McLennan SG. Chronic dry eye and regression after laser in situ keratomileusis for myopia. J Cataract Refract Surg. 2004;30(3):675–84. doi:10.1016/j.jcrs.2003.07.003 [published Online First: Epub Date].
29. Li XM, Hu L, Hu J, Wang W. Investigation of dry eye disease and analysis of the pathogenic factors in patients after cataract surgery. Cornea. 2007;26(9 Suppl 1):S16–20. doi:10.1097/ICO.0b013e31812f67ca [published Online First: Epub Date].
30. Belmonte C, Acosta MC, Gallar J. Neural basis of sensation in intact and injured corneas. Exp Eye Res. 2004;78(3):513–25.
31. Kuchle M, Cursiefen C, Nguyen NX, et al. Risk factors for corneal allograft rejection: intermediate results of a prospective normal-risk keratoplasty study. Graefes Arch Clin Exp Ophthalmol = Albrecht von Graefes Archiv fur klinische und experimentelle Ophthalmologie. 2002;240(4):580. doi:10.1007/s00417-002-0496-5 [published Online First: Epub Date].
32. Bucher F, Hos D, Matthaei M, Steven P, Cursiefen C, Heindl LM. Corneal nerve alterations after Descemet membrane endothelial keratoplasty: an in vivo confocal microscopy study. Cornea. 2014;33(11):1134–9. doi:10.1097/ICO.0000000000000250 [published Online First: Epub Date].

Chapter 16
Tissue Engineering of a Healthy Corneal Endothelium for FECD Patients

Isabelle Brunette and Stéphanie Proulx

16.1 Introduction

Corneal endothelial transplantation techniques have undergone significant evolution during the past decades, evolving from penetrating keratoplasty (PK) to deep lamellar endothelial keratoplasty (DLEK), to Descemet's stripping automated endothelial keratoplasty (DSAEK), and now to Descemet's membrane endothelial keratoplasty (DMEK). Each of these techniques has successively improved the functional outcome, resulting in negligible induced surface astigmatism, significantly better vision, and a decrease in the incidence of immune rejection [1].

Endothelial cell attrition and immune rejection, however, still figure among the list of potential complications following endothelial keratoplasty. Furthermore, human donor tissue shortage will be faced during the next decades. The cornea is one of the most transplanted tissues worldwide, with more than 53,000 corneal grafts performed in 2013 in North America alone [2]. It is however becoming difficult for eye banks worldwide to meet the increasing demand for transplantable tissue, which is in part due to population aging. According to the Eye Bank Association of America, the number of corneal transplantations in the United States has increased

I. Brunette (✉)
Centre de recherche de l'Hôpital Maisonneuve-Rosemont, Montréal, QC, Canada

Département d'ophtalmologie, Université de Montréal, Montréal, QC, Canada
e-mail: i.brunett@videotron.ca

S. Proulx
Centre de recherche du Centre hospitalier universitaire (CHU) de Québec – Université Laval, axe médecine régénératrice, Hôpital du Saint-Sacrement, Québec, QC, Canada

Département d'Ophtalmologie, Université Laval, Québec, QC, Canada

Centre de recherche en organogénèse expérimentale de l'Université Laval/LOEX, Québec, QC, Canada
e-mail: stephanie.proulx@fmed.ulaval.ca

C. Cursiefen, A.S. Jun (eds.), *Current Treatment Options for Fuchs Endothelial Dystrophy*, DOI 10.1007/978-3-319-43021-8_16

by more than 50 % since 2005, at a greater rate than the number of donors [2, 3]. Donor tissue shortage is therefore a growing concern globally [4–7], intensifying the need for alternatives to human donor corneas.

Tissue engineering might offer interesting alternatives for corneal endothelial replacement. The requirements for a tissue-engineered endothelium destined for transplantation should be at least the same as for standard eye bank native donor corneas. The ideal corneal endothelial substitute would allow safe replacement of the diseased corneal endothelium, without risk of disease transmission from the donor or risk of immune rejection. It would be highly cellular to compensate for the important cell loss known to occur after transplantation [8, 9]. The ideal substitute would be delivered on a biocompatible carrier, in a format suitable for the surgical techniques currently available for transplantation. It would allow for full and long-lasting rehabilitation of the corneal optical function and should be affordable and accessible within a reasonable time frame. A tissue engineering corneal endothelium could potentially fit these requirements.

In this chapter, we will review how tissue engineering currently allows to produce a healthy corneal endothelium from the normal corneal endothelial cells of a human donor. We will see how this technology could be used for allogeneic and/or autologous transplantation and how it could potentially be applied to patients affected by FECD. And finally, we will explain how tissue engineering can allow to develop promising experimental models of FECD in order to better understand the pathophysiology of this disease and develop new therapeutic alternatives.

16.2 Tissue Engineering of a Corneal Endothelium from Healthy Corneal Endothelial Cells

16.2.1 Postnatal Corneal Endothelial Cells

Corneal endothelial cells are non-mitotic in vivo. However, they retain proliferative capacity in vitro when cultured in the presence of serum and growth factors (media supplementation reviewed in [10, 11]). The number of passages they can undergo is limited. From our own experience and that of others [10, 12, 13], corneal endothelial cells generally retain their endothelial morphology up to the third passage (P3); after which, they either become senescent or transform into elongated fibroblast-like cells that have lost contact inhibition. The Descemet's membranes of two corneas of an adult donor usually yield up to 1 million cells from near-confluent P0 cultures. A 1:3 cell expansion can generate 3 million cells at P1, 9 million cells at P2, and 27 million cells at P3. If an endothelium is engineered using an initial cell density of 3,000 cells/mm^2 seeded on an 11 mm diameter substrate (thus requiring 285,000 cells/engineered endothelium), cell expansion from a single donor could treat up to 94 eyes. With a small improvement in culture conditions and if cells are used at the fourth passage, this number may increase to 284 eyes.

Not all donor corneas are equal in their ability to generate a culture of cuboidal endothelial cells. Using central Descemet's membranes, Zaniolo and colleagues [13] reported that 58 % of healthy corneas generated a culture, of which 43 % displayed cuboidal endothelial morphology. Recently, a paper reported an overall culture success of 32 % [12]. Successful samples were defined as having high cell adherence after isolation at P0 and cuboidal endothelial morphology at P1. Many variables can influence culture success, such as donor age, postmortem delay, isolation method, and culture conditions. Young donor age positively predicts the success of starting a culture of cells with an endothelial phenotype [12, 13]. The importance of culture conditions on the maintenance of a functional endothelial phenotype will be discussed in Sect. 16.2.3.

16.2.2 Corneal Endothelial Stem/Progenitor Cells

Stem cells are an interesting source of cells for tissue engineering because of their highly proliferative potential. The three main stem cell types are the embryonic stem (ES) cells, the induced pluripotent stem (iPS) cells, and the adult stem cells. Adult stem cells have been identified in many tissues of the adult body. They are responsible for the continual regeneration of tissues throughout life. The corneal epithelium, for instance, is maintained by a population of limbal stem cells. Amplification of these cells in vitro was shown to be a safe and effective source of epithelial cells for the treatment of patients suffering from limbal stem cell deficiency following a chemical burn [14]. One of the major advantages of using adult stem/progenitor cells over ES or iPS cells is that they are already committed to a cell lineage and are therefore more likely to differentiate into their tissue of origin. Contrary to ES or iPS cells, adult stem/progenitor cells do not have a tendency to produce multiple cell lineages both in vitro and in vivo.

The existence of corneal endothelial stem/progenitor cells has long been questioned, since the corneal endothelium is not continuously regenerating in vivo. There is growing evidence demonstrating the presence of corneal endothelial progenitor cells. Using a panel of stem cell markers, McGowan et al. [15] identified stem cells at the level of the trabecular meshwork and within the transitional zone between the trabecular meshwork and the corneal endothelial periphery (Fig. 16.1).

Following injury to the corneal endothelium, the authors showed activation of additional stem cell markers, suggesting that these stem cells could initiate an endothelial wound repair process. These progenitor/stem cells, however, were never isolated for culture purposes, the major difficulty being that the only successful method presently used to isolate corneal endothelial cells is by peeling Descemet's membrane (see Sect. 16.2.3). Stem cells peripheral to Descemet's membrane are thus not isolated.

The presence of slow-cycling cells (a characteristic of stem cells) and of cells expressing progenitor markers (such as nestin, leucine-rich repeat-containing G-protein-coupled receptor 5, Sox9, and nerve growth factor receptor p75) was

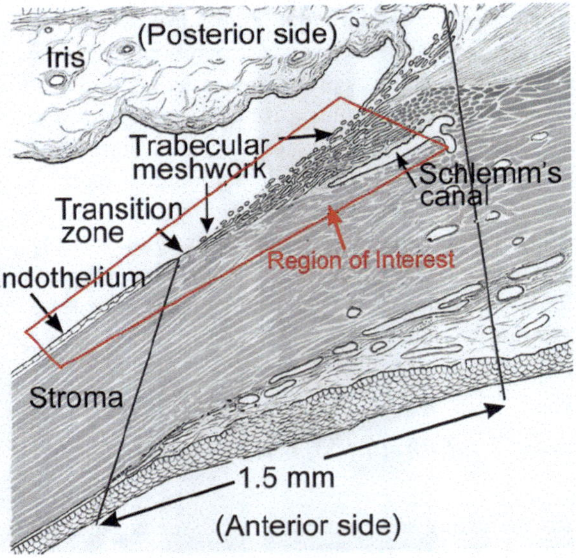

Fig. 16.1 Transverse diagram of the human cornea and limbus. The diagram illustrates the anatomic relationships of the tissues and regions discussed in McGowan's study (*outlined in red*). The posterior limbus is the region herein identified between the *solid vertical lines* and consists of the transition zone, the trabecular meshwork, and Schlemm's canal. The corneal endothelium is not part of the limbus (Reprinted from McGowan et al. [15]. Adapted from Histology of the Human Eye, Hogan, Alvarado, Weddell, The Limbus, p.113, 1971, with permission from Elsevier)

identified in the mature endothelium of murine eyes [16]. These cells were exclusively located at the extreme periphery of the endothelium, close to the transitional zone.

An efficient method to culture stem cells in vitro is by using the sphere-forming assay. This method is based on the principle that stem cells in suspension will continue to proliferate in vitro, forming spheres, contrary to differentiated cells that need adhesion to survive. Sphere-forming assays have been used to isolate human corneal endothelial progenitor cells [17–19]. A higher number of spheres were formed using cells from the periphery [18]. Some of the peripheral cells isolated using a sphere-forming assay expressed the stem cell marker nestin [17]. The number of cells expressing the stem cell-related markers GFAP, OCT3/OCT4, and nestin has been reported to be influenced by the composition of the cell culture media [17]. Progenitor cells have also been reported to be present at the center of Descemet's membrane. Using an approach different than the sphere-forming assay, Hara et al. showed that cells isolated from the periphery and from the center had the same colony-forming efficiency, suggesting that progenitor cells are present throughout the human corneal endothelium. This result is consistent with the presence of p75NTR-expressing cells both at the center and the periphery [20].

16.2.3 Cell Isolation and Growth of Corneal Endothelial Cells

A common strategy for the isolation of corneal endothelial cells consists of peeling off the Descemet's membrane (with the endothelial cells attached) and then to detach the cells using ethylenediaminetetraacetic acid (EDTA) [21] or enzymes such as collagenase [22, 23], trypsin [19], or dispase [24]. Alternatively, cells can grow out of Descemet's membrane using an explant method [25]. The comparison of different isolation methods showed that the explant and the collagenase (0.1 or 0.2 % collagenase II) methods were more successful in generating cultures [12]. Success rates were in the order of 30 % using the explant method, 32 % using 0.1 % collagenase, and 37 % using 0.2 % collagenase, compared to 8 % with the other methods (trypsin/EDTA or 0.1 % dispase II). These observations were consistent with another study in which collagenase A was better than trypsin for the isolation of bovine corneal endothelial cells [26].

Once the P0 cells have reached confluence, cell dissociation reagents (such as trypsin/EDTA) are used to separate the cells from the dish and from each other, which allows to seed them in new cell culture dishes, usually at a 1:3 ratio. The disruption of intercellular junctions that unavoidably happens when using trypsin/EDTA may activate canonical Wnt signaling and promote endothelial-to-mesenchymal transition (EndMT) [27]. Success in avoiding EndMT of cultured corneal endothelial cells could reside in the development of culture conditions in which confluence and gain of apical–basal polarity is rapidly achieved. For example, increasing cell seeding density has been shown to diminish the occurrence of fibroblastic transformation within human corneal endothelial cell culture [28]. The maintenance of a functional endothelial phenotype throughout cell expansion by finding ways to prevent EndMT is currently a research area of high interest [29]. Conditioned media obtained by NIH-3T3 cells or human bone marrow-derived mesenchymal stem cells (MSC) have been shown to help maintain a corneal endothelial phenotype during in vitro expansion [30]. The media conditioned by MSC was superior to the 3T3-conditioned media in terms of increasing proliferation and motility. The authors showed that the effect on proliferation was maximal using 10 % MSC-conditioned media [30]. SB431542, a selective inhibitor of the transforming growth factor-beta (TGF-ß) receptor, has also been shown to counteract the appearance of a fibroblastic phenotype [31]. Cells cultured in the presence of SB431542 generated a contact-inhibited monolayer of polygonal corneal endothelial cells that maintained the expression of function-related proteins [31].

Recently, a novel dual media culture approach has been proposed for the in vitro expansion of corneal endothelial cells. This method using two different culture media, one for proliferation and one for maintenance once cells reach 80–90 % confluence, showed consistent third-passage corneal endothelial cells with homogenous polygonal morphology. Cells expressed high levels of the sodium–potassium pump Na^+/K^+-ATPase, ZO-1, glypican-4, and CD200 [32]. The authors also combined this dual media approach with the use of 10 μM selective Rho-associated kinase (ROCK) inhibitor, Y-27632 [33]. They showed increased cell attachment of

P0 cells when using Y-27632. Also, in the presence of Y-27632, P0 cells retained a smaller cell size while maintaining their polygonal morphology. Finally, the Y-27632 treatment increased cell proliferation, with a 1–6 % overall increase for the 24-h 5-ethynyl-2'-deoxyuridine incorporation assay [33].

16.2.4 Determination of Cell Quality Prior to Tissue Engineering

In the absence of specific markers, the discrimination of cultured corneal endothelial cells from possible keratocyte/corneal stromal fibroblast contaminants is presently performed on the basis of cell morphology (polygonal cells at post-confluence) and the expression of ZO-1 and Na^+/K^+-ATPase proteins. Other corneal endothelial cell markers that can be used to discriminate between corneal stromal and endothelial cells include glypican-4, CD200, S100A4, S100A6, stress-induced protein immediate early response 3 (IER3), CD166, peroxiredoxin-6, and integrin subunit alpha 3 [34–37]. Cell quality should also be assessed prior to seeding, based on cell size, trans-endothelial resistance, and permeability.

16.2.4.1 Cell Size

Eye banks will only consider donor corneas for transplantation if the endothelial cell density is at least 2,000 cells/mm^2 [38, 39]. Therefore, engineering an endothelium with a high cell density is of high importance. Unfortunately, corneal endothelial cell size increases following successive passages. Different approaches have been proposed in order to generate an endothelium of high cell density, including selecting the smallest cells by density-gradient centrifugation [40]. The authors hypothesized that they could separate the enlarged and flattened cells from the smaller more potent cells according to their specific gravity using density-gradient centrifugation. They showed that the smallest cells from the pellet generated a mean cell density of 1,584 cells/mm^2, while those of the supernatant yielded a mean cell density of 828 cells/mm^2 [40], indicating that this approach could be used to separate the small cells from a culture of cells of heterogeneous sizes. Finding culture conditions that could maintain the small endothelial cell size throughout cell expansion would be ideal. Further research is needed in order to address this point.

16.2.4.2 Trans-endothelial Resistance and Permeability

In the living eye, the corneal endothelium is a leaky selective barrier that allows the diffusion of nutrients from the aqueous humor toward the stroma to nourish the keratocytes while limiting the entrance of fluid in order to maintain corneal stromal deturgescence. In vitro, the barrier integrity of an endothelium formed from expanded corneal endothelial cells can be assessed using trans-endothelial electrical resistance (TER). Its paracellular permeability can be measured using diffusion of sodium fluorescein or FITC–dextran [41, 42]. For example, Singh et al. showed that bovine corneal endothelial cells grown at three different cell densities (<1000, 1000–1999, and >2000 cells/mm^2) had TER measurements of 14 ± 5, 13 ± 3, and 14 ± 4 Ωcm^2, respectively. They also observed high paracellular permeability for the lowest cell density [41]. Thus, prior to cell seeding on a carrier, a sample of cells can be used to measure the capacity of the expanded endothelial cells to form a leaky barrier in vitro, allowing to select the best populations for transplantation.

16.2.5 Carriers

A monolayer of human endothelial cells can be obtained in vitro with the proper culture conditions (reviewed in [43, 44]). However, a monolayer of endothelial cells is too fragile to be transplanted on its own. The cells need to be seeded on a carrier. The optimal carrier should be thin, flexible, transparent, and strong enough to be manipulated. It should allow the development of a fully functional endothelial phenotype and of interactions between stromal and endothelial cells. Different carriers have been proposed for the engineering of a posterior cornea using cultured cells (reviewed in [11, 45]).

16.2.5.1 Thin Membranes

Thin membranes of the thickness of a Descemet's membrane offer the advantage of being "ready to use" without additional tissue preparation or stromal dissection prior to grafting. However, they can be difficult to handle as carriers. Because they are usually more fragile than a native Descemet's membrane, each fold or stretch in the carrier damages the overlying endothelial cells. Scrolling can also be bothersome if a Descemet's membrane is used as a carrier. In the context of the growing experience with DMEK, however, corneal surgeons are now ready to replace the diseased corneal endothelium by a thin lamellar posterior donor consisting of a tissue-engineered endothelium reconstructed on a thin carrier.

Proposed thin membranes include gelatin membranes [46–48], hydrogel lenses [49, 50], vitrigel (collagen sheets) [51], cross-linked collagen [52–54], isolated Descemet's membrane [55], and amniotic membranes [24, 56].

A thin carrier can also be tissue engineered in vitro using the self-assembly approach. The technique is based on the capability of mesenchymal cells to secrete and deposit their own extracellular matrix in the presence of ascorbic acid [57, 58]. Corneal stromal fibroblasts produce a "living" corneal stromal substitute, in which cells are embedded in an extracellular matrix composed of collagen types I, V, VI, and XII, as well as lumican and decorin [59, 60]. Human corneal endothelial cells, seeded on top of this substitute, formed a uniform endothelial monolayer [60–62] with a cell density of 966 ± 242 cells/mm^2 [60]. This endothelium expressed both the Na^+/K^+-ATPase and the sodium/bicarbonate cotransporter Na^+/HCO_3^-. To test the biocompatibility of these stromal carriers, they were transplanted in vivo (without endothelial cells) in the corneal stroma of feline eyes. Four months after transplantation, the stromal substitutes were transparent, functional, and well tolerated by the eye. All grafts remained avascular, with no signs of immune rejection, despite only a short course of low-dose topical steroids. Furthermore, corneal sensitivity returned to preoperative levels [59].

16.2.5.2 Native Stromas

Fresh native corneas denuded of their endothelium have also been used as carriers for the reconstruction of a corneal endothelium [63–80]. Prolonged periods of culture, however, are not possible with fresh corneas, due to the contamination of the endothelial cell culture by the proliferating corneal epithelial cells. Eliminating the native cells from fresh corneas before engineering a new endothelium would prevent contamination. Different techniques of corneal devitalization or decellularization have been described (reviewed in [81]). An endothelium engineered using cells seeded on a decellularized native cornea has been reported [70, 82, 83]. A main advantage of using a native stroma as a carrier is that cells are seeded on a Descemet's membrane, which is their natural substrate. Proulx et al. reported that endothelial cells seeded on decellularized native stromas and cultured for 2 weeks formed a highly cellular monolayer of normal endothelial morphology [82]. Endothelial cells were well adhered to Descemet's membrane and expressed the function-related proteins ZO-1, Na^+/K^+-ATPase, and Na^+/HCO_3^- (Fig. 16.2). Mean endothelial cell counts were 2272 ± 344 cells/mm^2 using feline cells [82].

16.2.6 In Vivo Transplantation of a Tissue-Engineered Endothelium on a Carrier

In vivo outcomes of these engineered endothelia have been assessed [83, 84]. Results showed that cultured endothelial cells seeded on a devitalized stromal carrier can recover an active pump function, restore and maintain normal corneal thickness, and yield crystal clear corneal transparency during 7 days after transplantation in the living feline eye. The reconstructed endothelium had a normal morphology and ultrastructure and expressed the function-related proteins Na^+/K^+-ATPase $\alpha 1$, Na^+/HCO_3^-, and ZO-1.

16.2.7 Injection of Corneal Endothelial Cells in the Anterior Chamber Without a Carrier

Cell injection in the anterior chamber as a means to replace the corneal endothelium is an old concept that has recently regained interest. Cell adhesion to the Descemet's membrane represents the first challenge and different strategies have been proposed

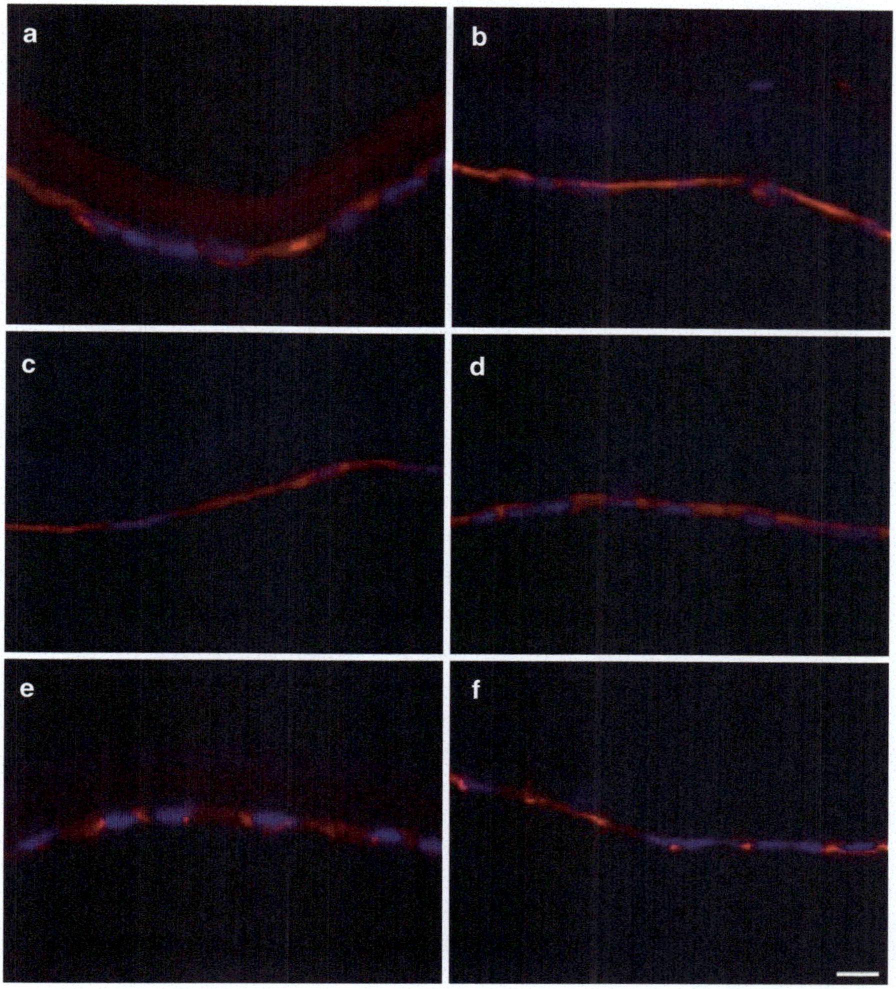

Fig. 16.2 Function-related protein expression in a feline endothelium engineered on a devitalized cornea. Immunofluorescence labeling showing that the engineered feline endothelium (**a**, **c**, **e**) and the native feline endothelium (**b**, **d**, **f**) expressed Na^{+}/HCO_3^{-} (**a**, **b**), Na^{+}/K^{+}-ATPase (**c**, **d**) and ZO-1 (**e**, **f**). Scale bar, 10 μm (Figure from Proulx et al. [82], with permission from Mary Ann Liebert)

to address it. Maintenance of an eye-down prone position, allowing cells to reach Descemet's membrane by gravity, has been shown to be helpful in reforming an endothelium in vivo, especially when the injected cells were precursors obtained by sphere-forming assay [85, 86]. Using a rabbit endothelial deficiency model, the authors showed that corneal transparency was restored when animals were kept in prone position for at least 6 h, contrary to the group positioned for only 1 h, which displayed focal edema and incomplete coverage of the endothelial defects in three out of six rabbits [85].

Another proposed strategy consists of the use of an extraocular magnetic field to attract injected endothelial cells loaded with magnetic particles such as iron [87, 88], magnetite oxide superparamagnetic microspheres [89], or superparamagnetic nanoparticles [90] toward the Descemet's membrane.

Finally, the addition of the selective ROCK inhibitor Y-27632 has been shown to increase the adherence of corneal endothelial cells to plastic tissue culture plates in vitro [33, 91, 92] and to the Descemet's membrane after injection in vivo [93]. The injection of cells and ROCK inhibitor Y-27632 in rabbit and monkey eyes resulted in the recovery of a transparent cornea with a monolayer of hexagonal endothelial cells expressing Na^+/K^+-ATPase and ZO-1 [40, 93]. In their recent paper, Koizumi's group [40] mentioned that corneal endothelial cell injections, combined with ROCK inhibitor, are presently being performed in bullous keratopathy patients, a first-in-man clinical trial at the Kyoto Prefectural University of Medicine. Clinicians around the world are anticipating the results of this trial, as it will confirm the feasibility of cell injection for the treatment of corneal endotheliopathies in human subjects.

16.3 Tissue Engineering of a Corneal Endothelium from FECD Corneal Endothelial Cells

16.3.1 FECD Endothelial Cell Morphology in Culture

The culture of FECD cells has initially been reported after transduction with the human papilloma virus E6 and E7 oncogenes [94]. Zaniolo et al. then showed that FECD endothelial cells can be successfully isolated and cultured without transduction, with the same isolation and culture conditions used for healthy cells [13]. The Descemet's membrane and endothelium specimens collected from 29 consenting patients having undergone Descemet's stripping automated endothelial keratoplasty (DSAEK) were used for this study. Of these 29 specimens, 18 successfully initiated a culture, corresponding to a 62 % success rate. Cell counts between 8.0×10^3 and 1.8×10^5 cells (mean ± SD, $9.0 \times 10^4 \pm 4.5 \times 10^4$) were obtained. Of these 18 cultures, 12 had an endothelial rounded, slightly elongated cell morphology and six had more of a fibroblastic-like morphology (thin and very elongated cells) (Fig. 16.3). Cultures initially showing an endothelial morphology maintained it after subsequent passages (Fig. 16.3). These differences in cell morphology were also observed with the normal human corneal endothelial cell cultures.

16.3.2 Conditions Favorable to FECD Cell Growth

This group also identified factors favoring the success of FECD cell culture [13]. Younger patient's age was the leading factor, as generally accepted for primary cell culture [12, 21, 95–97]. All specimens from patients aged 60 years or less successfully started a culture of endothelial morphology, while the success rate for patients

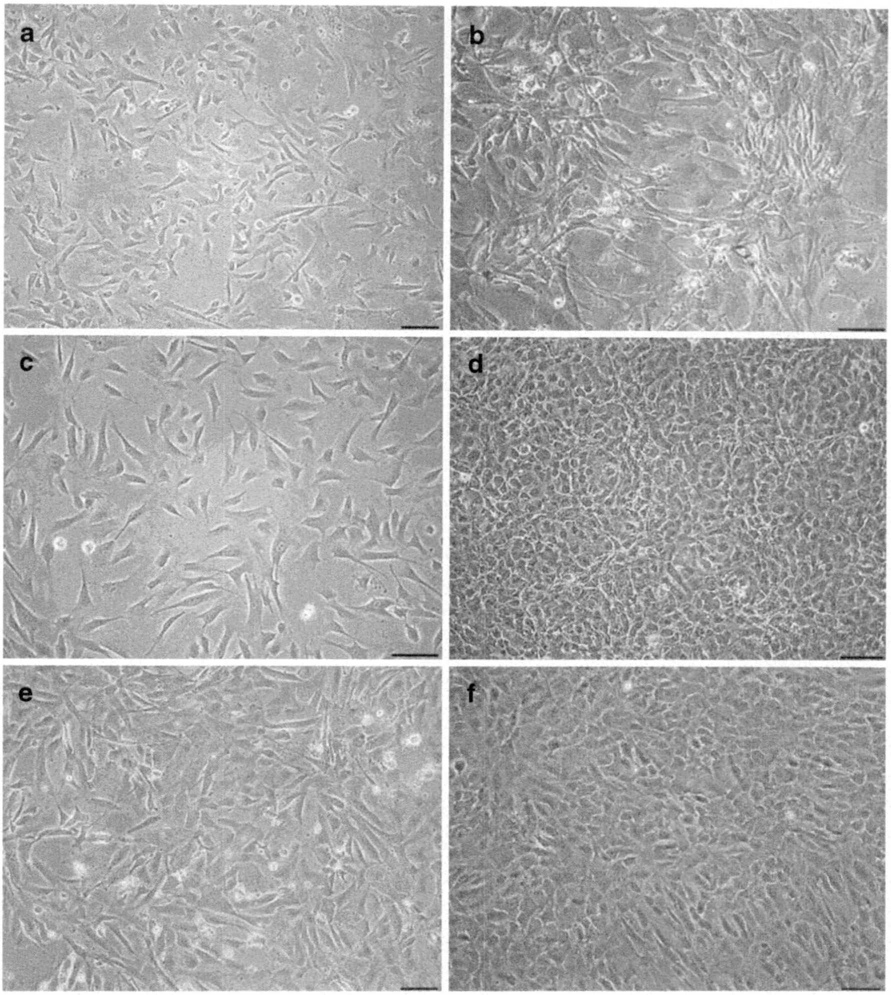

Fig. 16.3 Morphology of FECD and healthy corneal endothelial cells in culture. (**a–d**) FECD cells. (**e–f**) Healthy human cells. (**a**) Endothelial-like morphology of a primary FECD (P0) culture. (**b**) Mixed morphology of FECD corneal endothelial cells containing many thin and elongated cells growing on top of each other (fibroblast-like morphology) of another primary (P0) culture. (**c**) Second-passage FECD cells of the population shown in A. (**d**) Confluent third-passage FECD cells of the same population shown in (**a**) and (**c**). The culture formed a monolayer of polygonal cells. (**e**) Subconfluent culture of normal corneal endothelial cells in P0. (**f**) Confluent third-passage culture of healthy corneal endothelial cells. Scale bars, 100 μm (Reprinted from Experimental Eye Research, Zaniolo et al. [13], with permission from Elsevier)

aged 80 years and over was very low, with only one of six specimens generating a culture and none with an endothelial morphology. A negative correlation was found between age and the number of days to confluence in the group displaying an endothelial morphology.

The absence of a fibrillar layer covering the posterior aspect of the Descemet's membrane was also associated with a greater culture success rate. Among the 13 Descemet's membranes studied, none of specimens that allowed the establishment of a culture with an endothelial cell morphology had a fibrillar layer. The endothelial cells isolated from Descemet's membranes covered with a fibrillar layer ($n=6$) either did not generate a culture ($n=4$) or generated one with fibroblastic-like cell morphology ($n=2$).

The corneal edema, presence of guttae, pigmentation of the endothelium, specimen size, and donor gender were not predictive factors for culture success.

16.3.3 Short-Term In Vivo Functionality of a Tissue-Engineered Corneal Endothelium Using FECD Cells

Haydari et al. [84] were the first study to demonstrate that the diseased endothelial cells of clinically decompensated FECD corneas, when cultured and seeded on a devitalized stromal carrier, can recover active pump function and restore and maintain corneal transparency for 7 days after transplantation in the living feline eye. Fifteen healthy animals underwent full-thickness corneal transplantation, with a corneal endothelium tissue engineered from human FECD ($n=7$) or healthy ($n=2$) endothelial cells. Controls received a native full-thickness corneal graft ($n=2$) or a stromal carrier only (no endothelial cells; $n=4$). Seven days after transplantation, six of the seven tissue-engineered FECD grafts, all tissue-engineered healthy grafts, and all healthy native grafts were clear, while all carriers-only grafts were opaque. Tissue-engineered FECD grafts progressively became thinner, with a mean central thickness of 772 ± 102 μm (659–1023 μm) and an average endothelial cell count of 966 ± 165 cells/mm^2 on postoperative day 7; after which they were harvested for histopathology analysis. Transmission electron microscopy showed subendothelial loose fibrillar material deposition in all tissue-engineered FECD grafts, but no structures suggestive of guttae were observed. The tissue-engineered endothelium expressed Na^+/K^+-ATPase and $Na^+/HCO3^-$, however, with less intensity than in the normal native grafts.

16.3.3.1 Partial Rehabilitation

The major finding of this paper was that diseased endothelial cells of clinically decompensated FECD corneas were able to recover active pump function in culture and restore corneal transparency for 7 days after transplantation in the living eye. The endothelium tissue engineered from FECD cells performed better in the animal eye than the diseased FECD endothelium in the patient's eye. Proposed hypotheses for this partial rehabilitation include the beneficial effect of the culture conditions and/or the natural selection of the healthiest cells in culture. Removal of the diseased thickened Descemet's membrane may also have played a role in the recovery of these endothelial cells.

The partial recovery of these end-stage FECD endothelial cells harvested from the central and most diseased part of the cornea and the demonstration of their in vivo functionality open the door to a new horizon. Further studies are needed to evaluate if these first results can eventually lead to therapeutic strategies capable of delaying the course of the disease in FECD patients.

16.3.3.2 Rapidly Evolving FECD Progression

Despite this functional improvement, however, once transplanted back to a native living environment, the tissue-engineered FECD corneas rapidly developed a combination of signs typical of Fuchs dystrophy, including corneal edema, low endothelial cell counts, incomplete cell–cell attachments, intracytoplasmic filaments, and the accelerated and excessive production of Descemet's membrane-like loose fibrillar subendothelial material. These are the characteristics of a functional experimental model for FECD.

16.4 New Model for Studying FECD

The experimental short-term living model developed by Haydari et al., based on the culture, partial rehabilitation, and transplantation in the living eye of FECD corneal endothelial cells, offers several advantages: (1) It allows the rapid appearance of FECD signs over a 7-day period; (2) it offers quantifiable clinical and histopathological parameters for the characterization of endothelial function and structure; (3) it is polyvalent, in that it is not limited to one specific FECD mutation or cell line; (4) it allows selective assessment of FECD endothelial cells in the absence of diseased Descemet's membrane and guttae; (5) it allows for correlations between in vitro and in vivo endothelial cell behavior; (6) it was developed in the feline eye, which is similar to the human eye in several aspects (nonreplicating endothelial cells in vivo [98], comparable endothelial cell density [99–101], corneal thickness, a large corneal diameter that permits full-size grafts, using the same surgical and diagnostic techniques as for human subjects); and, finally, (7) short-term human-to-cat corneal xenografts are well tolerated [102, 103]. Additional improvements would include a longer follow-up, which in the context of xenografts would necessitate immunosuppression of the host.

This model opens the way to new research opportunities previously inaccessible through observations of end-stage surgical specimens harvested at the time of corneal transplantation, which were traditionally used to document this disease. This living model offers the opportunity of exploring the pathophysiology and of testing new therapeutic approaches at different stages of the disease.

16.5 The Future of Tissue Engineering for the Treatment of FECD

The concept of tissue engineering of a corneal endothelium for allogeneic transplantation is now conceivable, and significant work has been done in this direction during the past decades. The remaining challenges to be met include the capacity of generating highly cellular endothelia (with cell densities at least equal or superior to those currently obtained with human donor corneas), the choice of the ideal carrier, and the long-term in vivo assessment.

Autologous endothelial transplantation would eliminate the risk for immune rejection. Isolation of a sufficient number of healthy cells from the patient to initiate the culture would however be an additional challenge.

The fact that a subset of FECD endothelial cells were shown to have retained the potential of regenerating a functional endothelium represents a new avenue to be explored. Regeneration of an autologous endothelium in culture prior to its reimplantation in the host, with or without a carrier, would constitute an interesting option. A better understanding of the mechanisms resulting in the rehabilitation of the FECD endothelium in culture might also one day allow to investigate in vivo applications, with the aim of treating at least partially or delaying corneal endothelial failure in FECD eyes. Such nonsurgical therapeutic modalities would represent an exciting additional step toward improved management of this disease.

References

1. Anshu A, Price MO, Price Jr FW. Risk of corneal transplant rejection significantly reduced with Descemet's membrane endothelial keratoplasty. Ophthalmology. 2012;119:536–40.
2. Eye Bank Association of America, 2014. 2013 Eye Banking Statistical Report. Washington D.C.
3. Eye Bank Association of America, 2010. 2009 Eye Banking Statistical Report. Washington D.C.
4. Mack RJ, Mason P, Mathers WD. Obstacles to donor eye procurement and their solutions at the University of Iowa. Cornea. 1995;14:249–52.
5. Poinard C, Tuppin P, Loty B, Delbosc B. The French national waiting list for keratoplasty created in 1999: patient registration, indications, characteristics, and turnover. J Fr Ophtalmol. 2003;26:911–9.
6. Rasouli M, Caraiscos VB, Slomovic AR. Efficacy of routine notification and request on reducing corneal transplantation wait times in Canada. Can J Ophthalmol. 2009;44:31–5.
7. Reinhard T, Bohringer D, Bogen A, Sundmacher R. The transplantation law: a chance to overcome the shortage of corneal grafts in germany? Transplant Proc. 2002;34:1322–4.
8. Price MO, Giebel AW, Fairchild KM, Price Jr FW. Descemet's membrane endothelial keratoplasty: prospective multicenter study of visual and refractive outcomes and endothelial survival. Ophthalmology. 2009;116:2361–8.
9. Price MO, Gorovoy M, Benetz BA, Price Jr FW, Menegay HJ, Debanne SM, Lass JH. Descemet's stripping automated endothelial keratoplasty outcomes compared with penetrating keratoplasty from the Cornea Donor Study. Ophthalmology. 2010;117:438–44.
10. Peh GS, Toh KP, Wu FY, Tan DT, Mehta JS. Cultivation of human corneal endothelial cells isolated from paired donor corneas. PLoS One. 2011;6:e28310.
11. Proulx S, Brunette I. Methods being developed for preparation, delivery and transplantation of a tissue-engineered corneal endothelium. Exp Eye Res. 2012;95:68–75.

12. Choi JS, Kim EY, Kim MJ, Khan FA, Giegengack M, D'Agostino Jr R, Criswell T, Khang G, Soker S. Factors affecting successful isolation of human corneal endothelial cells for clinical use. Cell Transplant. 2014;23:845–54.
13. Zaniolo K, Bostan C, Rochette Drouin O, Deschambeault A, Perron MC, Brunette I, Proulx S. Culture of human corneal endothelial cells isolated from corneas with Fuchs endothelial corneal dystrophy. Exp Eye Res. 2012;94:22–31.
14. Pellegrini G, Rama P, De Luca M. Vision from the right stem. Trends Mol Med. 2011;17:1–7.
15. McGowan SL, Edelhauser HF, Pfister RR, Whikehart DR. Stem cell markers in the human posterior limbus and corneal endothelium of unwounded and wounded corneas. Mol Vis. 2007;13:1984–2000.
16. Espana EM, Sun M, Birk DE. Existence of corneal endothelial slow-cycling cells. Invest Ophthalmol Vis Sci. 2015;56:3827–37.
17. Noh JW, Kim JJ, Hyon JY, Chung ES, Chung TY, Yi K, Wee WR, Shin YJ. Stemness characteristics of human corneal endothelial cells cultured in various media. Eye Contact Lens. 2015;41:190–6.
18. Yamagami S, Yokoo S, Mimura T, Takato T, Araie M, Amano S. Distribution of precursors in human corneal stromal cells and endothelial cells. Ophthalmology. 2007;114:433–9.
19. Yokoo S, Yamagami S, Yanagi Y, Uchida S, Mimura T, Usui T, Amano S. Human corneal endothelial cell precursors isolated by sphere-forming assay. Invest Ophthalmol Vis Sci. 2005;46:1626–31.
20. Hara S, Hayashi R, Soma T, Kageyama T, Duncan T, Tsujikawa M, Nishida K. Identification and potential application of human corneal endothelial progenitor cells. Stem Cells Dev. 2014;23:2190–201.
21. Zhu C, Joyce NC. Proliferative response of corneal endothelial cells from young and older donors. Invest Ophthalmol Vis Sci. 2004;45:1743–51.
22. Li W, Sabater AL, Chen YT, Hayashida Y, Chen SY, He H, Tseng SC. A novel method of isolation, preservation, and expansion of human corneal endothelial cells. Invest Ophthalmol Vis Sci. 2007;48:614–20.
23. Zhu YT, Hayashida Y, Kheirkhah A, He H, Chen SY, Tseng SC. Characterization and comparison of intercellular adherent junctions expressed by human corneal endothelial cells in vivo and in vitro. Invest Ophthalmol Vis Sci. 2008;49:3879–86.
24. Ishino Y, Sano Y, Nakamura T, Connon CJ, Rigby H, Fullwood NJ, Kinoshita S. Amniotic membrane as a carrier for cultivated human corneal endothelial cell transplantation. Invest Ophthalmol Vis Sci. 2004;45:800–6.
25. Walshe J, Harkin DG. Serial explant culture provides novel insights into the potential location and phenotype of corneal endothelial progenitor cells. Exp Eye Res. 2014;127:9–13.
26. Su CC, Chen CW, Ho WT, Hu FR, Lee SH, Wang IJ. Phenotypes of trypsin- and collagenase-prepared bovine corneal endothelial cells in the presence of a selective Rho kinase inhibitor, Y-27632. Mol Vis. 2015;21:633–43.
27. Zhu YT, Chen HC, Chen SY, Tseng SC. Nuclear p120 catenin unlocks mitotic block of contact-inhibited human corneal endothelial monolayers without disrupting adherent junctions. J Cell Sci. 2012;125:3636–48.
28. Peh GS, Toh KP, Ang HP, Seah XY, George BL, Mehta JS. Optimization of human corneal endothelial cell culture: density dependency of successful cultures in vitro. BMC Res Notes. 2013;6:176.
29. Roy O, Leclerc VB, Bourget JM, Theriault M, Proulx S. Understanding the process of corneal endothelial morphological change in vitro. Invest Ophthalmol Vis Sci. 2015;56:1228–37.
30. Nakahara M, Okumura N, Kay EP, Hagiya M, Imagawa K, Hosoda Y, Kinoshita S, Koizumi N. Corneal endothelial expansion promoted by human bone marrow mesenchymal stem cell-derived conditioned medium. PLoS One. 2013;8:e69009.
31. Okumura N, Kay EP, Nakahara M, Hamuro J, Kinoshita S, Koizumi N. Inhibition of TGF-beta signaling enables human corneal endothelial cell expansion in vitro for use in regenerative medicine. PLoS One. 2013;8:e58000.
32. Peh GS, Chng Z, Ang HP, Cheng TY, Adnan K, Seah XY, George BL, Toh KP, Tan DT, Yam GH, Colman A, Mehta JS. Propagation of human corneal endothelial cells: a novel dual media approach. Cell Transplant. 2015;24:287–304.

33. Peh GS, Adnan K, George BL, Ang HP, Seah XY, Tan DT, Mehta JS. The effects of Rho-associated kinase inhibitor Y-27632 on primary human corneal endothelial cells propagated using a dual media approach. Sci Rep. 2015;5:9167.
34. Chen Y, Huang K, Nakatsu MN, Xue Z, Deng SX, Fan G. Identification of novel molecular markers through transcriptomic analysis in human fetal and adult corneal endothelial cells. Hum Mol Genet. 2013;22:1271–9.
35. Cheong YK, Ngoh ZX, Peh GS, Ang HP, Seah XY, Chng Z, Colman A, Mehta JS, Sun W. Identification of cell surface markers glypican-4 and CD200 that differentiate human corneal endothelium from stromal fibroblasts. Invest Ophthalmol Vis Sci. 2013;54:4538–47.
36. Ding V, Chin A, Peh G, Mehta JS, Choo A. Generation of novel monoclonal antibodies for the enrichment and characterization of human corneal endothelial cells (hCENC) necessary for the treatment of corneal endothelial blindness. MAbs. 2014;6:1439–52.
37. Yamaguchi M, Shima N, Kimoto M, Ebihara N, Murakami A, Yamagami S. Markers for distinguishing cultured human corneal endothelial cells from corneal stromal myofibroblasts. Curr Eye Res. 2015;40:1211–7.
38. Armitage WJ, Dick AD, Bourne WM. Predicting endothelial cell loss and long-term corneal graft survival. Invest Ophthalmol Vis Sci. 2003;44:3326–31.
39. Ehlers N. Corneal banking and grafting: the background to the Danish Eye Bank System, where corneas await their patients. Acta Ophthalmol Scand. 2002;80:572–8.
40. Okumura N, Kusakabe A, Hirano H, Inoue R, Okazaki Y, Nakano S, Kinoshita S, Koizumi N. Density-gradient centrifugation enables the purification of cultured corneal endothelial cells for cell therapy by eliminating senescent cells. Sci Rep. 2015;5:15005.
41. Singh JS, Haroldson TA, Patel SP. Characteristics of the low density corneal endothelial monolayer. Exp Eye Res. 2013;115:239–45.
42. Srinivas SP. Dynamic regulation of barrier integrity of the corneal endothelium. Optom Vis Sci. 2010;87:E239–54.
43. Peh GS, Beuerman RW, Colman A, Tan DT, Mehta JS. Human corneal endothelial cell expansion for corneal endothelium transplantation: an overview. Transplantation. 2011;91: 811–9.
44. Polisetti N, Joyce NC. The culture of limbal stromal cells and corneal endothelial cells. Methods Mol Biol. 2013;1014:131–9.
45. Mimura T, Yamagami S, Amano S. Corneal endothelial regeneration and tissue engineering. Prog Retin Eye Res. 2013;35:1–17.
46. Jumblatt MM, Maurice DM, Schwartz BD. A gelatin membrane substrate for the transplantation of tissue cultured cells. Transplantation. 1980;29:498–9.
47. McCulley JP, Maurice DM, Schwartz BD. Corneal endothelial transplantation. Ophthalmology. 1980;87:194–201.
48. Schwartz BD, McCulley JP. Morphology of transplanted corneal endothelium derived from tissue culture. Invest Ophthalmol Vis Sci. 1981;20:467–80.
49. Mohay J, Lange TM, Soltau JB, Wood TO, McLaughlin BJ. Transplantation of corneal endothelial cells using a cell carrier device. Cornea. 1994;13:173–82.
50. Mohay J, Wood TO, McLaughlin BJ. Long-term evaluation of corneal endothelial cell transplantation. Trans Am Ophthalmol Soc. 1997;95:131–48; discussion 149–51.
51. Koizumi N, Sakamoto Y, Okumura N, Okahara N, Tsuchiya H, Torii R, Cooper LJ, Ban Y, Tanioka H, Kinoshita S. Cultivated corneal endothelial cell sheet transplantation in a primate model. Invest Ophthalmol Vis Sci. 2007;48:4519–26.
52. Doillon CJ, Watsky MA, Hakim M, Wang J, Munger R, Laycock N, Osborne R, Griffith M. A collagen-based scaffold for a tissue engineered human cornea: physical and physiological properties. Int J Artif Organs. 2003;26:764–73.
53. Griffith M, Osborne R, Munger R, Xiong X, Doillon CJ, Laycock NL, Hakim M, Song Y, Watsky MA. Functional human corneal equivalents constructed from cell lines. Science. 1999;286:2169–72.
54. Mimura T, Yamagami S, Yokoo S, Usui T, Tanaka K, Hattori S, Irie S, Miyata K, Araie M, Amano S. Cultured human corneal endothelial cell transplantation with a collagen sheet in a rabbit model. Invest Ophthalmol Vis Sci. 2004;45:2992–7.

55. Lange TM, Wood TO, McLaughlin BJ. Corneal endothelial cell transplantation using Descemet's membrane as a carrier. J Cataract Refract Surg. 1993;19:232–5.
56. Wencan W, Mao Y, Wentao Y, Fan L, Jia Q, Qinmei W, Xiangtian Z. Using basement membrane of human amniotic membrane as a cell carrier for cultivated cat corneal endothelial cell transplantation. Curr Eye Res. 2007;32:199–215.
57. Auger FA, Rémy-Zolghadri M, Grenier G, Germain L. Review: the self-assembly approach for organ reconstruction by tissue engineering. e-biomed J Regen Med. 2000;1:75–86.
58. L'Heureux N, Paquet S, Labbe R, Germain L, Auger FA. A completely biological tissue-engineered human blood vessel. FASEB J Off publ Federation Am Soc Exp Biol. 1998;12:47–56.
59. Boulze Pankert M, Goyer B, Zaguia F, Bareille M, Perron MC, Liu X, Cameron JD, Proulx S, Brunette I. Biocompatibility and functionality of a tissue-engineered living corneal stroma transplanted in the feline eye. Invest Ophthalmol Vis Sci. 2014;55:6908–20.
60. Bourget JM, Proulx S. Characterization of a corneal endothelium engineered on a self-assembled stromal substitute. Exp Eye Res. 2016;145:125–9.
61. Jay L, Bourget JM, Goyer B, Singh K, Brunette I, Ozaki T, Proulx S. Characterization of tissue-engineered posterior corneas using second- and third-harmonic generation microscopy. PLoS One. 2015;10:e0125564.
62. Proulx S, d'Arc Uwamaliya J, Carrier P, Deschambeault A, Audet C, Giasson CJ, Guerin SL, Auger FA, Germain L. Reconstruction of a human cornea by the self-assembly approach of tissue engineering using the three native cell types. Mol Vis. 2010;16:2192–201.
63. Aboalchamat B, Engelmann K, Bohnke M, Eggli P, Bednarz J. Morphological and functional analysis of immortalized human corneal endothelial cells after transplantation. Exp Eye Res. 1999;69:547–53.
64. Alvarado JA, Gospodarowicz D, Greenburg G. Corneal endothelial replacement. I. In vitro formation of an endothelial monolayer. Invest Ophthalmol Vis Sci. 1981;21:300–16.
65. Amano S. Transplantation of cultured human corneal endothelial cells. Cornea. 2003;22:S66–74.
66. Amano S, Mimura T, Yamagami S, Osakabe Y, Miyata K. Properties of corneas reconstructed with cultured human corneal endothelial cells and human corneal stroma. Jpn J Ophthalmol. 2005;49:448–52.
67. Bahn CF, MacCallum DK, Lillie JH, Meyer RF, Martonyi CL. Complications associated with bovine corneal endothelial cell-lined homografts in the cat. Invest Ophthalmol Vis Sci. 1982;22:73–90.
68. Bohnke M, Eggli P, Engelmann K. Transplantation of cultured adult human or porcine corneal endothelial cells onto human recipients in vitro. Part II: evaluation in the scanning electron microscope. Cornea. 1999;18:207–13.
69. Chen KH, Azar D, Joyce NC. Transplantation of adult human corneal endothelium ex vivo: a morphologic study. Cornea. 2001;20:731–7.
70. Engelmann K, Drexler D, Bohnke M. Transplantation of adult human or porcine corneal endothelial cells onto human recipients in vitro. Part I: cell culturing and transplantation procedure. Cornea. 1999;18:199–206.
71. Gospodarowicz D, Greenburg G. The coating of bovine and rabbit corneas denuded of their endothelium with bovine corneal endothelial cells. Exp Eye Res. 1979;28:249–65.
72. Gospodarowicz D, Greenburg G, Alvarado J. Transplantation of cultured bovine corneal endothelial cells to rabbit cornea: clinical implications for human studies. Proc Natl Acad Sci U S A. 1979;76:464–8.
73. Gospodarowicz D, Greenburg G, Alvarado J. Transplantation of cultured bovine corneal endothelial cells to species with nonregenerative endothelium. The cat as an experimental model. Arch Ophthalmol. 1979;97:2163–9.
74. Insler MS, Lopez JG. Transplantation of cultured human neonatal corneal endothelium. Curr Eye Res. 1986;5:967–72.
75. Insler MS, Lopez JG. Extended incubation times improve corneal endothelial cell transplantation success. Invest Ophthalmol Vis Sci. 1991;32:1828–36.
76. Insler MS, Lopez JG. Heterologous transplantation versus enhancement of human corneal endothelium. Cornea. 1991;10:136–48.

77. Joo CK, Green WR, Pepose JS, Fleming TP. Repopulation of denuded murine Descemet's membrane with life-extended murine corneal endothelial cells as a model for corneal cell transplantation. Graefes Arch Clin Exp Ophthalmol. 2000;238:174–80.
78. Jumblatt MM, Maurice DM, McCulley JP. Transplantation of tissue-cultured corneal endothelium. Invest Ophthalmol Vis Sci. 1978;17:1135–41.
79. Mimura T, Amano S, Usui T, Araie M, Ono K, Akihiro H, Yokoo S, Yamagami S. Transplantation of corneas reconstructed with cultured adult human corneal endothelial cells in nude rats. Exp Eye Res. 2004;79:231–7.
80. Tchah H. Heterologous corneal endothelial cell transplantation–human corneal endothelial cell transplantation in Lewis rats. J Korean Med Sci. 1992;7:337–42.
81. Lynch AP, Ahearne M. Strategies for developing decellularized corneal scaffolds. Exp Eye Res. 2013;108:42–7.
82. Proulx S, Audet C, Uwamaliya J, Deschambeault A, Carrier P, Giasson CJ, Brunette I, Germain L. Tissue engineering of feline corneal endothelium using a devitalized human cornea as carrier. Tissue Eng Part A. 2009;15:1709–18.
83. Proulx S, Bensaoula T, Nada O, Audet C, d'Arc Uwamaliya J, Devaux A, Allaire G, Germain L, Brunette I. Transplantation of a tissue-engineered corneal endothelium reconstructed on a devitalized carrier in the feline model. Invest Ophthalmol Vis Sci. 2009;50:2686–94.
84. Haydari MN, Perron MC, Laprise S, Roy O, Cameron JD, Proulx S, Brunette I. A short-term in vivo experimental model for fuchs endothelial corneal dystrophy. Invest Ophthalmol Vis Sci. 2012;53:6343–54.
85. Mimura T, Yamagami S, Usui T, Seiichi, Honda N, Amano S. Necessary prone position time for human corneal endothelial precursor transplantation in a rabbit endothelial deficiency model. Curr Eye Res. 2007;32:617–23.
86. Mimura T, Yokoo S, Araie M, Amano S, Yamagami S. Treatment of rabbit bullous keratopathy with precursors derived from cultured human corneal endothelium. Invest Ophthalmol Vis Sci. 2005;46:3637–44.
87. Mimura T, Shimomura N, Usui T, Noda Y, Kaji Y, Yamgami S, Amano S, Miyata K, Araie M. Magnetic attraction of iron-endocytosed corneal endothelial cells to Descemet's membrane. Exp Eye Res. 2003;76:745–51.
88. Mimura T, Yamagami S, Usui T, Ishii Y, Ono K, Yokoo S, Funatsu H, Araie M, Amano S. Long-term outcome of iron-endocytosing cultured corneal endothelial cell transplantation with magnetic attraction. Exp Eye Res. 2005;80:149–57.
89. Patel SV, Bachman LA, Hann CR, Bahler CK, Fautsch MP. Human corneal endothelial cell transplantation in a human ex vivo model. Invest Ophthalmol Vis Sci. 2009;50:2123–31.
90. Moysidis SN, Alvarez-Delfin K, Peschansky VJ, Salero E, Weisman AD, Bartakova A, Raffa GA, Merkhofer Jr RM, Kador KE, Kunzevitzky NJ, Goldberg JL. Magnetic field-guided cell delivery with nanoparticle-loaded human corneal endothelial cells. Nanomedicine. 2015;11: 499–509.
91. Li S, Wang C, Dai Y, Yang Y, Pan H, Zhong J, Chen J. The stimulatory effect of ROCK inhibitor on bovine corneal endothelial cells. Tissue Cell. 2013;45:387–96.
92. Pipparelli A, Arsenijevic Y, Thuret G, Gain P, Nicolas M, Majo F. ROCK inhibitor enhances adhesion and wound healing of human corneal endothelial cells. PLoS One. 2013;8:e62095.
93. Okumura N, Koizumi N, Ueno M, Sakamoto Y, Takahashi H, Tsuchiya H, Hamuro J, Kinoshita S. ROCK inhibitor converts corneal endothelial cells into a phenotype capable of regenerating in vivo endothelial tissue. Am J Pathol. 2012;181:268–77.
94. He Y, Weng J, Li Q, Knauf HP, Wilson SE. Fuchs' corneal endothelial cells transduced with the human papilloma virus E6/E7 oncogenes. Exp Eye Res. 1997;65:135–42.
95. Joyce NC. Proliferative capacity of the corneal endothelium. Prog Retin Eye Res. 2003;22:359–89.
96. Joyce NC, Zhu CC. Human corneal endothelial cell proliferation: potential for use in regenerative medicine. Cornea. 2004;23:S8–19.
97. Konomi K, Zhu C, Harris D, Joyce NC. Comparison of the proliferative capacity of human corneal endothelial cells from the central and peripheral areas. Invest Ophthalmol Vis Sci. 2005;46:4086–91.

98. Van Horn DL, Sendele DD, Seideman S, Buco PJ. Regenerative capacity of the corneal endothelium in rabbit and cat. Invest Ophthalmol Vis Sci. 1977;16:597–613.
99. Bahn CF, Glassman RM, MacCallum DK, Lillie JH, Meyer RF, Robinson BJ, Rich NM. Postnatal development of corneal endothelium. Invest Ophthalmol Vis Sci. 1986;27:44–51.
100. Bahn CF, Glassman RM, MacCallum DK, Lillie JH, Meyer RF, Robinson BJ, Rich NM. Postnatal development of corneal endothelium. Invest Ophthalmol Vis Sci. 1986;27:44–51.
101. Giasson CJ, Gosselin L, Masella A, Forcier P. Does endothelial cell density correlate with corneal diameter in a group of young adults? Cornea. 2008;27:640–3.
102. Bahn CF, Meyer RF, MacCallum DK, Lillie JH, Lovett EJ, Sugar A, Martonyi CL. Penetrating keratoplasty in the cat. A clinically applicable model. Ophthalmology. 1982;89:687–99.
103. Ohno K, Nelson LR, Mitooka K, Bourne WM. Transplantation of cryopreserved human corneas in a xenograft model. Cryobiology. 2002;44:142–9.

The manufacturer's authorised representative in the EU is Springer
Nature Customer Service Centre GmbH, Europaplatz 3, 69115 Heidelberg,
Germany. If you have any concerns regarding our products, please
contact ProductSafety@springernature.com

Printed and bound by CPI Group (UK) Ltd, Croydon, CR0 4YY
25/09/2026
02222863-0004